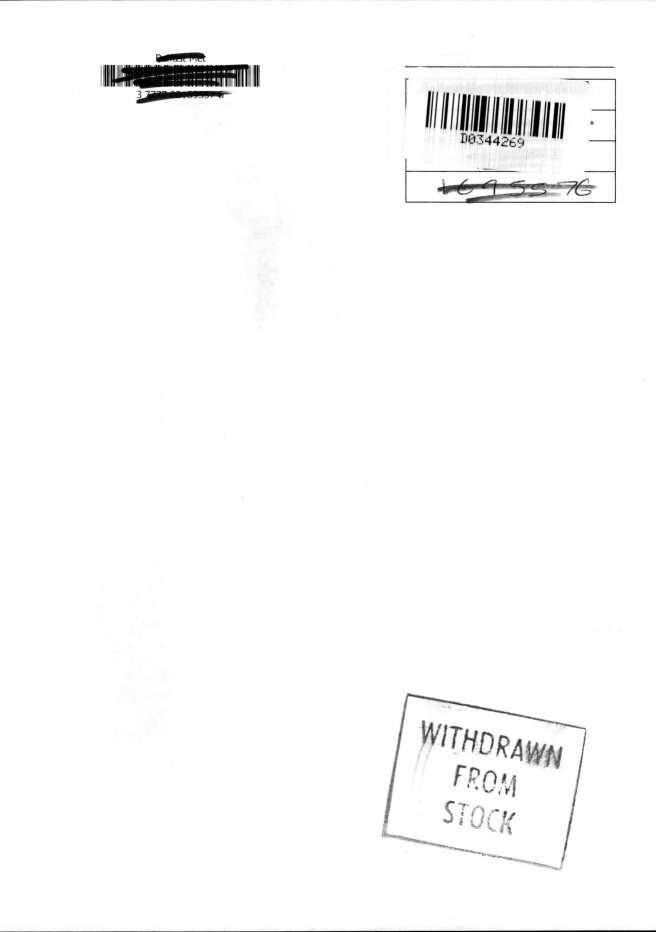

THE WOMEN'S GUIDE TO HERBAL MEDICINE

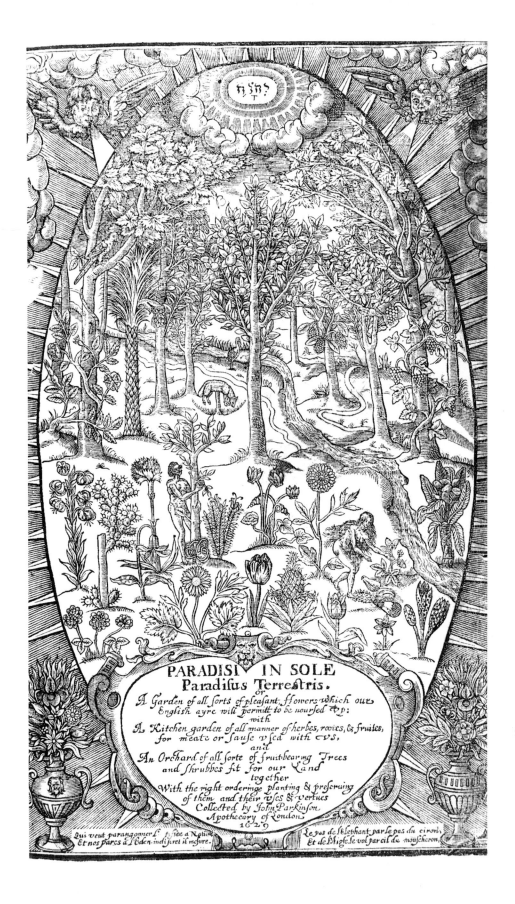

PARADISI IN SOLE
Paradisus Terrestris.
Or
A Garden of all sorts of pleasant flowers which our
English ayre will permitt to be noursed vp:
with
A Kitchen garden of all manner of herbes, rootes, & fruites,
for meate or sause vsed with vs,
and
An Orchard of all sorte of fruitbearing Trees
and shrubbes fit for our Land
together
With the right orderinge planting & preseruing
of them and their vses & vertues
Collected by John Parkinson
Apothecary of London
1629

Qui veut parangonner l'Espee a Nature,
Et nos parcs à s'Eden, indiscret il mesure.

Le pas de sElephant par se pas du ciron,
Et de sMigse se vol par cil du mousheron.

THE WOMEN'S GUIDE TO HERBAL MEDICINE

Carol Rogers

HAMISH HAMILTON · LONDON

To women everywhere,
especially my patients
from whom I have learnt
so much

HAMISH HAMILTON LTD

Published by the Penguin Group
Penguin Books Ltd, 27 Wrights Lane, London W8 5TZ, England
Penguin Books USA Inc., 375 Hudson Street, New York, New York 10014, USA
Penguin Books Australia Ltd, Ringwood, Victoria, Australia
Penguin Books Canada Ltd, 10 Alcorn Avenue, Toronto, Ontario, Canada M4V 3B2
Penguin Books (NZ) Ltd, 182–190 Wairau Road, Auckland 10, New Zealand

Penguin Books Ltd, Registered Offices: Harmondsworth, Middlesex, England

First published 1995   **188483**
10 9 8 7 6 5 4 3 2 1

Filmset in Linotron Palatino by Cambridge Photosetting Services
Printed in Great Britain by Butler & Tanner Ltd

A CIP catalogue record for this book is available from the British Library

ISBN 0-241-13347-5

Contents

Acknowlegements

I would like to thank all of the following for their generous help: Dr Andrew Lockie for his inspiration; Professor Peter O. Behan of the Department of Neurology, University of Glasgow, for kindly lending research papers: Dr Ilse Sommer, formerly of the Department of Neurology, University of Glasgow, for her helpful comments; Mary Kennedy, midwife and National Childbirth Trust antenatal teacher, for her invaluable comments, and Dr Helen Patterson, National Childbirth Trust breast-feeding counsellor; Alicia Melrose, Janet Hicks and Chanchal Cabrera, members of the National Institute of Medical Herbalists, for the benefit of their experience; Dr Nic Rowley for his overview; Liz Cole of the Student Advisory and Counselling Service of the University of Strathclyde for her information on eating disorders; Judy Howard of the Dr Edward Bach Centre; and Marian Pallister of the *Evening Times*.

For their sheer hard work, I am indebted to Jay Wild of Hypertype and Anne Mair.

I would also like to thank Stewart Jackson for his beautifully drawn herb illustrations; the Royal Botanic Garden, Edinburgh, for reproduction of the plates from L. Fuchs, *De Historia Stirpium*. (1542), and frontispiece from John Parkinson, *Paradisi in Sole Paradisus Terrestris* (1629); the Dr Edward Bach Centre for permission to reprint Dr Bach's Flower Remedies; and Dr Andrew Lockie for permission to reprint the diagrams from *The Women's Guide to Homeopathy* on pages 16 and 69.

Last, but never least, John O'Reilly for his encouragement, patience and support.

Introduction

Herbal medicine almost needs no introduction: it is common to all races, cultures and epochs. Dating from time immemorial, it is still extensively practised today: modern medicine is based on it, many drugs are still produced from plants, and our shops are full of products derived from them. The fact that the use of 'simple' herbs (herbs used for medicinal purposes) has survived in the Western world is proof of their continued popularity and validity.

This guide is about herbs for women. It is mainly concerned with gynaecology, dealing with the major developments and changes that occur during the natural course of a woman's physical passage through life; however, it also covers a wide range of everyday ailments.

The home medicine cupboard has long contained traditional herbal remedies for many common ailments. In the last twenty years the use of these has declined, and a visit to the local pharmacist or doctor is often thought necessary even for minor, self-limiting problems. However, a desire to return to greater self-sufficiency is reflected in the many self-help books now available on the subject of health. This guide aims to empower women to take responsibility for their own health with the use of herbs; it is the author's belief that healing should not be exclusive to professionals, whether medical doctors or herbalists, because often the most potent healing lies in what we do for ourselves towards recovery.

The Women's Guide to Herbal Medicine is written from a personal perspective and condenses years of experience into what hopefully the reader will find a sensible, practical and reliable source of herbal self-help. It is concerned less with the philosophical question of what herbal medicine is than with how it works in practice. Herbs work by supporting the body in the natural healing process. Holism is an important concept in natural healing; its basic tenets are as follows:

1 Viewing the body as a whole, with the mental, emotional and physical spheres intertwined, each affecting the other.

2 Treating the individual as a unique and subtle human being.
3 Using the whole herb in treatment and not an extract supposed to contain its active principle, or a synthesized equivalent.

This is what the guide means by a whole-person approach. It implies that factors affecting the health of the individual are (not necessarily in this order of priority): life-style and circumstances; emotional relationships and mental health; genetic and constitutional inheritance.

This multi-faceted approach to health care is diametrically opposite to what is known as the modern biomedical model, a mechanistic concept on which orthodox medicine has been based for the last 200 years, and according to which:

1 The body is compared to a machine consisting of separate parts working together; when it is functioning well, the person is healthy.
2 In ill health one of these parts is defective.
3 The body is easily reduced to its component parts for treatment of disease by repair or replacement.

This model implies that the patient puts herself into the hands of the practitioner and gives away responsibility for her own well-being. This is in marked contrast to the holistic model whereby the patient is an informed participant in her own recovery.

Women and herbal medicine

Women have always been healers and nurses for their families and communities in time of sickness. They have traditionally been birth attendants and last-passage helpers; there to assist their families into and out of life. The womanly qualities of nurturing, compassion, intuition, gentleness, kindness and patience all sit well with the practice of healing. They can be seen as qualities of the earth, epitomized by Mother Earth as worshipped by our forebears.

Knowledge of the healing power of plants and their use has been passed on by word of mouth through generations of women as well as in rare herbals. In the Middle Ages, women's knowledge was often profound, and professional healers such as Hildegard of Bingen made an important contribution to the development of medicine as we know it.

Sadly, many of these women have been written out of history. As the practice of medicine developed, teaching colleges were formed to which women were not admitted, and men took over as professional doctors. Women healers were denounced for their knowledge of nature and simple herbs – countless numbers of them were burnt as witches over a period of 200 years in Europe, and thus the lineage of European 'wise women' died out.

The use of simple herbs, being equated with women's medicine, was no longer recognized as significant. In the seventeenth and eighteenth centuries medicines became expensive, elaborate concoctions based on dubious medical dogma, and often worked less well than the herbal simples of the women healers. Medical treatment became a heroic and sometimes dangerous affair, with cupping, purging and blood-letting as standard procedures. The new medicine reflected the male, often martial, qualities of rationality, aggression and ambition in pursuit of disease. As professional decision-makers took over, patients became dominated by their doctors in a kind of power-game.

The scales have been weighted so heavily for so long in this direction, but the balance is finally being redressed. Women are emerging again in their own right as healers and doctors, and as patients they are once more taking responsibility for their own health. At the same time, a return to gentler remedies and natural ways of healing is gaining popularity in the West as the defects of the mechanistic medical model become evident.

Modern medicine has been successful beyond all expectations in some fields, especially in the treatment of infection and in surgery. However, it has not fulfilled its promise in other areas, for example in chronic conditions like arthritis and heart disease, and the adverse effects of medical treatment based on mechanistic assumptions have multiplied, leaving many problems with no solution.

Treating yourself

With the aid of a few herbal allies, that is, plants you have got to know really well, you can provide yourself not only with first aid for many common ailments but with a lasting source of healing. As with any self-treatment, if you decide to make herbal medicine your first choice of health care, you will probably want to consult a professional herbalist from time to time.

Every woman is unique and her case individual. It must be stressed that there is no substitute for knowing yourself well and knowing what makes you ill. If you always bear this in mind, you are more likely to treat yourself correctly when you are ill, and better when you are well. This may sound simple but in fact it can sometimes take years to get back in touch with what makes you 'tick'. Women are discouraged from childhood from listening to their rhythms and cycles, their needs and requirements. Try to see everything you do in daily life as affecting you for better or worse; it goes without saying that the psychological and the physical are inextricably intertwined. Look for underlying causes – a chronic illness always starts as an imbalance, becoming a disharmony and finally a 'dis-ease'.

The professional herbalist

The medical herbalist today is much like the old-fashioned general practitioner of forty years ago. She has studied the course and treatment of disease, is trained in orthodox diagnostic techniques and will use various standard tests in common with allopathic doctors. She is trained to recognize problems of a serious nature that need referral to a specialist and is happy to work closely with a patient's doctor if required.

During a consultation the herbalist relies to a great extent on her own experience and what she perceives from her careful questioning and examination of the patient. Some time is spent in building up a picture not only of the disease but also of the sufferer. This patient–practitioner relationship cannot be underestimated in the recovery process.

The practice of herbal medicine today

To see how herbal medicine can fit into a modern health service is not as difficult as one might think. In hospital a doctor wants to use fast-acting, powerful drugs as the first line of defence, whereas a general practitioner, seeing the same chronic ailments week after week, may choose gentler remedies. Certainly herbs are eminently suitable for minor, self-limiting conditions and in their treatment these herbal medicines could replace stronger drugs and certainly take precedence over surgery, except in an emergency such as acute appendicitis. Herbal medicine also has a part to play in preventive health – the watchword of medicine today – as chronic degenerative diseases sap available resources.

Training

The initials MNIMH or FNIMH after the practitioner's name indicate membership of the National Institute of Herbalists, which is conferred after completion of a recognized four-year course in herbal medicine. Colleges offering recognized courses at present are the School of Herbal Medicine (Phytotherapy) in Sussex and Middlesex University.

How to use this guide

Part One covers the main areas of health care which most concern women: menstrual problems, pregnancy and childbirth, weight control, menopause, fatigue, nutrition. Part Two lists specific ailments and conditions. Both parts are carefully cross-referenced, enabling the reader to seek further information as required. All conditions, etc. presented in SMALL CAPITALS can be found in the A–Z Directory in Part Two.

Under each ailment or condition there is a brief description of its symptoms, causes, possible outcome and orthodox treatment. Cross-reference is provided to other conditions characterized by the same symptoms when applicable. This is followed by common-sense and practical self-help information, suggesting the use of various simple natural methods. Life-style changes are often recommended on the premise that it is pointless to shore up a diseased body with herbal remedies if the basic problems besetting it are not addressed. Information on nutritional supplements is given where appropriate.

Each ailment concludes with herbal treatment: a choice of remedies is suggested following the guidelines previously given. Individual combination is important after all the aspects of the problem have been considered. The herbs suggested first are the author's own choice, but alternatives are given. All the combinations suggested under 'formulas' are included as a result of their use in years of practice. It is hoped that they may provide a starting-point for treatment.

NOTE: Dozens of herbs are mentioned in this guide; they have been indicated for each ailment where they are appropriate rather than each herb being listed according to everything that is known about it, as in some herbals, then leaving the reader to decide on this basis. The aim has been to make it simpler for the reader to choose. 'Directions for the use of herbs' at the end of the major chapters provides further indications for their use. Please refer to the Bibliography on page 204 for other recommended herbal books.

Part One

1   Green Pharmacy

This chapter provides an introduction to the way herbs work and gives directions for making herbal preparations yourself, from a simple standard infusion of herbs to your own herbal creams. Explanations of many herbal terms used throughout the book can be found here.

The Preparation and use of herbal remedies section (page 8) explains how to use the various preparations described throughout this guide. Finally, there are a few recommendations on the purchase, storing and harvesting of herbs.

Pharmacology of herbs

Pharmacology is the study of a chemical substance to find out its properties and hence possible actions in the body. The discovery of biochemical constituents within plants responsible for their medicinal effects is known as the science of phyto-pharmacology.

Modern practice of herbal medicine is based on sound principles according to the actions of herbs on the body. We know they work in certain specific ways: for example an anti-inflammatory remedy containing a substance known to be anti-inflammatory is used to calm heat, redness, swelling and pain; an example is aspirin, extracted from White Willow Bark.

In the last hundred years or so many herbs, generally very powerful ones, have found their way on to official drug lists or pharmacopoeias. They include morphine derivatives from Opium Poppy, hyoscine from Henbane and atropine from Atropa Belladonna among others; over the years, however, most have been replaced with synthesized equivalents not derived from the plant.

Recent research has proved that many plant medicines have a scientific basis for their actions, which has in some measure validated their use. Pharmaceutical companies are scouring the plant kingdom for cures for the worst diseases of our times, such as AIDS and cancer. Discoveries include the anti-leukaemia drugs vinblastine and vincristine, made from the Madagascar Rosy Periwinkle.

Plant chemistry is a growing science, but any reputable herbalist believes in the use of the whole plant and not in extracting individual promising constituents that may be chemically reproduced and investigated in the same way as synthetic chemical compounds. The pursuit of phyto-pharmaceuticals could become the Holy Grail of modern medicine, but there is more to medicinal herbs than this 'fast lane' approach.

Most herbalists would argue that the total sum of the parts of a herb represents more than the individual actions of any one part (a single plant sometimes has dozens of constituents, many of which can be unknown substances contributing to its medicinal effect). One could go one further and say that in common with other traditional philosophies such as that of Traditional Chinese Medicine, this is due not only to the complexity of phytochemistry but also to the phenomenon of vitalism; that is, the existence of an underlying life force as found in all living things. This concept implies both a directive intelligence and a sustaining energy which determine the well-being or ill health of an individual plant or person.

Phytopharmacology will probably only be of immediate interest to readers contemplating a career in medical herbalism. For general interest, however, an indication is given here of the possibilities its magic chemistry contains.

Of the dozens of identified plant substances, the better-understood ones are alcohols, resins, waxes, oils, volatile oils and carbohydrates (including sugars, starches, mucilage and pectins that have a healing role in the gut in particular). The following are especially important.

Phenols have strong antiseptic properties; Thyme is an example. *Flavones* or *flavone glycosides* belong to this group and are found in an enormous number of plants, whose common characteristic is their yellow colour. They have wide-ranging actions: for example some are stimulants, others are anti-spasmodic.

Bioflavonoids, found alongside Vitamin C in natural sources, are well known for their strengthening effect on the blood capillaries.

Tannins act as an astringent for the skin (see Astringent, page 6).

Anthraquinones have a laxative effect on the bowel, and herbs containing these are used with discretion.

Alkaloids include narcotics, painkillers and poisons and are found in the more powerful herbs not generally available to the public. They have given medicine many of its irreplaceable drugs.

Saponins are interesting in relation to treatment of female problems. Some contain steroidal rings, types of molecules that closely resemble the structure of our own hormones. Plant or phytosterols are discussed below (see page 7) under Hormonal agent.

Actions of herbs

In this guide herbal remedies for ailments are suggested according to their main actions. The main principle of herbal treatment – the whole herb to treat the whole person – is evident in the use of some terms explained below, such as bitters, emmenagogues, cholagogues and alteratives, which in their whole-body action have no equivalent in modern medicine. However, while these terms are exclusively herbal, others are used in common with orthodox medicine. The principal known actions of herbs are as follows:

Adaptogen; alterative; analgesic (or painkilling); anti-inflammatory; anti-microbial; anti-spasmodic; astringent; bitter; cholagogue; demulcent and emollient; diuretic; emmenagogue; expectorant; nervine (includes sedatives or anxiolytics for anxiety; and anti-depressants).

Other actions include tonic, meaning for improvement of general function or level of health, a concept lost to modern medicine.

Two other terms – trophorestorative, literally meaning to bring back tone or life to an organ, and thymoleptic, meaning to raise mood or sense of well-being – are specific to herbal theory.

Especially relevant to this guide is a more recently coined term – hormonal action, as applied to women's physiology, specifically progestogenic or oestrogenic.

Other terms used, such as anti-tussive (for coughs), anti-catarrhal (for upper respiratory passages), anti-emetic and anti-diarrhoeal (for digestive system), anti-allergic, anti-haemorrhagic, etc., are self-explanatory.

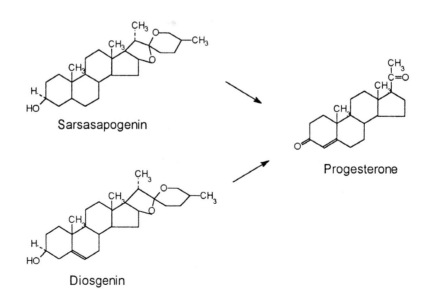

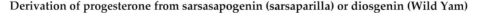

Derivation of progesterone from sarsasapogenin (sarsaparilla) or diosgenin (Wild Yam)

Classification

Another way to understand how herbs work is to group them according to the areas of the body or bodily systems they help most: nervous system, digestive system, etc. This principle will become clear when the treatment of individual ailments is described.

Many herbs have more than one action or use, and so work well when combined as a remedy – the 'two birds with one stone' approach. It is worth looking at their main individual actions in detail as understanding them is always the key to following treatment.

Principal actions

Adaptogen

This is a new concept in Western medicine, although it is part of traditional medicine such as the Chinese. An adaptogen is used to enhance or improve the function or general level of energy within the body. Panax Ginseng is a classic example of this, as are other 'imperial' Chinese tonic herbs. As their name suggests, these herbs are highly prized. Women's Ginseng or Dang Gui (Chinese Angelica) is particularly recommended for the female system.

Alterative

Herbs with this action have been used for 200 years or more, and have their origin in early North American herbal medicine, known as physiomedicalism. Many of them come from American Indian herbal lore; however, every country has its own. These herbs work by stimulating the digestion and assimilation of food and the elimination of waste and toxins from the body via the eliminative organs. They are sometimes called blood-purifiers. In some cases they are needed to start the process of healing and repair in a diseased organism. Their effects are widespread: according to physiomedical theory they can affect the whole body by reflex action, a unique concept whereby other organs are affected through their nervous connections. Alterative herbs include Garlic, Yellow Dock, Echinacea, Sarsaparilla and Red Clover.

Analgesic

Analgesia is pain relief. This action is provided by means of different herbs for disparate parts of the body, depending on the cause of the pain. For example, White Willow is most useful for osteoarthritis, whereas Devil's Claw is effective for rheumatism or rheumatoid arthritis. For menstrual pain Pasque Flower is the herb of choice if due to congestion; if due to spasm, Cramp Bark is superior. In digestive spasms nothing surpasses Chamomile for pain relief, although other herbs such as Peppermint work well for indigestion pain.

Anti-inflammatory

Herbs with this action reduce swelling, heat, redness and accompanying pain. Inflammation is part of the process of healing and it is important not to suppress it. The body uses inflammation to isolate and eliminate products of injury and infection. Anti-inflammatories are used in conjunction with other herbs such as diuretics and lymphatics to encourage this. There are anti-inflammatory herbs for all systems; some examples are anti-rheumatics such as Celery; digestive herbs include Chamomile, Liquorice and Meadowsweet; Marigold and Witch Hazel are used for treating the skin; and Wild Yam in gynaecology.

Anti-microbial

Also known as *antiseptics*, these are effective herbal alternatives to modern antibiotics if used judiciously. One of the most successful is Echinacea, which increases the production of white cells to fight the infection, particularly in respiratory illness. Those with a broad anti-microbial action on the body are Wild Indigo, Golden Seal, Marigold and Garlic. There are also specific anti-microbials for different bodily systems, illustrating the complexity of plants. Thyme and Garlic are superb for the lungs, and Barberry and Buchu for the bladder and kidneys. It should be mentioned that essential oils derived from many aromatic plants are highly anti-microbial, particularly Thyme, Lemon, Sage, Tea Tree and Marjoram. Indeed, so strong are they that in France they are matched to a bacterial culture in laboratory conditions to find the correct essential oil. Preparations may be used locally on the skin or as gargles, etc. Being so strong, oils must be used very sparingly and well diluted.

Some herbs may also be considered anti-viral in their ability to help the immune system hold its own against invaders. Important new additions to the herbal pharmacopoeia with this action are being found, such as Pau D'arco. It seems that as humankind develops different diseases, so we discover new wonders of the plant world to help us remedy them.

Anti-spasmodic

These are herbs that ease cramps or spasms any-where in the body. Again, they are specific for dif-ferent areas; in the uterus when there is period pain, for example, Black Haw Bark or Wild Yam is used; and for intestinal colic, Cramp Bark or Peppermint. Many essential oils are superb at relieving these types of pain, for example Aniseed, Dill and Fennel. These also have a carminative

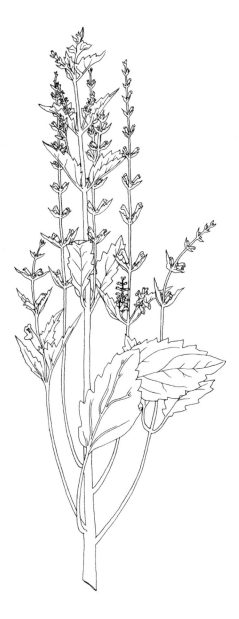

Skullcap *(Scutellaria laterifolia)*

action which calms wind and dyspepsia (indiges-tion) by relaxing musculature in the gut.

Astringent

Herbs with this action contract and tighten tissue through their tannin content, precipitating cells to coalesce. They are used for injuries and for exces-sive exudation of fluid or mucus from tissue. The stronger ones stop bleeding and are known as styptics when this takes place externally (examples are Yarrow and Witch Hazel); or they may stop bleeding internally, in the case of a stomach ulcer for example, when Geranium might be used. For heavy uterine bleeding, anti-haemorrhagics such as Birth Root are used. For diarrhoea, milder astringents such as Agrimony or Raspberry Leaf are usual. Other uses of astringents in the digestive system include protecting against stomach acidity, neutralizing toxins, and protecting delicate nerve endings from damage. Many herbs combine astrin-gency with other actions.

Bitter

These are herbs that have a bitter taste, of course, but to a herbalist a bitter action means stimulating taste-buds in the mouth and improving digestion. They also work by stimulating the nerves to pro-duce more digestive secretions and mobilizing the gut. They can have a reflex action on the whole body, by improving appetite and nutrition, and should ideally be taken fifteen minutes before a meal. Small amounts of strong bitters are used for general debility and recovery after illness. Well-known examples are Wormwood (*absinthium*, from which French absinthe is made) and Gentian. Many herbs have secondary bitter actions, espe-cially *hepatics* which work on the liver, such as Dandelion Root or Milk Thistle. Sedative Hops has a bitter principle, so is useful in nervous digestive disorders.

Bitters should not be doctored with sweet drinks to make them more palatable, as they then lose their effectiveness. Although their taste is strong, only small amounts at a time are needed.

Many bitters are also cholagogues (see below). Note that they can have a stimulating effect on the uterus, which is why many of them are contra-indicated in pregnancy.

Cholagogue

This term was coined to describe the function of stimulating the gall-bladder, which stores bile for the digestion of fats. Herbs with this action are important in herbal medicine as treatment of so many conditions starts in the gut. They cause the gall-bladder first to produce more bile for better digestion of fats, and second to contract strongly so that the bile can be poured into the gut when needed. Herbs with this action are taken ten to fifteen minutes before a meal. Among those commonly used are Golden Seal, Barberry and Gentian.

Demulcent

These contain soothing elements that are used to treat inflamed tissue internally. The external equivalent for the skin is called an emollient. Some plants contain large amounts of a gel-like substance or mucilage, usually in the leaf or root and occasionally in its bark. Those with strong demulcent action are Marshmallow and Slippery Elm, used for digestive problems; Irish Moss for cough preparations; and Aloe Vera for skin. Although a time-honoured remedy, Comfrey Root can now only be used externally.

Diuretic

Herbs with this widely understood property cause increased urination through several different actions which do not need to be detailed here. In common with orthodox preparations, some of these herbs, such as Dandelion Leaf, are used in the cardiovascular system to reduce blood pressure; others, such as Couchgrass and Parsley Piert, in the urinary system to relieve cystitis and urinary retention. Diuretics can relieve pre-menstrual and menopausal symptoms of fluid retention: examples are Fennel and Cleavers. The herbal uses of a diuretic are numerous, from treatment of arthritis with Meadowsweet to any condition where elimination is needed before healing can start.

Emmenagogue

This term, used exclusively by herbalists these days, covers the action of many herbs on the female reproductive system. It means to stimulate and promote menstruation, but some herbs with this property also have a wider hormonal action. This guide considers the emmenagogue herbs mainly in relation to menstruation, and where herbs work in other ways they are credited with a special hormonal action, oestrogenic or progestogenic (see Hormonal agent, below). Because they are so stimulating to the uterus, they are also known as abortifacients and are contraindicated in pregnancy. Examples are Penny Royal (as tea or tincture – *never* take the oil), Wormwood, Angelica Root and Rue.

Expectorant

Used to treat the lungs, an expectorant clears out mucus. It breaks up a dry and irritating cough and produces phlegm or removes existing catarrh. It does this in several ways, most commonly by irritating the mucous lining of the bronchial passages. It is excellent in treatment of chest infections in tandem with herbal anti-microbials, as an alternative to modern antibiotics which kill infection but do not allow pus and other products of bacterial infection to escape. Good examples are Garlic, which is particularly suited for the purpose by being mainly eliminated by the lungs, Coltsfoot, White Horehound, Elecampane and Thyme.

Galactagogue

This action encourages production of milk in the nursing mother. Sterling herbs are Borage, Goat's Rue, Milk Thistle, Chaste Berry and Vervain. Fennel Seed, Aniseed and Dill make excellent and delicious teas to drink when breast-feeding.

Hormonal agent

Herbs that contain phytosterols, or hormones used by the plant for its own growth, are compatible with female hormones and appear to work as building-blocks to provide ready-made material for hormonal production. In some cases the two chemical structures of steroidal rings are almost identical, and need only a little biochemical adjustment in the body. Some herbs, such as Chaste Berry, are thought to work on the level of the pituitary gland (the mother of the female hormones), and can produce either an oestrogenic or progestogenic effect as the body turns it to its own use. Those known as oestrogenic are used to treat oestrogen deficiency problems and are certainly effective: a prime example is False Unicorn Root.

Wild Yams provide the only natural plant source of progesterone available on the market at the present time, although work is in progress to produce it from the soya bean. Wild Yams reproduce the steroidal structure closest to progesterone, and in the 1950s a chemist effected the necessary change and produced natural-source progesterone, the basis for the contraceptive pill. However, this was used to develop a synthetic form which was better absorbed orally. Doctors in the USA are currently rediscovering natural progesterone and are making great claims for its efficacy when absorbed transdermally as a cream.

It is not known what side-effects, if any, the phytosterols have in the long term, and more research is clearly needed. Herbalists know from their use in practice over the years that they are effective, albeit more gentle, and no adverse effects have been reported.

Laxative

This well-used term for treating mild to chronic constipation covers herbal actions from aperient, a mild stimulant to the bowel like Liquorice and Dandelion Root, to true laxatives like Cascara, cathartics such as Senna, and purgatives which should rarely be used and then always under the guidance of a medical herbalist; only the milder ones are suggested in this guide. Anti-griping agents such as Ginger or Fennel are prescribed with strong laxatives. In any case, laxatives should only be used in conjunction with other treatment and the first matter to attend to is always dietary. Relaxing the bowel with anti-spasmodics may sometimes be all that is needed.

Nervines

These cover a range of actions from calming and nourishing to stimulating the nervous system. They are used to treat problems of physical origin affecting the emotional/mental sphere and vice-versa.

They fall into two main categories: sedative nervines and anti-depressant nervines. Herbs are not easily categorized, however, and many of them are used interchangeably, particularly for nervous and emotional problems. Sedatives have the ability to tranquillize gently; they have no side-effects, and no 'half-life', like tranquillizer drugs, to cause them to stay around in the body, leaving a drowsy feeling the following day. Examples of sedatives, which are best used in conjunction with relaxation techniques, etc. are Californian Poppy and Passion Flower. An anti-depressant action is self-explanatory and covers herbs such as Rosemary and Lavender, most often used in conjunction with nourishing tonics as depression is a bodily as well as mental condition.

Herbs to treat insomnia, which include Valerian and Hops, are described as hypnotic. They work best when taken regularly, and you may need to take them during the day as well, to help you relax sufficiently to sleep at night.

Some plants are described as having a trophorestorative effect, which is an all-embracing term meaning to restore tone and health to an organ, in this case the nervous system; a thymoleptic effect improves the emotional state. Although their names are old-fashioned they are so typical of the subtle nature of herbal medicine that there is really no substitute for them. Examples of trophorestoratives are Oats, Alfalfa and Vervain, and thymoleptics include St John's Wort and Damiana. Both cross over with the tonic herbs (see below).

Tonics

These provide sustenance for the nervous system and the body generally. An excellent tonic herb for women is Siberian Ginseng, which is not actually a true ginseng at all but is so called because it could be considered an adaptogen. Its action is typical of herbal medicine, gently restoring energy and strength after illness or childbirth, or during the menopause. There is no comparable action among modern chemical drugs, whose effectiveness is based on identifying and treating symptoms of disease, not preventing them. Chinese herbal medicine includes many tonics, such as *chi* tonics and blood tonics. Among the best-known blood tonics for women is Chinese Angelica (Dang Gui) frequently recommended in this guide.

As seen above, bitters also have a tonic action: the proprietary preparation known as Swedish Bitters contains a mixture of these valuable herbs.

Cola and Capsicum were much used in the past as very stimulating tonics, but in our busy contemporary Western life-style, women are so overstimulated that these tonics are not needed. Depression and debility are frequently connected with stress and tension and so these remedies would be inappropriate.

Preparation and use of herbal remedies

Preparation

The active constituents that provide the medicinal effect have to be extracted in some way from the plant material. Occasionally, the type of preparation recommended in this guide depends on the active constituents of a plant, being extracted only in water or oil/alcohol. With most herbs you can choose which method of preparation you prefer, keeping to the guidelines below.

Dried herbs for use in the preparations described below come commercially ready-cut, usually coarsely unless finely is specified, or as a powder when very finely cut and sieved.

Standard metric measures are used in the guide. If you still think in imperial measures, you may find it useful to bear in mind the following approximate equivalents:

1 ounce = approx. 30g or 300mg
1 pint = approx. 600ml.
(The old measure of 'a handful' of herbs to roughly a pint of water is useful in the absence of scales.)
Also useful: 1g = 1ml and 20 drops = 1ml.

For accuracy with small amounts, scales showing grams, designed for slimmers, are useful.

Infusion

This is the simplest method of preparing a herb to take either medicinally or as a refreshing tea. Chamomile, Lime Flowers, Rose Petals and Lemon Balm make especially pleasant infusions. Aniseed, Fennel and Peppermint are good as digestives after meals. The delicate parts of the plant are used in the infusion: dried or fresh leaves, flowers, or a combination of both, and in some cases seeds. Double the quantity for freshly gathered herbs. The strength is approximately 1:20.

Directions for 2–3 cups:
1 Pour 600ml boiling water over 30g herbs in a teapot or other container. Leave to stand for five to ten minutes. The longer it stands the stronger it will be.
2 Strain, sweeten to taste with honey if desired. It is taken by the cupful, usually three times a day, and can be kept for up to three days if refrigerated.

Decoction

This is used for the hard or woody parts of the plant or tree, such as dried roots or bark, whose medicinal benefits are not extracted by the infusion method. Decoctions are strong-tasting so are often sweetened, or a piece of Ginger or Liquorice is added during simmering.

Directions:
1 Place 30g root in 1 litre cold water in a saucepan and bring to the boil. Simmer for ten minutes or more until reduced by half.
2 Cover and strain. It is taken by the cupful and can be kept for up to three days if refrigerated.

Note: to preserve an infusion or decoction glycerol (available from chemists) or cider vinegar may be added. Proportions are 50 per cent herbal infusion/decoction to 50 per cent preservative.

To make a syrup, add 350g sugar to ½ litre herbal infusion/decoction and heat until the sugar dissolves. This is very good for cough mixtures.

Cold decoction

This is made using cold water and is suitable for plants containing a lot of mucilage such as Marshmallow or Comfrey. Comfrey, as mentioned above, should only be used externally.

Directions:
1 Proceed as for decoction, above, but steep in cold water overnight and then bring to the boil the following day.
2 Cool, strain and preserve if necessary.

Comfrey mucilage (after Dr Christopher)

This is suitable for applying as a poultice to inflamed skin or for VARICOSE VEINS or phlebitis (inflamed veins).

Directions:
1 Soak 100g chopped Comfrey Root in 2 litres water for twelve hours.
2 Bring to the boil in a saucepan, cover and simmer for thirty minutes. Strain, then filter and squeeze through a piece of muslin.
3 Return the liquid to a clean pan and add 300g honey and 100ml vegetable glycerine. Simmer for five minutes, then remove from the heat and set aside to cool.
4 Pour into a wide-necked container and store in a cool place.

Maceration or tincture

This preparation is usually made with a mixture of water and alcohol, extracted over a period of standing. The result is called an alcoholic tincture. The proportions are one part herb to five parts liquid so it is much stronger than an infusion and is taken by the teaspoonful. Tinctures come ready-made in various strengths depending on the dilution necessary to extract their particular constituents. They can be purchased from herbal suppliers. Make your own as follows:

Directions:
1 Allow 200g dried herb/root to 1 litre of liquid consisting of 250ml vodka or gin and 750ml water. The alcohol needs to be 30 per cent proof.
2 Pour the liquid over the herbs in a large jar or other container. Seal tightly and leave for ten to

fourteen days in the dark, shaking the jar once a day to mix the contents.

3 Strain and press the maceration: a press used for home wine-making, which comes with a thin mesh bag, is ideal.

4 Bottle in dark glass, well capped. It will keep for a year.

Note: If you wish to remove most of the alcohol before taking the tincture, pour a little boiling water on and leave until cool.

Tincture should be diluted with a little water before taking. Doses vary between 1 and 10ml three times a day, but 5ml is standard. See individual ailments for directions.

Pills or tablets
These are difficult to make at home, even with experience. Over-the-counter brands often contain a fluid extract, which is a stronger preparation than the above tincture, being 1:1.

Capsules
If you cannot obtain tincture or need to avoid alcohol, powder herbs in an electric coffee grinder until very fine, then sieve finely. Put into size 00 vegetable gelatin capsules (obtainable from mail order suppliers of supplements, see page 203). Capsules have the advantage of being more palatable than tincture, and even woody bark or root can be taken this way.

Suppository or pessary
A suppository is a solid bolus used anally and a pessary is used vaginally for introducing herbs for treatment in certain cases; they melt in contact with body heat. The simplest type is made with cocoa butter as a carrier for the herbs.

Directions:
1 Make as many funnels out of aluminium foil as you need, about the size of your index finger.
2 Melt cocoa butter (obtainable from herbal suppliers), allowing 5g to each pessary. Add the herbs, allowing 5mg herbs, powdered or finely sieved, or ½ml tincture to each pessary. (You may want to evaporate the alcohol from the tincture first, as described below.)
3 Pour the mixture quickly into the foil moulds as it sets fast. (If you are using very fine powdered herbs, add 1g or more until you get a pliable mixture, then roll into shape before it sets.)
4 Refrigerate until required. Peel off foil and insert. They are usually used overnight.

Ointment or cream
Ointments are oil-based and semi-solid; creams are water-based and soft. The fatty nature of an ointment keeps it from being absorbed into the skin; it acts on the surface and also has protective qualities. Creams are moisturizing and are absorbed into the skin taking the herbs with them. Ointments are much easier to make. A standard ointment is made from oil or fat with an agent added to set it, usually beeswax.

To make a warm infused oil
Dried or fresh herbs are added to oil and gently warmed in the oven for an hour or more. The oil will be brightly coloured when the process is completed. Marigold Flowers for cuts, burns and sore skin and St John's Wort for skin irritation are ideally suited for this. Allow 50g or a large handful of flowers to 200ml oil (almond oil is ideal, olive is cheaper but stronger-smelling). Remember that twice as much fresh herb is needed.

An alternative method is to add tincture to oil in the ratio 2:25ml/g. It is preferable to evaporate the alcohol first by heating. Use a snugly fitting bowl over a pan of boiling water and allow to evaporate until reduced by half.

To make an ointment
For the oil method, strain the herbs out of the oil through fine muslin such as is used in wine-making. Add 25g beeswax (obtainable from herbal suppliers), grated up into small pieces, and heat gently, until melted. Pour into jars before it starts to set, cap when cool.

Other ingredients that can be used instead of almond oil are wheatgerm oil, Jojoba oil, Cocoa butter and lanolin. Drops of essential oils (see below) can be added.

Specialist ingredients are needed for creams, or you can buy emulsifying cream from chemists, melt it and add oil or tincture as above.

To preserve ointments and creams add oil of Benzoin, allowing 2–5 drops to 50g.

To make a cold infused oil
Using measures as above for warm infused oil, steep the herbs in the oil in a tightly sealed container for three weeks in the sunlight. Make sure all the herbs are covered by the oil, otherwise they may go mouldy. Turn gently every day to mix. Press out the herb and strain through very fine

mesh or muslin. St John's Wort makes a beautiful rich red oil used for skin healing.

Essential oil

Also known as volatile oils and perhaps most familiar as aromatherapy oils, these are different from the oils made by simple oil infusion above. They are distilled from flowers and are very concentrated, giving off a strong scent as they break down when exposed to air. They cannot be made at home without specialist equipment and are best purchased. Well-loved examples are Peppermint, Chamomile and Lavender.

These oils have been used since ancient times and have a whole therapy devoted to them today. Apart from their use in carrier oils for massaging the body, they are often added to ointments, herbal douches or washes. Added to a bowl of hot water, they are used as an inhalation for catarrh, sinus problems or colds: Thyme and Eucalyptus in particular are used in this way. Essential oils, especially Tea Tree oil, are used by herbalists for their antiseptic and antimicrobial action. Being concentrated, very small amounts are sufficient. Do not exceed 1 per cent dilution in most cases (1 drop: 10ml).

These oils are not generally recommended for taking internally without advice. They must be of top quality and certified pure for internal use. If taken, they should be dissolved in a little alcoholic spirit such as brandy before diluting with water (they will not dissolve in water otherwise). When adding 1 drop to a douche containing tincture, it is recommended to add it to the tincture first before diluting the solution. In the bath, agitate the water well to disperse before getting in.

For an inhalation or to fragrance a room, 1–2 drops of essential oil can be added to a little water in an essential-oil vaporizer or burner.

Applications

Poultices

These are made by placing the fresh crushed or pounded herb (traditionally done in a pestle and mortar) between two layers of gauze or clean cotton for application to the affected part. First paint the part with olive oil, then apply the poultice and cover with plastic to prevent evaporation. You may also need to bind it on with a bandage. Herbs giving superb results when used fresh include Comfrey Leaf for bruising and Marigold Flowers for sprains. Soaked dried herbs can also be used. Comfrey mucilage (see above) makes an excellent poultice.

A traditional drawing poultice for boils to bring out the pus is made with Marshmallow Root powder and Slippery Elm powder in 50:50 quantities made into a stiff paste with water and applied to gauze as above. In this case heat is applied over the part as well (a hot-water bottle will do).

Other uses for poultices include treating acute skin inflammation and itching, as in eczema, when softening Oatmeal may be used, or Chickweed, Ribwort Plantain or Cleavers.

Compress

Known also as a fomentation when used hot. This is made from a pad of clean cotton, gauze or lint soaked in a strained herbal infusion or decoction (see page 9) which is then applied as hot as possible

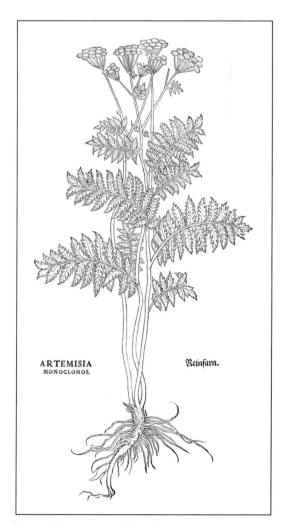

Tansy *(Tanacetum vulgare)*

to the part. Wrap as above, keep warm and replace as necessary. Uses include relief of pain, cramps and internal inflammation; anti-spasmodic herbs such as Chamomile and Penny Royal are applied to the lower abdomen for menstrual pain and pain during childbirth. Cold compresses are also used for headaches or bleeding; they should be ice-cold and replaced as soon as they become warm. Astringents make good cold compresses, for example Witch Hazel for VARICOSE VEINS.

Douche

Used to introduce herbs into the vagina. These are made from herbal infusions (see page 9), or occasionally decoctions, strained carefully when still warm and applied to the vagina at blood heat. A douche kit (obtainable from chemists) is recommended, although some women find a jug and a small funnel acceptable. (If using a kit, do not place the bag too high, or the force will be too great; you do not want to force the douche into the uterus, especially if there is infection.) Use about 50ml at a time and leave in for ten to fifteen minutes depending on directions for ailment. It is easier to keep it in if you raise your legs against a wall, using a pillow to support your back. Usually administered once a day, or twice if the problem is acute, for a week or until it clears up.

Used for many gynaecological problems due to inflammation, infection etc. See under individual ailments.

Enema

Used to introduce herbs into the rectum. Make as for douche, above, but up to 500ml is used. An enema kit (obtainable from chemists) is recommended. This consists of a bag or small bucket and has a nozzle with a tap that allows the fluid out a little at a time. The enema is best applied in an empty bath as the liquid tends to leak out. Suspend the bag above you, lie comfortably on a towel, insert the nozzle and start by holding 100ml in, working up to 500ml as the bowel gets used to it: initially the urge to pass it will be overwhelming. Raise legs as above. Used in Colon cleansing (see page 146), and for chronic CONSTIPATION (Dandelion Root is ideal) and to introduce the healing powers of herbs to the area.

Baths

Herbal baths are used for their soothing properties for skin, for example Chamomile Flowers for itching and Oatmeal for dryness and soreness. They are also relaxing for tension: try adding 1–3 drops essential oil of Lavender to warm, not hot, water and disperse well before getting in. For pain and muscle aches, anti-spasmodic herbs such as Cramp Bark are used.

Directions:
Make 1–2 litres of herbal infusion or decoction (see page 9), strain and add to warm bath-water. Dried herbs may also be put in a small muslin or thin cotton bag, securely tied at the top, and soaked in the bath. Infuse the bag first in boiling water and add the infusion to the bath as well. This is the preferred method for Oatmeal.

Hot sitz bath
Also known as hydrotherapy, a sitz bath is an old-fashioned but effective method of treating problems in the gynaecological area.

Directions:
For a sitz bath the water should cover the hips. A smaller hip bath is traditional but as most people do not have one nowadays, a large plastic bowl or old baby bath may be used. A back-rest is needed and a smaller bowl for a foot bath at the same time. Place a towel under the knees and behind the back. The room should be warm. Begin with a water temperature of 104°F and rapidly increase to 110°–115°F with jug of hot (not boiling) water, with foot bath at 115–120°F, for two to three minutes. Cool the bath to 40°F by adding cold water before getting out.

To add herbs to a sitz bath, see under individual ailments, and prepare as for baths above.

A sitz bath may be used for pelvic pain and inflammation, such as menstrual pain (see page 22) or Endometriosis (see page 24), painful urination, for treating CANDIDIASIS (thrush) or VULVAL PROBLEMS, or local bruising after childbirth (see pages 62–3), using the appropriate herbs. For local treatment, use as hot as possible and stay in the bath until it cools. The herbal infusion may be used twice if reheated on the same day. For piles follow with a cold sitz bath (see below).
Note: Always follow a hot sitz bath with a cool shower for full effect.

Cold sitz bath
This stimulates circulation in the pelvic area and tones up the bowels, bladder and uterus. It is considered helpful for pelvic congestion seen in many chronic female complaints, such as congestive menstrual pain (see page 22) and FIBROIDS. It is

taken for several days prior to menstruation each month. In cases where the uterus has not returned to normal size after childbirth and the flow is profuse, it should be used daily until improvement. It is helpful for constipation when the bowel is weak and relaxed, but needs to be taken daily for several weeks.

Directions:
Prepare equipment as above. The temperature should be cool – 60–70°F – and the foot bath 104–110°F or as hot as can be borne. Start with two minutes and work up to ten, rubbing the hips vigorously with a loofah or friction mitt. The temperature at the beginning of the series of baths should be around 85°F and lowered by 5° with each successive daily treatment until the suggested temperature of 60°F is reached.

Buying herbs

According to vitalistic theory the freshness of the plant and any treatment it has received are of the utmost importance. It cannot be stressed too often that your herbs should be as fresh as possible, and if they are dried, as many are, then you should be sure that they are not more than a year old and have preferably been grown with a minimum of interference, or picked in the wild (wild-crafted). A few reputable suppliers (see page 203) guarantee this. Take advice on sources from a friendly medical herbalist.

If recently harvested and properly dried and stored, dried herbs should not be uniformly brown. If there are flowers they should still have some of their colour, and the same applies to leaves.

Other herbal preparations available include specific tinctures made from freshly picked plants and preserved with an alcoholic solution, the same method used by homoeopaths for the 'mother tinctures' which are the basis of their remedies. Herbal juices made from freshly squeezed plants are an alternative. Of course it is ideal to use only the best, but if your herbs do not fulfil all the criteria it does not mean they will not work, just that they will probably not work as well.

Where to purchase herbal remedies
Some health-food shops stock dried herbs, but the range varies, as does the quality, and they do not usually stock tinctures. Shops specializing in the sale of herbs are few and far between but they usually provide a mail-order service. Reputable herbal mail-order health companies are recommended as they are quick, offer a wide range and are usually no more expensive than shops. As their turnover is higher they are likely to have fresher supplies.

A wide range of proprietary herbal tablets is available over the counter, in health-food shops and chemists. These carry product licences, which means they have been approved by the Department of Health for standardization. They are often well-established remedies but clinical trials have not been carried out to test their efficacy or safety. Compare their constituents against those recommended in this guide if you are taking them for a particular ailment.

See list of suppliers on page 203.

Harvesting herbs

There are many excellent books on growing herbs, which is too large a subject to cover satisfactorily here. However, if you have your own herb garden or want to gather in the wild, you may find the following on harvesting helpful.

- Correct identification of plants is essential, as some may be poisonous. Refer to a good wild herb field guide which has a key for herb identification (see page 205).
- Do not gather protected species in the wild. Do not decimate the area you are cropping: even with common plants, always leave enough for them to reproduce.
- Beware of plants growing within 500 metres of roads, especially motorways, as they are likely to have a high lead content. Be careful of picking near agricultural fields that are sprayed with chemicals as they are also likely to be polluted.

Fresh herbs
When using fresh plant material take just enough for your immediate needs. Cut off any dead leaves, wash in cold water and dry with a clean towel. Use right away as a standard infusion or make a fresh tincture; you will need twice the weight of fresh as you would of dried herbs.

Drying herbs
Herbs should be dried naturally at a warm, not hot, temperature, spread out thinly on trays or

ideally on a slatted base. (Airing cupboards with shelves lined with brown paper are perfect.) They may take several days to a week to dry.

If they turn mouldy, they are taking too long or the air is too humid and you need to dispose of them and start again. An alternative is to dry them outside in the sun if the weather is sufficiently good, or to hang them in bunches from the ceiling in a dry room indoors (not the kitchen, where the herbs would absorb cooking odours).

Storing herbs

Herbs should be kept in a cool, dry place, out of the light. A cupboard is ideal, otherwise store in dark glass or tins. Do not use plastic containers or clear glass. Do not store in paper bags as the aromatic oils will eventually disperse. The total shelf life of herbs is about a year, including the time prior to purchase, so buy small quantities and replace as necessary.

2   Pre-menstrual and Menstrual Problems

I am about to sing this song of yours,
This song of long life
Sun, I stand here on the earth with your song,
Moon, I have come in with your song.

Puberty Rite Dance Song – Apache Indian

Attitudes towards menstruation

At the time of menarche young girls talk together about the approaching change. For most it is an emotional event, approached with trepidation and excitement – becoming a woman. As girls sense their budding femininity it can be a time of blossoming of self-confidence, but in the absence of good role-models among older sisters or other women, it can be a source of anxiety instead. This may be a factor in development of Anorexia nervosa (see page 78) and other eating disorders.

Very often, due to Western society's taboo on discussion of the subject, the exciting first menstruation is spent secretly, alone. We are not geared to assisting girls and women through the physical passages they face during their lives. In fact, women are expected to ignore the monthly sexual rhythm of their lives from the beginning. The message girls are given encourages them to ignore the language of their bodies and instincts. Only older women can change this for their younger sisters.

By contrast, the period of monthly bleeding has been regarded as a special time in some cultures. According to anthropologists, in certain primitive societies it may have been perceived as unclean and been connected with superstitious beliefs; on the other hand, a woman segregated from the rest of the tribe in a hut set aside for that purpose may have been enjoying a break rather than enduring a punishment! For some aboriginal peoples of North America this time was honoured by the tribe as sacred and the women seen as having special abilities or powers. This was especially true where the line of descent was matriarchal, or the shaman or healer a woman. Indeed, as women were often

healers and sometimes keepers of knowledge they were accorded a special respect. In this type of society the young girl's menarche was seen as a rite of passage and celebrated by everyone, in the same way as attaining puberty was celebrated for boys.

Special rites for the time of the month have largely been lost in the West, as women endeavour to go about their normal work and leisure activities during menstruation. Old wives' tales persist as a source of inaccurate information in most cases; one being that a woman should not wash her hair during her period.

Strong negative attitudes to menstruation exist among women and men alike. It is often described as 'the curse', being 'on the rag', and is considered at best an inconvenient event. Pre-menstrual tension is the butt of many jokes. It seems bleeding should be discreet and sanitized to be acceptable in our society, and that if women suffer, they should do so in silence. Certainly that is the advertising message, as evidenced by the use of the internal sanitary tampon and personal hygiene products. Women almost never have periods in novels or films – certainly never when making love. It is still a taboo subject.

From a woman's intimate view, she may find this a special time of renewal and reflection, when her womb is getting ready again to prepare for the possibility of an egg being implanted and growing into a baby. It could also be a time of grieving as the womb loses its potential for childbearing for another month. The flow is even experienced as pleasant by some women if allowed to pass naturally. Either way, menstruation can provide space to look at one's life, to rest, read and dream. Many women do feel more creative and sensitive, and can be more in touch with their feelings at this time. If periods are painful and difficult it helps to let others, especially other women, know to ensure kind treatment at this time. Some women wear a red ribbon to let others in their circle know that they are menstruating.

The menstrual cycle

Normal female reproductive function involves the complex interplay of hormones and the reproductive organs. The part of the brain containing the hypothalamus produces hormone-releasing substances and the pituitary gland produces the hormones LH (luteinizing hormone) and FSH (follicle-stimulating hormone). These in turn stimulate the ovaries to produce the hormones oestrogen and progesterone. Oestrogen induces the growth of breasts and other female sexual characteristics and also has its own feedback effect to control the production of hormones from the brain.

This process creates the cycle of menstruation, inducing maturation of the egg in the ovary; its release down the fallopian tube in preparation for fertilization; the thickening of the uterine lining to receive it; and if it is not fertilized, its disintegration and discharge with the endometrial wall of the uterus, resulting in the flow of blood.

The average cycle lasts twenty-eight days (though it can be as short as eighteen days, and as long as forty) and the bleeding for three to seven days. Starting with the bleed (day one), the early part

of the cycle is characterized by slowly increased production of oestrogen to mid-cycle (days fourteen to eighteen) when the egg is released from the ovary by stimulation of LH and FSH. These reach a peak at day twenty-one approximately, then both decline. Progesterone levels increase towards the end of the cycle to maintain any fertilized ovum. Bleeding occurs fourteen days after the release of the egg if it is not fertilized, as a result of falling progesterone levels.

Awareness of this hormonal progression helps you to understand the problems that can occur during the menstrual cycle, and to work out your most fertile period, whether for the purpose of conception or contraception.

Pre-menstrual syndrome (PMS)

Some tiredness and feeling somewhat emotional before a period is normal, and could be characterized as 'pre-menstrual awareness' rather than a problem. If you experience this, it is probably wise to decrease your expectations of yourself around the time of your period. Slowing down a hectic lifestyle and being more aware of your body's needs may be all that is required to cope.

When the symptoms are exaggerated the condition becomes known as PMS. It may be very mild, or it may present a constellation of unpleasant emotional and physical symptoms that can make a woman's life a misery for part of every month. It appears to be an ever more frequent occurrence for

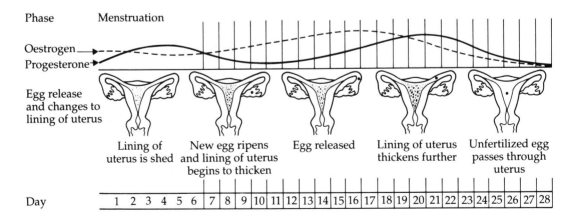

The menstrual cycle

women in Western society today. With its rising incidence, PMS has attracted more attention and has finally been recognized as a genuine medical problem, an altogether happier situation than previously.

Research has shown PMS to be the result of a quite complex hormonal imbalance. Why it should be on the increase is not yet known, although the fast pace of modern life may have something to do with it. Although heredity may also play a part, it seems that stress and emotional factors can upset the delicate balance of female hormones.

PMS affects up to 75 per cent of all women of menstruating age at some time and may occur from two to fourteen days before the period starts, although in some women it can cover as many as twenty-one days of the cycle. In some cases symptoms persist into the period as well.

These symptoms range from the mental and the emotional to the physical. Common denominators are unusually high oestrogen and low progesterone levels, or more rarely a relatively low oestrogen level mid-cycle and progesterone which is relatively high for five to seven days before the period. When women have low post-ovulation levels of progesterone, known as luteal deficiency syndrome (LDS), they have longer cycles; LDS may also lead to recurrent miscarriage.

(See chart above for normal hormonal patterns.)

Other hormones involved in PMS are FSH, prolactin, and aldosterone, which regulates water balance in the body.

PMS can be classified into four types, each with specific symptoms, hormonal profiles and metabolic ill-effects. Often women experience more than one of these types.

Classification of PMS symptoms

Type	Symptoms	Mechanisms
PMS(A)	Anxiety	High oestrogen (leads to excess adrenaline and serotonin)
		Low progesterone
	Irritability	
	Mood swings	
PMS(C)	Food cravings	Similar to hypoglycaemia
	Headache	
	Fatigue	
	Dizziness	
	Palpitations	

PMS(D)	Depression	Low oestrogen
	Crying	High progesterone
	Forgetfulness	High aldosterone (controls fluid balance)
	Confusion	
	Insomnia	
PMS(H)	Fluid retention	High aldosterone
	Weight gain	High oestrogen
	Breast tenderness	
	Abdominal tenderness	
	Swollen hands and feet	

PMS(A): 65–75 per cent of pre-menstrual women suffer from this type. The excess of oestrogen in relation to progesterone causes an imbalance in brain chemicals (adrenaline, serotonin and dopamine), which overstimulates and brings about the symptoms of ANXIETY, nervous tension, etc. Mental relaxation is inhibited. It also blocks the metabolism of Vitamin B_6 and leads to poor metabolism of the essential fatty acids in the body. In this case the minerals magnesium, zinc and chromium will be depleted and there is an increased need for Vitamins C and B_3, as well as B_6. Because of this, it is difficult to maintain normal blood-sugar levels, especially if nutrition is poor, so symptoms of HYPOGLYCAEMIA with associated mood changes may be present. Magnesium and zinc supplements may help, as may a well-balanced wholefood diet.

PMS(C): The main symptoms of this type are similar to HYPOGLYCAEMIA. It affects 25–35 per cent of pre-menstrual women. The exact mechanism is not known, but increased sensitivity to insulin pre-menstrually (with less insulin produced) may be due to deficiency of a hormone-like substance, prostaglandin, PGE1. This means that blood-sugar level swings between high and low. Intake of high levels of coffee, tea, chocolate and alcohol in an attempt to help the situation will only escalate it, especially if combined with a poor diet high in refined carbohydrate and sugar. In the absence of caffeine and other stimulants the body produces excess adrenaline which also causes anxiety, palpitations, sweating and shakiness. Supplements of Evening Primrose oil (500mg twice daily) and magnesium (600mg daily) may help.

PMS(D): This type appears to be due to a relative excess of progesterone in relation to oestrogen, with the progesterone acting as a depressant. It affects 25–37 per cent of pre-menstrual women. It is often associated with PMS(A) which it usually follows, causing symptoms of depression, weepiness, confusion, clumsiness and lack of concentration. The low levels of oestrogen are thought to aggravate the symptoms by breaking down mood-enhancing brain chemicals. A feature of this type of PMS is a tendency towards an excess of lead in the blood plasma and in the hair, which blocks oestrogen uptake. (This may be the result of exhaust fumes and other pollutants and is compounded by a deficiency of magnesium that allows the deposit of lead in the body.) Supplementation with magnesium, zinc and iron may help excrete the lead. Vitamins B1 and B6 help counteract the symptoms.

PMS(H): This type, of which the main symptom is fluid retention, affects 65–72 per cent of pre-menstrual women. There may be weight gain, abdominal bloating, breast swelling and tenderness, swollen ankles and facial swelling. High oestrogen level disrupts the normal output of aldosterone which regulates fluid balance, causing salt and water retention. It is worsened by high excretion of magnesium from the kidneys. Daily supplements that may help include magnesium, Vitamin E (400–800 IUs), Evening Primrose oil (up to 1000mg) and Vitamin B_6. Salt in the diet should be strictly avoided.

A woman may have symptoms from one or two of the sub-groups, or symptoms from all of them. There is a lot of variation. Other less common symptoms of PMS include lack of sex drive, panic attacks, agoraphobia, suicidal feelings, extreme aggression, BACKACHE, genital herpes, vaginal CANDIDIASIS and IRRITABLE BOWEL SYNDROME.

Self-help
PMS can be prevented in many cases by dietary measures, as follows:

- All refined carbohydrates (sugars, sweets and white flour products as in cakes and biscuits) should be limited and all concentrated carbohydrates (dried fruit, maple syrup, fruit juice and honey) eaten in moderation. Use unrefined, preferably organic wholegrain products such as wholemeal bread, wholemeal flour for cakes, biscuits, etc, wholemeal pasta and brown rice.

- If you have a tendency to bloat, eliminate wheat and all wheat products for a month, then reintroduce them and monitor the effects.
- Vegetable protein intake (nuts, beans and pulses, including soya products) should be increased.
- Dairy foods and eggs should be decreased or avoided altogether. Dairy animals are injected or fed with artificial hormones which will disrupt natural hormone levels, and the high fat content in dairy foods may disrupt the prostaglandin balance.
- All animal fats should be decreased, while polyunsaturated vegetable oils should be increased to boost intake of essential fatty acids.
- Use only hormone-free organic meat and chicken. Increase intake of fish.
- Increase intake of green leafy vegetables to boost dietary fibre and promote hormone clearance. Eat as much as possible of your vegetables and fruit raw.
- Avoid pre-packed and ready-made meals.
- Restrict intake of alcohol, coffee, tea, chocolate and cocoa. Follow the 'twice a week rule' for each, but if you are severely affected avoid these drinks altogether during the pre-menstrual period.
- Reduce salt intake; add during cooking but not after serving. If you suffer severely from water retention, avoid altogether during the pre-menstrual period.
- Don't snack, but if you do, eat nuts or fresh fruit instead of sugary snacks, or have a protein snack. Limit fruit intake to two pieces a day in PMS(C).
- Read all food labels as many ready-made foods are padded out with sugar, even savoury ones such as soups and baked beans.

These dietary measures are suggested with the aim of regulating blood sugar and correcting nutritional imbalances. Supplementation may also be necessary to correct existing PMS.

Supplements
Evening Primrose oil: 500mg two or three times daily.
B complex vitamins: 50mg daily.
1 multi-mineral, including zinc, magnesium and chromium daily.
(See also above under each type of PMS.)
For further help contact The Women's Nutritional Advisory Service (see page 202).

Life-style changes are important. Take exercise regularly if you do not already do so, as this will reduce stress and help weight control (excess fat can interfere with metabolism of sex hormones). Good gynaecological health depends of course on overall good health. The importance of sensible eating, plenty of exercise, rest, sleep and space to be ourselves, and caring for ourselves generally, cannot be overemphasized. This is *vital* good health as opposed to the absence of disease.

Herbal treatment of PMS

First, it is important to promote optimum function of the liver, as this organ detoxifies the body, breaking down the hormones for excretion. Second comes the herbal treatment of hormone imbalance. Poor liver function may not be reflected in liver-function tests, as these only show when function is severely disrupted. However, less than optimum liver performance is not uncommon, especially where enhanced demands are made on the liver. This is often the case when there is a history of dieting or food disorders such as Bulimia nervosa (see page 81). Alcohol should be cut down or avoided altogether, recreational drugs cut out, and unnecessary over-the-counter drugs (such as paracetamol) avoided.

A suggested regime to follow would include detoxification: see Colon cleansing (page 146). If you think that you may have put your liver under strain in the past, or feel tired and sluggish most of the time, try the Liver diet (page 148) for four weeks followed by Liver herbs (below) for six to eight weeks. It will also be of benefit to fast on juices for one day a week for six months.

Liver herbs

There are many of these – the following are the author's choice: Dandelion Root, Milk Thistle, Barberry, Wormwood, Golden Seal. Where the bowels do not move regularly, Blue Flag, Yellow Dock Root. (See Directions for use of herbs, at end of chapter.)

Any one of these is ideal combined with the hormonal herbs (see below) for the first one to two months of treatment.

Hormonal herbs

Herbs with a hormonal action contain steroidal glycosides which have a similar structure to the steroid hormones that are present in the human body. Because they have a similar biological basis

they are compatible with our bodies and appear to work by either boosting or stimulating our systems. There are many plants containing these phytosterols. Wild Yam from Mexico, for example, was used in the synthesis of the hormonal contraceptive pill.

A six-month study of thirty women suffering from PMS was carried out by the author, in the course of which the results of various treatments were noted. One of the conclusions was that the traditional herbal treatment of Chaste Berry is only of help where the symptoms are mainly those of PMS(A), (where progesterone is low). Other hormonal herbs need to be added in the right combination in order to relieve other symptoms. Again, it must be stressed that prescription in practice is individual: guidance is given along the lines that were found helpful to the greatest number of women.

As a result of the study and years of practice, the

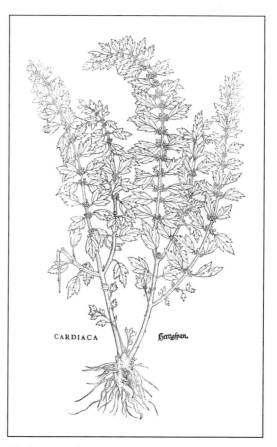

Motherwort (*Leonorus cardiaca*)

following herbs are suggested for the various sub-groups of PMS:

PMS(A)

Progestogenics: Chaste Berry, Sarsaparilla, Wild Yam.

Oestrogenics and hormonal balancers: Chinese Angelica (Dang Gui), False Unicorn Root.

Nervines or sedatives: Skullcap, Valerian, Passion Flower, Lime Flowers, Vervain.

PMS(C)

Evening Primrose oil and Borage (Starflower) tincture or oil, as these contain essential fatty acids (EFAs). Liquorice to balance blood-sugar levels and support adrenal glands: this also contains oestrogenic substances.

Nervines and circulatory balancers: Valerian, Skullcap, Hawthorn.

PMS(D)

Oestrogenics: False Unicorn Root, Red Clover, Sage, Liquorice, Black Cohosh, Motherwort if coming up to menopause.

Anti-depressants: Vervain, St John's Wort, Damiana, Rosemary.

PMS(H)

Herbal diuretics: Dandelion Leaf, Cornsilk, Cleavers, Fennel Seed, Juniper.

Progestogenics: Chaste Berry, Wild Yam.

Kidney-supporting remedies: Pellitory-of-the-Wall, Parsley Piert.

For further information see Directions for use of herbs, at end of chapter.

Formula for PMS

A suggested combination for the most common type, PMS(A), with some symptoms of fluid retention, would be the following:

Skullcap	25 per cent
Chaste Berry	25 per cent
Dandelion Leaf	25 per cent
False Unicorn Root	25 per cent

Total: 100ml/g a week. Dose: tincture, 5ml, three times daily; or infusion/decoction of dried herb in equal parts, 1 cup three times daily from the onset of symptoms, e.g. day twenty-one of cycle, to start of period.

If symptoms of depression are present towards the time of the period, add some of the herbs recommended under PMS(D) (see above) as an infusion and take 2 or 3 cups daily. (See recommended doses at end of chapter.) Follow this principle for PMS(C) as well.

In order to rebalance the cycle it is necessary to carry on the treatment for a minimum of six months, otherwise the symptoms will often return within a month or two. The intricate balance of hormones is easily upset and overriding stress is the most common reason for the return of symptoms of PMS. After you have helped yourself to better health it pays to nurture yourself. You will probably be the best judge of the areas in your life that need adjustment and the steps you can take to bring about a more harmonious life-style; but if you find this difficult, ask for referral to a counsellor.

There are herbal proprietary brands purporting to treat PMS. Some are mainly diuretics, so check the constituents. Chaste Berry and False Unicorn Root can be purchased individually as tablets over the counter. If in any doubt consult a medical herbalist.

Menstrual problems

The process of maturation

The average woman is fertile for about thirty years, and has some 300 to 400 periods in her life, with 20,000–40,000 possible eggs present in her ovaries at first menstruation. One egg is shed at each period. The remaining egg cells never come to maturity and simply degenerate in the ovary, demonstrating nature's prolific providence. The actual mechanisms for initiating puberty are not known, but puberty occurs at around ten to fifteen years in girls, with the first period or menarche sometime around 13½ years. However, in the West, the age of the menarche is decreasing with every decade. There is some suggestion that the presence of growth hormones in meat, and in water and other environmental sources, may be a contributory factor. Whatever the reason, girls are maturing earlier. (Interestingly, menopause is also starting earlier. The average age is usually taken as fifty, but early to mid-forties is not uncommon.)

Some girls start their periods easily, others become depressed or otherwise emotionally upset before the menarche. Moodiness for some time before its onset in girls of nine or ten is not uncommon and may be a first sign that periods are imminent. Some girls may experience cramping pains from the beginning, and others heavy bleeding, but in most cases abnormal bleeding settles down after a few cycles. For help with cramps see Painful periods (page 22).

Periods are part of a normal healthy cycle and any abnormality shows a loss of balance and good health. Period pain and pre-menstrual symptoms are not illnesses but represent a chronic state of imbalance. Deeper loss of balance is shown in the more serious internal disturbances connected with the monthly bleed.

Self-help for menstrual problems

Normal blood loss is small, just a few tablespoons, and is composed of blood, mucus, water and tissue fragments. It may be more if something is amiss. Extra iron may be needed during this time if you are not already taking enough iron-rich foods, as about 15–30mg of iron are lost during each period, although this should be made up again naturally by the body. Natural sources of iron are best, as it is most easily absorbed (see pages 134–5). Adolescent girls need 18 per cent more iron than adolescent boys; many girls are mildly iron-deficient in the Western world, and much more so in the developing countries. Add this to chronic deficiencies of other minerals, such as zinc, among young girls, and you have a recipe for hormonal disruption in later life.

It is wise to be cautious about sanitary protection used as there have been increased reports of the incidence of Toxic Shock Syndrome, caused if internal tampons are left in for too long, or are used when there is internal abrasion. It is suspected that the use of non-cotton fibres may also be a cause. If you are prone to vaginal thrush it is not a good idea to wear internal tampons. If you do use them, change them frequently. It is more comfortable and ecologically sound to use cotton washable sanitary towels, which can be purchased from specialist firms, or made at home. All sanitary protection should he frequently changed for hygiene reasons.

Menstruation should not be painful. However, there seems to be an increasing trend for young girls to regularly experience painful periods (see page 22) so regularly that these are beginning to be considered normal. Pain during periods is a puzzle, but may be linked to the decline in health of the population in other areas, or to general toxicity in the body.

Exercises are beneficial to release painful menstrual cramps. One of these is the pelvic rock (see Abdominal and pelvic exercises, page 195). Lying on a special slant-board or with the legs up over the arm of a sofa of the edge of a bed is helpful. Breathing through pain as in labour is very beneficial. Massage between mothers and daughters, sisters and friends, or by a willing sexual partner is wonderful for relaxation and release at this time. The incidence of pre-menstrual tension (PMT) (see page 16) is growing at the same time, and many younger women are experiencing it. It used to be a problem suffered more by older women, due to hormonal fluctuations more common in this age group.

Of course it cannot be repeated too often that good gynaecological health is not possible without good general health.

Herbal treatment of menstrual problems

In herbal treatment of menstrual problems many of the same herbs are used in different conditions. It is the way in which they are combined that produces success. If in doubt, take professional advice from a medical herbalist. See also directions for use of herbs at the end of this chapter. If you cannot find the symptom bothering you in the following list of ailments, look it up in Part Two: A–Z Directory of Other Conditions (pages 151–92).

Caution: If you are going to self-medicate, you should take the following into account:

- Have your symptoms diagnosed by a general practitioner or gynaecologist. Do not attempt to self-diagnose as this can be very misleading. Discuss your progress with a practitioner if possible as the course of an illness can also be confusing. Very few run according to the textbooks. Report any new symptoms. The following are *danger signs* to be aware of:
    Unusual bleeding, especially between periods.
    *Any *unusual pains* in the abdomen or on intercourse.
    *Other vaginal *discharges*, especially blood-stained.
    Swellings or lumps appearing anywhere in breasts, pelvis or labia.
- Do not mix herbs with drugs such as the contraceptive pill, those used in hormone replacement therapy (HRT), anti-epileptic drugs, insulin, cardiac drugs or steroids.

• Do not take *any* of the following herbs if you are pregnant or trying to become pregnant, unless on expert advice.
(See Medicinal herbs contra-indicated in pregnancy, page 41.)

Painful periods (dysmenorrhoea)

Two types of pain are recognized, spasmodic and congestive pain.

Spasmodic pain

These are due to uncoordinated contractions of the opposing muscles of the uterus causing cramp and are most common in young women, usually disappearing after childbirth. The pain usually starts just before menstrual bleeding, or with it, and may continue for one to three days, varying from mild to excruciating. Other symptoms may be bowel problems, shivering or sweating, general weakness and tiredness, aching all over, back and leg pain or nausea and faintness. Far from being a minor problem, some women may feel really ill for a few days.

Self-help
Exercise is beneficial, especially yoga exercises as they increase the circulation to the pelvis. Sitting upright with the knees bent and the soles of feet together and hugged into the body is particularly helpful, as is the pelvic rock (see Abdominal and pelvic exercises, page 195). Slant-board exercises help (try making your own board from a plank); dry land swimming on the floor over a pile of cushions is particularly good for abdominal aching. Frequent hot baths help as heat reduces spasmodic cramps; add essential oils for extra relief. See also Self-help for menstrual problems, page 21.

Low levels of calcium may lead to cramping. Try taking a supplement of 500mg daily for ten days before a period. It could be worth looking into possible psychological reasons for persistent menstrual pain, especially in young girls. Talking with a therapist or counsellor may help.

Herbal treatment
Anti-spasmodic and analgesic herbs provide relief of symptoms but longer-term treatment would include uterine toners and hormonal balancers. It would be advisable to consult a medical herbalist, but in the meantime you could try the following for a couple of cycles.

Formula for spasmodic menstrual pain

Squaw Vine	30 per cent
Blue Cohosh	25 per cent
Black Cohosh	20 per cent
False Unicorn Root	25 per cent

Total: 100ml/g a week. Dose: tincture, 5ml three times daily, or infusion/decoction of dried herb, 1 cup three times daily.

Anti-spasmodic herbs: Black Haw Bark, Cramp Bark, and analgesic herbs Pasque Flower, Roman Chamomile, White Willow Bark, Jamaican Dogwood, Valerian.
Uterine toners: Raspberry Leaf, Mugwort, Yarrow.
These may be used in longer-term treatment.
(See Directions for use of herbs, at end of chapter.)

Warm compresses: Cloths soaked in a hot infusion and applied to the abdomen are pain-relieving. Try Penny Royal, Chamomile, Ginger, Black Haw: make as a standard infusion (see page 9).
Bath oils: Chamomile or Lavender essential oils: 1 drop well dispersed in hot water.

Some proprietary brands of herbal tablets for menstrual pain are available over the counter. Check the constituents against the above.

Congestive pain

Pain that starts well before the period is often due to inflammatory problems with the uterus such as endometriosis (see page 24), FIBROIDS, PELVIC INFLAMMATORY DISEASE or problems with the ovary, such as OVARIAN CYSTS.

Pain is due to congestion in the pelvic area. It usually occurs later in reproductive life, after the age of thirty, or after childbirth. The major symptoms are feelings of aching heaviness in the lower abdomen and legs; the thighs may be especially painful. Accompanying diarrhoea is not uncommon. The discomfort is usually relieved once bleeding starts. If it persists, you should consult a practitioner to rule out any more serious causes.

Herbal treatment
Herbal decongestants are used and hormonal balancers if there is PMT as well. See a medical herbalist for advice.

For a longer-term treatment include the following:
Decongestants: Yarrow, or White Deadnettle, Blue Flag, Golden Seal, Stone Root.
Anti-inflammatories: Chamomile, Liquorice, Wild Yam.

Hormonal balancers: Chaste Berry, Wild Yam, Blue Cohosh, Vervain.

Circulatory stimulants: Ginger, Prickly Ash.

(See Directions for use of herbs, at end of chapter.)

Try this helpful formula for a couple of months:

Formula for congestive menstrual pain

Chamomile	30 per cent
White Deadnettle	20 per cent
Yarrow	20 per cent
Blue Cohosh	20 per cent
Ginger	10 per cent

Total: 100ml/g a week. Dose: tincture, 5ml three times daily, or infusion/decoction of dried herb, 1 cup three times daily.

Anti-spasmodic herbs and analgesics mentioned for spasmodic pain above will give symptomatic relief.

Loss of periods (amenorrhoea)

A girl who has not menstruated at all by the age of sixteen is described as having primary amenorrhoea. Secondary amenorrhoea is the absence of a menstrual period of bleeding for over two normal cycles in a woman who has previously had normal periods. The medical term for scanty but regular periods is hypomenorrhoea, but these are not considered to be a problem.

Loss of periods may be due to hormonal change or the breakdown of a normal endocrine system, or they may have a pathological cause, such as abnormal structure of the uterus, vagina or Fallopian tubes. Normal physiological causes are either Pregnancy and Breast-feeding (see pages 35 and 63), (the most usual causes of a missed period), or Menopause (see page 85).

If prior to puberty insufficient hormones are produced to stimulate the ovaries to function, amenorrhoea will result. Other signs are usually present, such as lack of pubic and axillary hair. Other causes are obesity (see page 70), anorexia nervosa (see page 78), excessive exercise, especially in vegetarians, stress, emotional distress and post-contraceptive pill.

Herbal treatment

Secondary amenorrhoea can be treated by hormonal balancers. These are herbs that contain hormone precursors, substances which are used in the manufacture of hormones in the body. Used in conjunction with emmenagogues (see page 7) they have the ability to re-establish a normal cycle.

Hormonal balancers: False Unicorn Root, Liquorice, Chaste Berry, Wild Yam, Blue Cohosh, Motherwort, Sage.

Emmenagogues: Penny Royal, Southernwood, Mugwort, Angelica, Yarrow.

(See Directions for use of herbs, at end of chapter.)

Note: As amenorrhoea can be complex it is best to take advice from a medical herbalist if you have not had a period for more than three months or if the following formula does not lead to two normal cycles in succession.

Formula for amenorrhoea

Liquorice	20 per cent
Chaste Berry	20 per cent
Wild Yam	20 per cent
Blue Cohosh	20 per cent
Penny Royal	20 per cent

Total: 100ml/g a week. Dose: tincture, 5ml three times daily, or infusion/decoction of dried herb in equal parts, 1 cup three times daily.

Abnormal bleeding

Bleeding may be prolonged, or it may occur in the mid-cycle; it may be too frequent or irregular in other ways; or it may be abnormally heavy due to the menopause. Bleeding in pregnancy accompanied by pain should always be treated seriously as it may be a miscarriage (see page 39), ectopic pregnancy (see page 42) or other emergency.

Abnormal bleeding is usually due to an abnormality in the hormonal relationship between the brain (hypothalamus and pituitary gland) and the ovaries. Age is a factor too: it is more common during the early menstrual years and in women over forty-five.

In older women of reproductive age, abnormal pathological conditions need to be ruled out: these include blood disorders, cervical erosion and cervical cancer (see under CERVICAL PROBLEMS), and, though rarely, tumours of genital origin. Another cause is Endometriosis (see page 24) which accounts for painful, abnormal bleeding in up to 88 per cent of affected women. Other causes are thyroid disorders, use of oral contraceptives, and IUDs and certain drugs. Less serious spotting may be due to prolonged stress or travel.

Irregular or dysfunctional uterine bleeding (menorrhagia)

This is the most common type of abnormal bleeding (50 per cent of women affected are over forty-five), and of these cases 70 per cent are associated with periods where there is no ovulation. This results in hyperplasia or excessive thickening of the lining of the uterus. Bleeding is irregular and breakthrough bleeding common. You should find out the underlying cause, however, and have that treated. There is no substitute for professional prescription in hormonal cases.

Herbal treatment
Anti-spasmodic: Cramp Bark tincture, 5–10ml three times daily.
Uterine astringents: Shepherd's Purse, Cranesbill Root, Greater Periwinkle, Greater Burnet.
Total: 100ml/g a week. Dose: tincture, 5ml, or infusion/decoction of dried herb in equal parts 1 cup, three to five times daily during bleeding.

Any of these astringents will usually stop the bleeding or slow down the flow considerably. Sometimes two in combination are more effective. Tincture made from fresh Shepherd's Purse is most successful if you can obtain it.

Formula for excessive bleeding (menorrhagia)

Cranesbill Root	20 per cent
Greater Periwinkle	20 per cent
Golden Seal	20 per cent
Lady's Mantle	20 per cent
Black Haw	20 per cent

Total: 100ml/g a week. Dose: tincture, 5ml three times daily, or infusion/decoction of dried herb in equal parts, 1 cup three times daily.

As menorrhagia may also be due to pelvic congestion (see page 22) or inflammation, a herbalist would use in addition herbs such as Yarrow, Ginger, White Deadnettle, Stone Root, Horse Chestnut, Golden Seal.

Self-help
Daily pelvic and abdominal exercises and yoga, as well as remedies for the liver (see PMS above) help tone and cleanse and thus remove congestion.

Blood capillary fragility may be a contributory factor as the result of lack of Vitamin C or bioflavonoids, of free-radical damage, or occasionally of blood disorders: in which case add Buckwheat and Parsley to the diet.

Supplements
Vitamin C with bioflavonoids, Vitamin E and Vitamin A combined, and natural sources of iron such as herbal iron tonic. (See page 134 for sources.) Two Rutin tablets three times daily.

Frequent periods (polymenorrhoea)

If periods are coming more frequently than every twenty-six to thirty days, it is advisable to take the expert advice of a medical herbalist unless you have a very good working knowledge of the hormonal actions of herbs.

Those that are useful are: Birth Root, Chaste Berry, False Unicorn Root, Red Sage, Wild Yam. See Directions for use of herbs, at the end of this chapter.

Infrequent periods

These last the normal length of time but occur less frequently than every twenty-six to thirty days. They are common as menopause approaches. If due to other causes, they can be normalized with hormonal herbs if necessary. Seek the advice of a medical herbalist.

Delayed periods

Some cycles drag on for longer than a month, and the symptoms accompanying this can be very uncomfortable.

Herbal treatment
The herbs known as emmenagogues (see page 7) can be helpful in resolving this problem. The most effective are the following:

Penny Royal as tincture or infusion (*never* the oil). Do not take this if you are pregnant, or think you may be.
Mugwort or Tansy as a warm infusion, drunk copiously.
Other herbs are: Angelica, Rue, Black Cohosh, Blue Cohosh.
Chaste Berry may be taken as a hormonal regulator in small quantities: 10–20 drops on rising in the morning in the second half of the cycle.
(See also PMS, above, for treatment of symptoms, and Directions for the use of herbs, at the end of this chapter.)

Caution: You should *never* attempt to bring about an abortion by using these herbs. It is unlikely to work, and an incomplete abortion is very dangerous. (See also List of herbs contra-indicated in pregnancy, pages 41–2.)

Endometriosis

This pathological condition occurs when particles of the lining of the uterus (endometrium) appear in the pelvic cavity around and attached to the organs. Common sites are the ovaries and Fallopian tubes, the ligaments supporting the uterus, the uterus itself, the pelvic peritoneum, the bladder, between the uterus and the bowel, and sometimes the bowel itself. It is not known how or why this happens, but current theory suggests that the particles pass up the Fallopian tubes during a period. A poorly functioning immune system may allow the development of the condition. Hyperfolliculinaemia (the overproduction of the hormone oestrogen from the ovary) also seems to be implicated. These small abnormal sites are stimulated by the hormones oestrogen and progesterone every month and respond by proliferating during the cycle and bleeding during the period, causing irritation and pain and leaving scar tissue behind.

Symptoms include severe pain during the period which remains unrelieved by over-the-counter analgesics. The pain often spreads to the back and down the thighs. It may get worse towards the end of the period. Bleeding is often heavy and prolonged. If the bowel is involved, passing motions may be painful, and either CONSTIPATION or DIARRHOEA may be a problem too.

Endometriosis is most common among childless women, especially between the ages of thirty and forty, although it also occurs in adolescent girls. It has been suggested that it may be even more common than is thought, and that as many as one in six women may be affected in some way. It may have been the unrecognized cause of many menstrual problems in the past.

It is usually diagnosed by laparoscopy, when a small fibre-optic viewing instrument is inserted into the abdomen via a tiny incision. Orthodox treatment may be either by surgery or laser to remove the patches of endometriosis, or by prescription of the drug Danazol to inhibit ovulation (this drug has strong side-effects, however). Unfortunately endometriosis tends to recur after treatment in many women. Complete HYSTERECTOMY may be recommended if the problem spreads and becomes severe.

Apart from during menstruation, pain may also occur during ovulation at mid-cycle. Other associated symptoms may be a heavy or prolonged period, painful intercourse, infertility, aggravated PMS, pain from the bladder on urinating, difficult or painful bowel movements, backache and bloating. In some rare cases no pain is experienced with endometriosis, even though it may be widespread.

Other causes of acute gynaecological abdominal pain are PELVIC INFLAMMATORY DISEASE (see page 179), ectopic pregnancy (see page 42), ovaralgia, OVARIAN CYSTS, or adhesions following surgery.

(See also ABDOMINAL PAIN.)

Herbal treatment
A herbalist uses hormonal herbs, astringents, decongestants and analgesics, drawing on general support for the immune system and treating the liver and other symptoms, such as PMS, as appropriate. Raising general health and treating any underlying problems, particularly emotional, are also very important.

Hormonal herbs: Chaste Berry (as a progestogenic to counter oestrogen dominance, providing a braking action on hyperfolliculinaemia), Lady's Mantle or False Unicorn Root (the latter in small quantities as an oestrogen regulator), Saw Palmetto, Blackcurrant Leaf and Liquorice (as a hormonal balancer). Wild Yam is an anti-inflammatory and anti-spasmodic for pain, specifically ovarian and uterine. Progestogenic-type substances have been isolated from it.

Astringents and anti-haemorrhagics: From the time of ovulation onwards, herbal uterine astringents and toners: Agrimony, Yarrow, Lady's Mantle, Cranesbill Root, Shepherd's Purse, Witch Hazel, in ascending order of strength. As always, use only that which is necessary.

Decongestants and uterine toners: Stone Root, Yarrow, Golden Seal, White Deadnettle, Raspberry Leaf, Hawthorn Berry.

Pelvic analgesics and anti-inflammatories: Pasque Flower, Black Haw, Wild Yam, Jamaican Dogwood.

Immune system: Echinacea.

Chinese herbs: Astralagus, Codonopsis.

Nervous system tonics: Skullcap, Vervain, St John's Wort, Damiana.

For more information, see Directions for use of herbs, at the end of this chapter, or try the formula below. The effectiveness of any formula depends to a great extent on a woman's particular symptoms and case history; the following has proved helpful for a number of women.

Formula for Endometriosis

Witch Hazel	20 per cent
Echinacea	20 per cent
Golden Seal	20 per cent
Chaste Berry	20 per cent
Pasque Flower	20 per cent

Total: 100ml/g a week. Dose: tincture, 5ml three times daily, or infusion/decoction of dried herb in equal parts, 1 cup three times daily, for the whole month. Two to three cycles should see an improvement.

Note: In a severe case a herbalist would advise taking appropriate herbs before the mid-cycle and others afterwards, as well as more anti-haemorrhagics and analgesics prior to the period. As always, take advice on your own case if in any doubt.

Self-help

Meditation, relaxation, aromatherapy massage. Choose from the following essential oils: Rose Geranium, Cypress, Clary Sage, Chamomile, Lavender – 1–2 drops to a carrier oil such as almond. Life-style changes are often needed as there is evidence to suggest that stress contributes to the problem. A woman most likely to have endometriosis was traditionally supposed to be over thirty, childless, career-minded and ambitious. This may of course have been because these were the women most likely to demand treatment! However, the fact that stress levels for most working women and especially working mothers are high may well be a contributory factor. A link has been suggested between endometriosis, environmental and food ALLERGIES, and CANDIDIASIS.

Supplements

Vitamin B complex: 50–100mg daily (take professional advice if long-term).
Evening Primrose oil: 500–1000mg daily.
Vitamins A, C and E combined formula (for adhesions and inflammation).
Multi-minerals including selenium: 200mcg daily and zinc: 25–30mg daily.
Calcium: 500mg daily and magnesium: 250mg daily in second half of cycle.
See also supplements for PMS symptoms (page 18).

Directions for use of herbs for menstrual problems

Dried herbs are either powdered and put into capsules (buy or powder your own, see pages 10 and 13, or taken as dried leaf, flowers, etc. as a standard infusion or decoction (see page 9). The dose given is per cup and 1 (small) cup = approx. 100ml. In

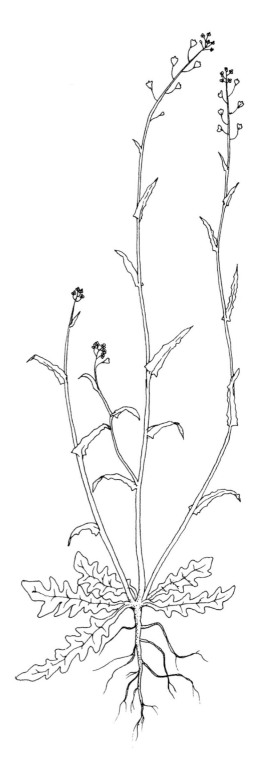

Shepherd's purse (*Capsella bursa-pastoris*)

measuring quantities, as a rough guide 5g of dried flower or leaf = 1 × 5ml medicine spoon or a teaspoon; dried root and bark weighs more, so halve the quantity. It is easier to make 300ml at a time, which is sufficient for a day. A general rule is 30g dried herb to 600ml of water.

Tinctures of herbs are available ready-made. They contain alcohol, usually in the proportion of 1:5, and are a concentrated form of herbal medicine. Doses below are given for tincture of this strength. Herbal tinctures are taken with water in the proportion of 1:8.

See page 9 for further directions on preparation of the above.

General guide to dosage

Total: 100ml/g a week. Dose: tincture, 5ml three times daily, or infusion/decoction of dried herb in equal parts, 1 cup three times daily. (Suggested dosages are *three times daily* unless otherwise stated. These are all within safe margins. *Do not exceed.)*

After consideration of the actions of the herbs listed below it is recommended to combine four or five in equal parts to make a balanced prescription. The actions referred to are those with a particular affinity with the female reproductive system. If in any doubt follow suggested formulas or consult a medical herbalist.

See List of Principal Herbs (page 198) for explanation of terms. Latin as well as common names are given for easy identification.

Key: **A = 1–2 ml/g; B = 3–4ml/g; C = 5ml/g; D = 6–10ml/g**

Agrimony (*Agrimonia eupatoria***)** Leaf
Dose: Tincture B. Dried herb or infusion B.
Actions: Mild astringent, mild uterine toner.
Indications: For excessive menstrual flow.

Angelica (*Angelica archangelica***)** Root
Dose: Tincture B. Dried herb or decoction B.
Actions: Anti-spasmodic. Bitter and aromatic. Emmenagogue. Tonic.
Indications: For delayed menstruation. Indigestion with flatulence.

Barberry (*Berberis vulgaris***)** Bark
Dose: Tincture A–B. Dried herb or decoction A.
Actions: Liver tonic, hepatic. Cholagogue, increases digestive secretions. Beneficial reflex action on lower digestive tract, kidney, uterus and other organs.
Indications: Liver congestion, jaundice, gallstones.

Birth Root or Beth Root (*Trillium pendulum***)** Root
Dose: Tincture A. Dried herb or decoction A.
Actions: Antihaemorrhagic. Uterine astringent.
Indications: Dysfunctional and heavy bleeding. Strengthens uterine contractions in childbirth.

Black Cohosh (*Cimicifuga racemosa***)** Root
Dose: Tincture A (works best in alcohol). Dried herb or decoction A.
Actions: Anti-spasmodic, anti-inflammatory, sedative. Restorative action on pelvic organs. General tonic for the nervous system.
Indications: Cramps of toxic origin. To relieve pain of menstruation and childbirth.

Blackcurrant (*Ribes nigrum***)** Leaf and Root
Dose: Tincture C. Dried herb or infusion C.
Actions: Diuretic, eliminator of uric acid, decongestant, hormonal regulator.
Indications: PMS. Endometriosis.

Black Haw (*Viburnum prunifolium***)** Bark
Dose: Tincture D. Dried herb or decoction B.
Actions: Uterine sedative, anti-spasmodic, indicated for period pain, threatened miscarriage and after-birth pains.
Indications: Period pains, threatened miscarriage, after-birth pains.

Blue Cohosh (*Caulophyllum thalictroides***)** Root
Dose: Tincture A. Dried herb or decoction A.
Actions: Anti-spasmodic. Uterine tonic and stimulant but has a long-term relaxant effect. Emmenagogue. Increases contractions in childbirth.
Indications: Period pains, painful cervical spasm.

Blue Flag (*Iris versicolor***)** Root
Dose: Tincture B. Dried herb or decoction A.
Actions: Anti-inflammatory. Cholagogue. Decongestant. Stimulating and detoxifying action on gall-bladder and liver.
Indications: PMS, congestive period pain and endometriosis with other herbs.

Borage (*Borago officinalis***)** Leaf and Flower or Seed Oil
Dose: Tincture C. Dried herb or infusion C–D. Oil in capsules 500–2000mg daily.
Actions: Contains essential fatty acids (EFAs), particularly gamma-linolenic acid (GLA) which is essential for biochemical actions in the body, forming prostaglandins. Anti-inflammatory action. Positive immune system action.
Indications: PMS, period pain, endometriosis, menopausal symptoms.

Chamomile (German) (*Chamomilla recutita***).** Flower
Dose: Tincture B–D. Dried herb or infusion A–B.

Actions: Mild sedative. Anti-inflammatory. Anti-spasmodic.

Indications: Restlessness. Irritability. Insomnia. Digestive spasms. Local use externally as anti-spasmodic for period pain.

Chamomile (Roman) (*Chamaemelum nobile*) Flowers

Dose: Tincture A–C. Dried herb or infusion A–B.

Actions: Sedative. Anti-spasmodic. Carminative.

Indications: Mental stress and anxiety-related period pain, endometriosis, loss of appetite, anorexia.

Chaste Berry (*Vitex agnus castus*) Berry

Dose: Tincture A. Dried herb or decoction A.

Actions: One of the most important herbs for women. Works on the pituitary hormone LSH to increase progesterone levels in menstrual cycle. Probably has a balancing and potentiating effect on other hormones. Regulates menstrual cycle.

Indications: Irregular periods, painful periods, heavy bleeding, endometriosis, lack of periods, Pre-menstrual syndrome, especially PMS(A). Enhances lactation. Menopausal symptoms.

Chinese Angelica (Dang Gui) (*Angelica sinensis*) Root

Dose: Tincture C. Dried herb or decoction C.

Actions: Blood tonic, in Chinese terms, for 'deficient blood', it both tones and moves blood at the same time.

Indications: Menstrual irregularity and pain, where the woman is debilitated, cessation of periods and period pain (with other herbs), anaemia, PMS.

Caution: Do not use in cases of high blood pressure or in inflammatory conditions.

Cleavers (*Galium aparine*) Leaf and Flower

Dose: Tincture D. Dried herb or infusion A–B. Fresh juice up to 15ml daily.

Actions: Astringent. Diuretic. Aids removal of toxic by-products in the body.

Indications: Enlarged lymph glands and sluggish lymphatic circulation.

Cramp Bark (*Viburnum opulus*) Bark

Dose: Tincture C. Dried herb or decoction B.

Actions: Powerful anti-spasmodic. Sedative. Astringent.

Indications: Cramps, especially of uterus, in menstrual pain, other uterine and ovarian pain, threatened miscarriage, heavy bleeding. Tones uterus, so is used prior to childbirth.

Cranesbill (*Geranium maculatum*) Root

Dose: Tincture B. Dried herb or decoction A.

Actions: Astringent.

Indications: For heavy bleeding and spotting between periods.

Damiana (*Turnera diffusa*) Leaf

Dose: Tincture B. Dried herb or infusion A–B.

Actions: Nerve tonic. Thymoleptic (improves mood). Balancer for hormonal system.

Indications: Depression and nervousness. Reputed to be an aphrodisiac.

Dandelion (*Taraxacum officinale*) Root and Leaf

Dose: Tincture C. Dried herb or decoction B–C. Leaf C.

Actions: Hepatic. Cholagogue. Bitter tonic to digestive system with reflex action on whole body. Gentle detoxifying agent. Leaf is diuretic for fluid retention.

Indications: Detoxification, constipation, debility, hormonal fluid retention.

Echinacea or Cone Flower (*E. angustifolia* or *purpurea*). Root

Dose: Tincture A. Dried herb A.

Actions: Anti-microbial and anti-viral. Positive immune system action.

Indications: Infection. Taken internally and used externally.

Evening Primrose (*Oenothera biennis*) Seed oil

Dose: Oil = 1000–3000mg daily.

Actions: Contains EFAs which are essential for biochemical actions in the body, forming prostaglandins. Anti-inflammatory action. Positive immune system action.

Indications: Hormonal problems, including PMS(A) and menopausal symptoms. Oil as local application for skin problems.

False Unicorn Root or Helonias (*Chamaelirium luteum*) Root

Dose: Tincture B. Dried herb or decoction A.

Actions: Important female herb. Oestrogenic. Hormonal balancer. Uterine and general tonic.

Indications: Hot flushes, PMS, endometriosis (small amounts), ovarian pain, threatened and recurrent miscarriage, infertility and cessation of periods.

Fennel (*Foeniculum vulgare*) Seed

Dose: Tincture A–B. Dried herb or infusion A.

Actions: Diuretic. Anti-inflammatory. Carminative.

Indications: Fluid retention, especially pre-menstrual bloating. Beneficial for digestion.

Ginger (*Zingiber officinale*) Root

Dose: Tincture A. Dried herb or decoction A. For nausea A repeated hourly up to 6 hours.

Actions: Gentle warming stimulant for all internal organs.

Indications: Relieves flatulence and colic. Poor

circulation and pelvic congestion. Dried preparation relieves nausea.

Golden Seal (*Hydrastis canadensis*) Root
Dose: Tincture A–B. Dried herb or decoction A.
Actions: Anti-haemorrhagic. Toning to uterus and other internal organs. Stimulates uterine contractions.
Indications: Long-term treatment of period pain, heavy periods and endometriosis.

Greater Burnet (*Sanguisorba officinalis*) Leaf and Flower
Dose: Tincture B–C. Dried herb or infusion B–C.
Actions: Astringent. Anti-haemorrhagic.
Indications: Heavy periods.

Greater Periwinkle (*Vinca major*) Leaf and Flower
Dose: Tincture C. Dried herb or infusion C.
Actions: Astringent and Anti–haemorrhagic.
Indications: Heavy periods and bleeding between periods.

Hawthorn (*Crataegus oxyacanthoides*) Berry, or Leaf and Flower
Dose: Tincture A. Dried herb or infusion A.
Actions: Circulatory tonic and restorative to heart. Leaf and flower indicated for circulatory insufficiency and high blood pressure.
Indications: Improves blood circulation. Pelvic congestion.

Herb Bennet or **Avens (*Geum urbanum*)** Leaf and Flower
Dose: Tincture C. Dried herb or infusion C.
Actions: Anti-haemorrhagic. Indicated for passive uterine haemorrhage.
Indications: Heavy periods and menopausal bleeding.

Horse Chestnut (*Aesculus hippocastanum*) Seed
Dose: Tincture A. Dried herb or decoction A.
Actions: Astringent and blood anti-coagulant.
Indications: Thrombophlebitis, varicose veins, haemorrhoids.

Jamaican Dogwood (*Piscidia erythrina*) Root and Bark
Dose: Tincture A–B. Dried herb or decoction A–B.
Actions: Sedative. Analgesic for neuralgic-type pain
Indications: Insomnia, period pain, migraine.

Juniper (*Juniperus communis*) Dried Fruit
Dose: Tincture A. Dried herb or infusion C.
Actions: Diuretic and antiseptic for kidneys.
Indications: Fluid retention and bladder infection where there is no kidney inflammation.
Note: Do not take for longer than two to three months.

Lady's Mantle (*Alchemilla vulgaris*) Leaf and Flower
Dose: Tincture C. Dried herb or infusion C.
Actions: Anti-haemorrhagic. Hormonal balancer. Organ restorative for the uterus in many conditions.
Indications: Specifically for regulating menstrual cycle, relief of menopausal symptoms (with Motherwort), heavy periods. Locally as wash for vaginal/vulval itching.

Lime Flowers (*Tilia europea*) Flower
Dose: Tincture C. Dried herb or infusion B.
Actions: Sedative. Anti-spasmodic. Hypotensive.
Indications: Nervous tension, PMS(A), insomnia, palpitations, migraine.

Liquorice (*Glycyrrhiza glabra*) Root
Dose: Tincture B. Dried herb or decoction A–B.
Actions: Adrenal agent. Anti-spasmodic. Anti-inflammatory.
Indications: Mild laxative. Indicated for PMS(C) and as an addition to other herbs in endometriosis. Where there is imbalance works synergistically with other hormones. Benefits any female condition where there is debility or exhaustion.
Caution: Liquorice should not be taken if there is high blood pressure.

Liquorice Chinese (Gan Cao) (*Glycyrrhiza uralensis*) Root
Dose: As for Liquorice above.
Actions: As above, but as it is roasted in honey, it is much more gentle and demulcent, and less stimulating. In Chinese terms it enters all the energy channels of the body and is used in very many formulas. Reputed to balance blood sugar problems (hypoglycaemia).
Caution: Liquorice should not be taken if there is high blood pressure.

Marigold (*Calendula officinalis*) Flower
Dose: Tincture 0.2–1.5ml. Dried herb or infusion A–B. Douche or cream.
Actions: Anti-inflammatory, anti-fungal, vulnerary. Externally and internally for inflammation.
Indications: Cuts, burns, ulcers, candidiasis, trichomonas infection, atrophic vaginitis.

Milk Thistle or Marian Thistle (*Carduus marianus*) Seed and Fruit
Dose: Tincture B. Dried herb or decoction A.
Actions: Hepatic. Organ restorative for liver. Bitter stimulant.
Indications: Chronic pelvic congestion. Hormonal problems related to poor liver function.

Mugwort (*Artemisia vulgaris*) Leaf and Flower
Dose: Tincture A. Dried herb or infusion B.

Actions: Emmenagogue.

Indications: For delayed, irregular or ceased periods and period pain. *Note*: Avoid large doses.

Parsley Piert (*Alchemilla arvensis*) Leaf and Flower

Dose: Tincture B–D. Dried herb or infusion B–C.

Actions: Diuretic.

Indications: Fluid retention, kidney and bladder problems.

Pasque Flower (*Anemone pulsatilla/A. vulgaris*) Leaf and Flower

Dose: Tincture of *dried herb* A. Dried herb or infusion 0.50mg.

Actions: Analgesic. Sedative. Anti-spasmodic. Anti-microbial.

Indications: Painful conditions of reproductive tract, endometriosis, pelvic inflammatory disease, ovaralgia, painful periods. Specifically where these conditions are associated with tension.

Passion Flower (*Passiflora incarnata*) Leaf and Flower

Dose: Tincture A–B. Dried herb or infusion A.

Actions: Sedative. Analgesic. Anti-spasmodic.

Indications: Insomnia, neuralgic-type pain, nervous tension.

Pellitory-of-the-Wall (*Parietaria diffusa*) Leaf and Flower

Dose: Tincture C. Dried herb or infusion C.

Actions: Diuretic. Indicated for fluid retention. Organ restorative for kidneys.

Indications: Pain of cystitis and oliguria (stoppage of urination).

Penny Royal (*Mentha pulegium*) Leaf and Flower

Dose: Tincture A–B. Dried herb or infusion A–B.

Actions: Emmenagogue. Spasmolytic.

Indications: Delayed and irregular periods, colic.

Note: Avoid in pregnancy.

Prickly Ash (*Zanthoxylum americanum*) Bark

Dose: Tincture A–B. Dried herb or decoction A–B.

Actions: Circulatory stimulant.

Indications: Poor peripheral circulation where there is sluggishness. Cold extremities and poor pelvic circulation. Relieves menstrual cramps.

Raspberry (*Rubus idaeus*) Leaf

Dose: Tincture B–C. Dried leaf as infusion C–D. Capsules or tablets B.

Actions: Hormonal precursor. Rich in minerals.

Indications: Specifically in preparation for childbirth; found traditionally in many birthing formulas. Nausea in pregnancy, threatened miscarriage, period pain. Encourages lactation. High in calcium for prevention of osteoporosis.

Rosemary (*Rosmarinus officinalis*) Leaf

Dose: Tincture C. Dried herb or infusion A–B.

Actions: Gentle circulatory stimulant. Anti-depressant. General tonic. Anti-spasmodic. Anti-microbial.

Indications: For depression, exhaustion, headache, PMS(D).

Sage (*Salvia officinalis*) Leaf

Dose: Tincture A–B. Dried leaf as infusion A–B.

Actions: Hormonal precursor. Reputed to be oestrogenic. Antiseptic.

Indications: PMS late in life. Any condition where antisepsis needed internally or externally.

Sarsaparilla (*Smilax spp.*) Root

Dose: Tincture B–C. Dried herb or decoction A–B.

Actions: Hormonal precursor. Reputed to be progestogenic. General tonic.

Indications: PMS, tiredness.

Saw Palmetto (*Serenoa serrulata*) Fruit

Dose: Tincture A. Dried herb or as decoction A.

Actions: Reproductive system stimulant. General tonic. Endocrine agent. Reputed to be progestogenic.

Indications: PMS, late sexual development, infertility.

Shepherd's Purse (*Capsella bursa-pastoris*) Leaf and Flower

Dose: Should be used *fresh,* or tincture made from fresh plant. Tincture A–B or A undiluted under tongue, in emergency. Fresh leaf infusion D.

Actions: Anti-haemorrhagic (vasoconstrictor and blood coagulant).

Indications: Uterine haemorrhage, post-partum haemorrhage.

Skullcap (*Scutellaria laterifolia*) Leaf and Flower

Dose: Tincture B–C. Dried herb or infusion A–B.

Actions: Sedative.

Indications: Nervous tension and anxiety. Combines well with Valerian.

Southernwood (*Artemisia abrotanum*) Leaf and Flower

Dose: Tincture A–B. Dried herb or infusion A–B.

Actions: Emmenagogue.

Indications: Delayed and irregular periods.

Squaw Vine (*Mitchella repens*) Leaf and Flower

Dose: Tincture B. Dried herb or infusion B.

Actions: Uterine toner and relaxant. Preparation for birth (week thirty-four of pregnancy onwards) and during first stage of labour.

Indications: Period pain, irregular periods.

St John's Wort (*Hypericum perforatum*) Leaf and Flower

Dose: Tincture B. Dried herb or infusion A–B.

Actions: Sedative. Analgesic and antiseptic locally.

Indications: Nervous tension and stress-related problems.

Caution: Possible photosensitive skin reaction in susceptible people, so do not apply before going out in strong sun.

Stone Root (*Collinsonia canadensis*) Root

Dose: Tincture C–D. Dried herb or decoction A–B.

Actions: Diuretic. Stimulates removal of uric acid and congestion. Tones all mucous tissues in the body.

Indications: Urinary stones. Liver congestion.

Valerian (*Valeriana officinalis*) Root

Dose: Tincture A–C. Dried herb or decoction A.

Actions: Tranquillizer. Anti-spasmodic. Hypotensive.

Indications: Stress, anxiety, nervous exhaustion, colicky pains, period pain, stress headaches, palpitations, high blood pressure.

Vervain (*Verbena officinalis*) Leaf and Flower

Dose: Tincture C–D. Dried or infusion A–B.

Actions: Gentle sedative. General nervous system tonic. Liver tonic.

Indications: Depression and exhaustion. Beneficial added to many herbal formulas for women to potentiate their action.

White Deadnettle (*Lamium album*) Leaf and Flower

Dose: Tincture C–D. Infusion C–D.

Actions: Uterine anti-spasmodic. Anti-inflammatory. Catarrhal conditions of all mucous tissues.

Indications: Cystitis, leukorrhoea and other vaginal discharges. After miscarriage, surgical abortion or childbirth.

White Willow (*Salix alba*) Bark

Dose: Tincture: A. Dried herb or as decoction A.

Actions: Anti-inflammatory. Analgesic.

Indications: Symptomatic relief for painful conditions. *Note:* aspirin was originally extracted from this herb.

Wild Yam (*Dioscorea villosa*) Root

Dose: Tincture C. Dried herb or decoction A–B.

Actions: Progestogenic. Anti-inflammatory. Anti-spasmodic.

Indications: Period pain. Uterine and ovarian pain, as a long-term treatment.

Yarrow (*Achillea millefolium*) Leaf and Flower

Dose: Tincture A–B. Dried herb or infusion C–D. Fresh juice D.

Actions: Anti-haemorrhagic. Emmenagogue. Anti-spasmodic. Haemostyptic. General circulatory tonic.

Indications: Painful periods, with Pasque Flower. Heavy bleeding and delayed periods (with other herbs). Atonic conditions of female reproductive system.

3 Pre-conceptual Care and Fertility

Pre-conceptual care

For the baby's sake, it makes sense to be in the best possible health before conceiving, and this applies not only to prospective mothers, but to fathers as well. Research has proved that steps taken to secure optimal health and nutritional condition in both parents not only improves the chances of conception but reduces the possibility of perinatal death and many congenital anomalies. As a rule, six months of excellent nutrition and nutritional supplements before conception are recommended by clinicians in pre-conceptual care. This may seem a big commitment but it is well worth persevering for the joy of a happy, healthy baby.

Should you have been unfortunate enough to miscarry in the past, now is the time to put it behind you and start again, in the knowledge that you are doing your very best for your future baby.

Any pathology must be ruled out and blood tests for abnormalities should be performed, to rule out chronic infections, including those that are sexually transmitted; mineral evaluation and allergy tests should be carried out if necessary. Prospective fathers should have a genito-urinary examination and semen test and mothers a gynae-cological examination. If you are unable to attend a private practitioner specializing in pre-conceptual care, many of these tests can be arranged with the help of your doctor or hospital. In a recent study at Surrey University, 89 per cent of couples following this type of programme went on to conceive, and all had healthy, normal babies after previous histories of reproductive problems, mainly infertility and miscarriage.

It is important to avoid exposure to anything known or thought to cause foetal abnormalities. The following guidelines are recommended.

- Avoid the contraceptive pill and IUD for six months prior to conception. (After discontinuation of the pill abnormal abortuses are increased, with a significant rise in chromosomal abnormalities.) Use barrier methods of contraception in the meantime.
- Avoid pollutants and chemicals at work and at home. (This includes fumes from paints, thinners, solvents, wood preservatives, varnishes, glues, spray adhesives, dry cleaning fluids, vinyl chloride, rubber tuolene, PCBs from decomposing plastics and handling cat faeces.)
- No smoking or drinking alcohol. Stop all drugs and medicines unless essential. (This includes antacids, haemorrhoid preparations, motion sickness drugs, sulphonamides, aspirin, acne medication, mercury in dental fillings, herbal laxatives and other herbs contra-indicated in pregnancy: see pages 41–2.)
- Other possible risks may be use of VDUs, ultrasound investigation, amniocentesis, electronic foetal monitoring and incompatible rhesus factors.
- Life-style changes may be necessary so that plenty of fresh air and exercise are taken and stress levels reduced.
- Improve nutrition. Your diet should be based on wholefoods, not refined foods, with a large proportion of fresh vegetables and fruit, organically grown if possible, with good protein and clean water. All food should of course be freshly prepared and cooked (see page 126).

Predisposing deficiencies in vitamins and minerals need to be corrected and the following are recommended:

Daily supplements for pre-conception

Vitamin A 2500–5000 IUs; Vitamins B_1, B_2, B_3, B_6 10–20mg each and folic acid 400mcg; choline and inositol 10–20mg; Vitamin C 100–500mg; E 100–200 IUs; essential fatty acids; and minerals: calcium 400–800mg; chromium 50–100mcg; copper 0.5–1mg; iron 10–20mg; magnesium 200–400mg; manganese 5–10mg; selenium 25–50mcg; trace elements: phosphorus, potassium, silicon iodine and vanadium.

Note: The above dosages are based on recommended daily allowances in pregnancy and you should check the amounts needed in your particular case. Cantassium produce a supplement designed for pre-conception, available from Larkhall (see page 203).

For further information on pre-conceptual care there are a number of organizations that can be consulted. One is Foresight: Association For Pre-Conceptual Care; although it does not adopt a holistic, herbal approach, none the less it has some good practices to offer. See page 201.

Infertility

Infertility is defined as failure to conceive after a year of regular, unprotected intercourse. Statistics show that one in eight couples is infertile. There may be many causes; these are the common functional ones:

1 The position of the womb may be abnormal (i.e. retroverted).
2 There may be insufficient hormonal activity.
3 The Fallopian tubes may be blocked.
4 The vaginal mucus may be too viscous.
5 There may be gynaecological pathology such as ovarian cysts or endometriosis.

A greater proportion of infertility occurs in women whose reproductive function is otherwise normal than as a result of any of these abnormalities, which suggests that the psyche may have a bigger effect on conception than was previously thought. Another factor in Western societies is that there is a far greater incidence of mental disorders in women than in men. Women bring to the experience of motherhood their whole socialization as women, with all that implies, aspects of which they may have been rejecting for years. Small wonder there may be conflict! This raises big issues outside the scope of this book, which cannot be resolved without radical changes in the way society perceives and values women's roles. The individual woman can only work on solving her own dilemmas.

You should be sure that you want a baby for itself and not for other reasons, such as pleasing your partner or family. Sort out any ambivalence by talking with friends with children or spending time with children. Baby-sit as much as possible.

Women are often told that more relaxation, less stress and anxiety about conceiving will help; cases are often cited where a woman conceives after adopting a child. However, it is an anxious and heart-rending time if a woman is longing to have a child, she may become depressed, particularly at menstruation. In this case, she should seek help: Infertility counselling should be available to any couple that requires it, and herbal remedies may also play an important part in emotional healing as well as assisting fertility. (See EMOTIONAL PROBLEMS.)

Fertility herbs

Herbs have an excellent reputation for enhancing fertility. They appear to do this both by balancing the hormones and by creating a favourable condition in the uterus. They have been known to help where there is no pathological reason for infertility.

Over 500 hundred plants contain phytosterols or plant hormones. The best-known hormonal agents used in women's ailments come from North American Indian women; these are True Unicorn Root, False Unicorn Root, Squaw Vine, Blue and Black Cohosh. False Unicorn Root is considered by herbalists to be so potent that women wishing to avoid pregnancy are advised not to use it. Another is Wild Yam from Mexico, originally used as a progestogen for the contraceptive pill. Natural plant hormones work directly or indirectly on the human female hormones in a beneficial way and are an exciting potential area of research for gynaecological medicine. Many Chinese tonic herbs for women do wonders for the reproductive system. Emmenagogues, or herbs promoting menstruation, help to regulate cycles where the period is scanty and/or prolonged (see page 24).

Regulation of ovulation can be achieved by use of herbal hormonal normalizers, particularly Chaste Berry which makes timing sexual intercourse for conception easier. This may take two to three cycles.

The author has had considerable success in recommending programmes for infertility where there is no pathological cause. These programmes are tailored to individual needs but follow the same broad pattern. It is important to follow advice for pre-conceptual care as well.

First, hormonal normalizers are prescribed until the cycle is regular. Then nourishing herbal tinctures or teas are taken for several months, and finally uterine tonics for two months or so until conception. The programme takes around six months in all. It is advisable not to try to conceive for at least the first three months of taking herbs, to allow your body to come to peak condition. After herbal nourishment of all the tissues involved, the uterine tonics appear to provide the catalyst for conception.

The principles of treatment are as follows:

Hormonal normalizers: Chaste Berry, Wild Yam, False Unicorn Root.

Nourishing tonics: Alfalfa, Nettles, Red Clover, Raspberry Leaf, Peony Root, Rehmannia (Shu Di Huang), Schizandra (Wu Wei Zi), Chinese Angelica (Dang Gui). High levels of minerals, particularly calcium and magnesium, thought to be necessary in bringing about a successful conception are found in Red Clover and Raspberry Leaf.

Uterine tonics: False Unicorn Root, Squaw Vine, True Unicorn, Blue Cohosh, Golden Seal.

(See Directions for use of herbs for menstrual problems and Directions for use of herbs for menopause problems, pages 26 and 101 for doses.)

Caution: All herbal remedies should be stopped at once if you become pregnant.

Supplements

A combination of Vitamin E and Vitamin A has the reputation of increasing fertility in both men and women. (See also Daily supplements for pre-conception, page 32.)

The male partner

As half of all cases of infertility are due to male sperm abnormalities, treating the male partner is often necessary. In the Surrey University study mentioned on page 32, 42 per cent of male partners had a reduction in sperm quality. General ill health, stress, overwork, tiredness, poor diet, overindulgence in alcohol and tobacco are all contributory causes to male infertility. Vitamin A deficiency lowers fertility in men. When Vitamin E is increased, sperm quality increases markedly. Zinc and manganese are essential. Zinc is found in larger amounts in the sperm, testicles and prostate than anywhere else in the body. Up to 50mg of zinc supplementation daily may be required for a short period of time, or until conception. There are herbal tonics for the male reproductive area that work well to enhance sperm potency. These include Panax Ginseng, Schizandra, He Shou Wu, Saw Palmetto and some of the nourishing herbs used for women as well.

Self-help

Changing the pH of the vagina so that it is more acid and the mucus more hospitable to sperm, by douching before intercourse with vinegar or lemon juice diluted in the proportion of 1 tablespoon to 1 litre of water, may help. Following a mucus-free diet for a month may also help. The Billing's method of natural contraception will teach you to 'read' your mucus and establish where you are in your cycle. Plan to have intercourse around the time of ovulation, i.e. 2 days before it is expected and 2 days after. The fertile period lasts for up to 72 hours, depending on the length of time the sperm remains alive.

It is also useful to keep a temperature chart. A thermometer is used to pinpoint ovulation, as there is a small temporary rise in temperature just before this takes place. However, this does mean taking your temperature every morning before rising. Home ovulation prediction kits are also available over the counter.

Being underweight or very overweight can be a barrier to conception. Be prepared to lose weight if necessary or to build yourself up by eating more nourishing foods. Being fit obviously plays a part in conception too; nature may sometimes select those bodies that are most suited to reproduction.

Orthodox tests and treatment

You will have to wait a long time for these unless you are prepared to go privately, but once accepted for infertility treatment you will be offered mucus sampling after intercourse, semen testing and blood tests for hormone levels at different times of the month. Laparoscopy may be offered to view the Fallopian tubes and ovaries through a small incision in the abdomen wall.

Orthodox treatment is by fertility drugs initially, and if this fails you may be offered either GIFT (an artificial implantation technique whereby your eggs and your partner's sperm are put into your Fallopian tubes for fertilization) or artificial insemination and implantation technique (IVF). Obviously a lot of careful thought needs to go into the decision to go ahead with artificial fertilization. The chances of success on a first try are very low, it is a long and costly process, and a heartbreaking experience if ultimately unsuccessful. You should be offered infertility counselling before making a decision, and if the treatment is unsuccessful, counselling is even more important.

4 Pregnancy

'Pregnancy . . . a daily song of triumph and thanksgiving in a woman's mind and heart.'
Juliette de Bairaclai-Levy, Herbalist

Taking good care of yourself and your developing baby in pregnancy is essential. So of course is professional ante-natal care, but it is vital not to lose sight of the natural process. For the mother this is a time of respect and awe for the new life growing inside her, for the baby a time of peace, stillness and security, when they are totally dependent. As it is believed that the energy of thoughts and feelings can affect the growing baby in the womb, being at peace with your world is as important as your life-style.

Special care can be taken with any minor health problems that arise by following a natural regime of diet, exercise and rest, and nature supplies many gentle remedies for pregnancy and birthing.

A full-term pregnancy is calculated at forty weeks from the first day of your last period: however, the World Health Organization (WHO) definition is thirty-eight to forty-two weeks. It is divided into *three trimesters* of three months each for convenience.

1 *Early* one to twelve weeks: The embryo becomes established as a foetus and grows very rapidly; all the major organs are being formed and it is at its most vulnerable.
2 *Middle* twelve to twenty-four weeks: Development continues of the recognizably human foetus, with maturation of the major systems of the body.
3 *Late* twenty-four to thirty-eight weeks: where growth is more gradual to full term when the baby is ready for birth and survival outside the womb.

Early signs of pregnancy

The first sign of pregnancy is usually a missed period. The standard urine pregnancy test provides a positive diagnosis after four to six weeks,

although new ones that show results earlier can be bought over the counter.

Other signs are breast tenderness and enlargement, an increased desire to pass water, and possibly nausea. Emotionally you may feel more sensitive, mentally vague and physically tired. Bear in mind that most of these discomforts pass by the fourteenth week and you will usually feel a good deal better in the second trimester. Indeed

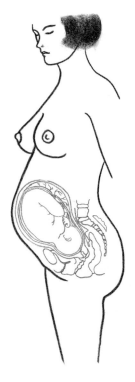

Third Stage of Pregnancy

women feel full of health and well-being then, showing the 'bloom' of pregnancy, perhaps nature's reward for being fruitful!

Various minor discomforts that arise during the second and third trimesters are hardly surprising as your body undergoes profound changes to cater for the growth of a new human being inside you. Your metabolic rate, respiratory rate, heart rate and volume of blood all increase, as does relaxation of the tendons and joints to allow for suppleness during birth. Your body is designed to cope with all this, so unless you have pre-existing heart disease or diabetes, in which case extra care will need to be taken, your organs will not be over-strained.

Pre-natal diagnosis

The increasing use of medical technology in pregnancy means that unless you are classed as a 'low-risk' mother (in good health, aged under thirty, of average weight, average blood pressure and with no family history of congenital abnormality) you are likely to be offered pre-natal tests.

Ultrasound scanning

Even low-risk mothers are offered an ultrasound scan which enables them to 'see' the baby, for on-the-spot monitoring in the uterus. The average number of ultrasound scans per woman in the UK has increased from two in one study in 1984 to three in a recent report. Ultrasound is commonly used in the first trimester for dating the foetus as well as for detecting early abnormalities, but if you are sure of your dates and the pregnancy is proceeding normally, an ultrasound scan is not necessary.

The efficiency of ultrasound detection is dependent on highly trained personnel, and it decreases markedly when handled by inexperienced staff. The WHO recommendation is that until long-term scientific evaluation is carried out, ultrasound should not be used routinely. They say that in the meantime it is sensible to use ultrasound only when necessary and not to subject the entire pregnant population to it. If there are long-term effects, the minimum number of mothers and babies will have been put at risk. Against this it must be said that it is almost certain that ultrasound does not cause any gross defects or problems, so if you have to have one for a good reason, do not worry.

The problem, however, is that experts still have no idea about the possible long-term subtle effects that ultrasound might have on babies. Low birth-weight, pre-term babies and dyslexia have been suggested in several studies.

CVS or amniocentesis test

You may be offered a chorion villus test (ten to twelve weeks) or an amniocentesis test (at sixteen to eighteen weeks). The CVS test takes a sample of cells from the baby's cord and can be performed via the vagina through the cervix; it has the advantages of taking place earlier and being slightly less invasive than the later test.

Amniocentesis aspirates some fluid from around the baby via a needle inserted in the mother's abdomen.

These tests are done to test for anomalies such as spina bifida and Down's syndrome and other chromosomal problems. The indications are if you have an abnormal or borderline blood test, an abnormal child previously, a family history of congenital defects, or if you are over thirty-five. However, the age limit is clearly going down, having decreased from forty to thirty-five in the fifteen years since it was introduced. Neither of these tests is 100 per cent safe. Amniocentesis carries a miscarriage risk of 1:100.

The triple test

The triple test or maternal serum alpha, foetoprotein (MSAFP) has been introduced recently, using blood taken from mothers at sixteen to eighteen weeks of pregnancy. This provides a calculation of the chance of Down's syndrome or neural tube defects (spina bifida) based on the measurement of markers for alpha, foetoprotein (AFP), human chorionic gonandotrophin (HCG), and unconjugated oestrial (UOE). Accurate knowledge of the gestational age of the baby is essential. The results of the test can be ambiguous and an amniocentesis test is often needed for clarification. Bad news is not uncommon with a first AFP screening. If the AFP is higher than average it may indicate a neural tube defect, but it may also indicate a twin pregnancy or incorrect dating of the pregnancy. The triple test is supposed to give a better prediction and about 5–8 per cent of women will go on to have a second screening after MSAFP.

Although the new test is non-invasive and in itself carries no risk of miscarriage, there are drawbacks which some may feel outweigh the benefits: first, false negatives or missed cases – MSAFP identifies about 80–90 per cent of anomalies;

second, routinely false positive results, as the test is predictive and not diagnostic, so women with normal pregnancies may be labelled high risk with all the increased possibilities of intervention that this involves.

New information is emerging all the time about these tests. For help or more information contact AIMS, the Association for Improvements in the Maternity Services (page 201).

Information screening

Prior to screening, couples should be informed of the voluntary nature, limitations and implications of the test, and of the possible need for further screening. Before taking tests you may want to prepare questions to discuss with the health professionals concerned. You may wish to know the particular risk for your age group, for instance, compared to the risk of an invasive test. You may need to know more about chromosome disorders. Couples should be offered the opportunity of pre-natal diagnosis counselling to have it explained in comprehensible language, to receive written information and have time to go away and think about it. A counsellor should provide objective information and not direct towards a particular decision. Pre-natal diagnosis poses agonizing choices for parents at risk as abortion is an integral part of this new technology. Parents may need information to decide if they can cope with a handicapped child or not. They may feel that they would wish to have the child whatever was wrong, but would prefer to have time to prepare and information to deal with it. Most couples, of course, receive reassurance that all is well.

Remember that with pre-natal tests mothers have to live with the anxiety of a tentative pregnancy for four or five months, taking into account several weeks' waiting for the result, so that their commitment to their baby remains uncertain until the all-clear is given. The increasing trend towards all mothers being offered pre-natal blood tests in future may lead to a tentative pregnancy as the norm, a horrifying scenario with unknown consequences for mothers and babies, and as far from a natural pregnancy as is possible to imagine. As Sally Inch says in *Birthrights: A Parent's Guide to Modern Childbirth*:

The techniques which are developed to provide benefits for specific groups of people gradually tend to be used for more and more people, on wider and vaguer indications (on the ground that what is beneficial for some must be beneficial to all) to the point where people who do not require any treatment at all are being given it. As the latter group will have nothing to gain from the technique, they will be worse off if it carries any risk than they would be if left alone.

If you are interested in a natural pregnancy and childbirth, it is as well to be aware of this.

Preparing for childbirth

Ensure you receive good-quality ante-natal care where you can be monitored for normal progress, either at home, in a local clinic, doctor's surgery or hospital.

Do attend ante-natal classes as well, which should prepare you and your partner for parenthood, childbirth and breast-feeding, and teach you relaxation methods to cope with pain. NHS hospitals often provide these classes for women, or the National Childbirth Trust (see page 201) runs very good classes that usually both partners can attend.

Exercise

Regular exercise is important, but do not start training for the Olympics if you were not in the habit of doing so previously! Skiing, climbing and horseriding are not advisable, nor is anything else that may lead to a fall. An hour's walk every day is healthy, and swimming exercises all the muscles gently and is especially beneficial later on when you feel heavy and clumsy, as it provides buoyant relief.

Yoga exercises are very beneficial, but again should be taken gently if you were not practising them before. Some yoga positions are particularly recommended for pregnancy and are aimed at developing the muscles used in childbirth, especially the pubococcygeal muscles. These are very important, so even if you exercise nothing else, remember these. Identify the muscles to begin with by trying to stop yourself passing water in midflow. If you can stop with no problem then they are in good condition. Practise with an empty bladder. While inhaling, hold them as tightly as possible for a few seconds, then let go in several stages, exhaling, until relaxed again. Try to imagine a lift going down and stopping on several floors. Try repeating three or four times, several times a day. A good way to remember is to do it after passing water. It becomes second nature after a while!

YOGA FOR PREGNANCY

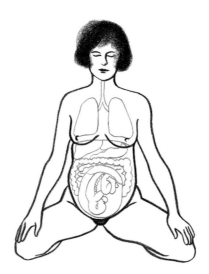

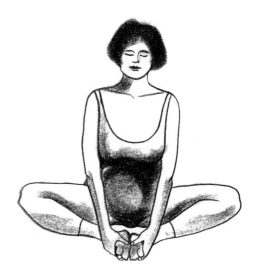

Meditation Pose
Sit upright on your heels, knees apart with back straight and arms relaxed.

The Cobbler
Sit upright with legs apart, knees bent and pull your feet towards you. Hold in a position that is comfortable.

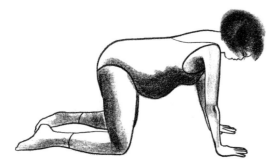

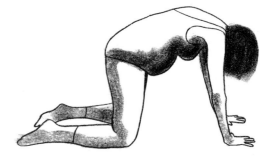

The Cat
1 Rest on all fours with hands and knees apart, and back straight.

2 Arch your back gently, tucking in your head and behind; feel the stretch along your back. Raise your head as you relax back to normal position. Repeat 2–3 times.

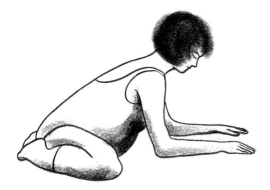

The Frog
Starting from a kneeling position, stretch forward on to your elbows and lower yourself until your tummy rests comfortably on the floor. Stretch forward as far as you comfortably can.

Diet

Your diet should be as well balanced as possible (see pages 43–4). Many problems in pregnancy are attributed to poor diet. In addition you will need extra calcium, and foods containing iron and protein. The bulk of protein should come ideally from fish, pulses, cereals, nuts and seeds rather than from meat and dairy foods. Fresh foods should be of the best quality: organic produce is best, eliminating the dangers of agro-chemicals. Resist snacking on chocolate, fizzy drinks and other empty calories. If you feel very hungry have small meals frequently instead of main meals. Junk foods and fast foods are out!

Eat for two in terms of quality but not in terms of quantity or you will gain too much weight. Vitamin and mineral supplementation may be necessary at certain stages of your pregnancy, but take advice from your practitioner. The UK Department of Health recommends a folic acid supplement from the B group of vitamins of 400mcg daily pre-conceptually and up to the fourth week of pregnancy to prevent congenital abnormalities such as spina bifida. Vitamin and mineral supplement formulations that are specially balanced for pregnancy can be purchased over the counter.

Avoid the following:

- Alcohol, as this has been proved to have an adverse effect on the baby.
- Vitamin A (Retinol), although beta-carotene from orange-coloured vegetable and fruits is all right as a supplement. It can cause birth defects in large quantities, however.
- Liver, as one portion of liver or liver pâté contains up to twelve times the RDA of Vitamin A.
- Coffee, as this is too stimulating for both mother and baby. Even weak tea may not be a good idea in early pregnancy. Stick to mild herbal teas, including Rosehip, Chamomile and Lime Flowers, or fruit teas, fruit juices and mineral water. Coffee substitutes can be bought in health food shops.
- Unpasteurized milk and cheese as they may contain the listeria bacteria.

Miscarriage

One in three first pregnancies end in miscarriage, and this is a very upsetting event for all concerned. One in nine women will have two miscarriages; one in twenty-seven women will have three, and after that miscarriage is termed 'habitual abortion', fortunately rare (see Recurrent miscarriage, below, for treatment). The term abortion for miscarriage is unfortunate: it does not imply that you are in any way to blame, but simply means the loss of the 'products of conception' before twenty-four weeks. Most losses occur in the first twelve weeks or trimester. A miscarriage is not caused by normal lifting and carrying, or even minor falls, as the fluid around the foetus provides cushioning. Contrary to popular belief, neither do emotional shocks.

Threatened miscarriage

This starts as slight bleeding which usually resolves spontaneously. A brown discharge or scanty bleeding may occur monthly at the expected time of the period in early pregnancy and is nothing to worry about. The classic treatment is bed-rest until it stops, although recent thinking is that this does not make much difference. Still, it is wise to take it easy for a few days. Herbal treatment has traditionally been used to stop the bleeding and settle the pregnancy down, but it will not maintain a pregnancy where miscarriage is due to abnormalities of development in the embryo.

Herbal treatment

Black Haw and False Unicorn Root are classic remedies. Use the former if there is much anxiety and tension. It is anti-spasmodic and a sedative for the uterus. False Unicorn Root is specifically for downward pressure sensations. Skullcap can be added as a general sedative if needed.

Dosage
Add 600ml boiling water to 30g of either Black Haw or False Unicorn Root, or both if indicated, in which case 15g of each. Simmer for 10 minutes, covered. Drink 1 cup every hour, sipping slowly. Tincture: 2.5ml of each every hour in water.
Note: Vitamin E (500 IUs) twice daily for a month is thought to help prevent miscarriage.

Spontaneous abortion

If bleeding does not resolve and cramping pains similar to period pains start, then a spontaneous abortion may be imminent. Contact your GP as any heavy bleeding is potentially serious in pregnancy.

Herbal treatment

While you wait for professional help you can take the following remedies. Combine Cramp Bark (indicated where there are pains in the lower back and thighs as well) for its powerful anti-spasmodic properties and Squaw Vine. Follow directions for herbs under Threatened miscarriage above. After the bleeding has stopped, continue the dose for each waking hour for a day, then three times a day for three weeks. (If you have had a miscarriage before it is as well to keep a small stock of these herbs in case of emergency.)

Sometimes solid tissue may be passed, which should ideally be kept for investigation. An ultrasound examination is usually made in hospital to confirm the presence of an intact gestational sac and rule out an incomplete miscarriage, which is dangerous. In the latter case a surgical evacuation or D & C is performed because of the risk of continued bleeding and infection.

If the foetus dies in the womb without any sign of bleeding, this is a missed abortion: the uterus stops growing, morning sickness stops and the breasts diminish in size. If you suspect this you should get a medical check-up without delay.

After miscarriage a tea of White Deadnettle,

1 heaped teaspoon to a cup, should be taken several times daily for two weeks.

Recurrent miscarriage

A woman who has had three or more miscarriages will obviously experience anxiety over conceiving again. The main causes of miscarriage are foetal abnormality (50 per cent), hormone deficiency, genetic incompatibility, uterine abnormalities and incompetence of the cervix. Generalized maternal illness is also a factor. However, women who have had repeated miscarriages are more likely to have normal aborted foetuses, which suggests that the cause is a failure of the implantation mechanism or of the mother's ability to support the foetus, assuming she is in good health otherwise. The prognosis will generally be good following herbal treatment which works on healing and nourishing the uterus and rebalancing the mother's hormones.

Research has shown that poor nutritional condition has a part to play in foetal abnormality and miscarriage, as well as other factors such as radiation, chemicals, heavy metal toxicity, drugs, smoking, viruses and stress.

Herbal treatment

This treatment is aimed at restoring normal uterine function before trying to conceive again.

Caution: Stop taking the herbs a few weeks before you try to conceive again.

Formula for uterine weakness
Combine the following: False Unicorn Root, Raspberry Leaf, Golden Seal, Blue Cohosh, Squaw Vine. Total: 100ml/g a week. Dose: tincture 1ml of each three times daily, or infusion/decoction of dried herb in equal parts, 1 cup three times daily.
Herbal tonics: Herbs are good for increasing vitality and health, so in addition the following could be taken to optimize your health for conception: Dandelion Root or Blessed Thistle to optimize liver function.
Verbena is a nervous system tonic specially good for women.
Doses as above.
Chinese Herbal tonics: Dang Gui (Chinese Angelica) and Wu Wei Zi (Schizandra), as tonics for the reproductive system, Siberian Ginseng (*Eleutherococcus*) as general tonic. Dose: 5ml of one twice daily, or one-third of dose for all three.
Ginger Root, fresh or dried, may be added to all the above herbs as it increases circulation to

the pelvic area and improves the general circulation. Dose: 2–3ml to 100ml of tincture, or it may be made into an infusion: a little fresh or dried ginger is very pleasant added to China tea.

The uterine weakness formula can be taken for up to six months and other herbs added as necessary. It is best to take advice from a medical herbalist on the most appropriate for you.

Loss of a baby

After twenty-four weeks loss of a baby is termed a stillbirth, if after birth the baby neither breathes nor shows any sign of life. After twenty-four weeks a live birth is a pre-term baby which has a chance of survival, with intensive care. If a baby dies before twenty-four weeks there is no legal obligation to issue a death certificate and no statutory obligations about what happens to the baby's body. Many parents find this deeply upsetting.

The death of a baby at any stage is a severe shock, and it helps if the parents are able to see and hold the child if they wish, or have a photograph, to be able to acknowledge and grieve for the loss. Naming the child may help. Most hospitals can arrange for a cremation from eighteen weeks and some as early as thirteen weeks. A baptism with a funeral or a memorial service can also be held. It is worth making inquiries. Some hospitals have a chapel, or will advise you where to go, and most provide counselling support. The Stillbirth and Neonatal Society and the Miscarriage Association are very helpful, and the latter has a network of support groups (see page 201). Health visitors will visit parents who have suffered a miscarriage if asked to do so, although this is not routine.

Emotional devastation may be followed by a sense of unreality or numbness. It is important to go through a mourning process: women who do not may take longer to accept the reality of the loss and to recover. Understanding the medical reasons for the death is also helpful in coming to terms with it and not suffering guilt afterwards.

Use of herbs in pregnancy

The herbs mentioned in this chapter are mild in their action and safe in the dosages recommended. In practice, I have found that women are more sensitive physically as well as psychologically when carrying their children, and smaller doses of herbs work well too.

Most authorities recommend that no herbal medication be taken internally in the first trimester (three months) unless for threatened miscarriage. It is best to keep to this rule apart from the case of morning sickness where only well-proven gentle remedies are suggested. Herbal remedies work best and are safest in the last trimester.

Herbalists prefer not to treat any long-standing illnesses in pregnancy unless they are interfering with the progress of the baby in some way. Do not try to self-medicate in such instances. If in any doubt at all it is advisable to seek help before taking herbal medication in pregnancy: ask your doctor or medical herbalist.

In most cases herbs are safer than many drugs available over the counter. They have been used for many hundreds of years and stand the test of time. The author believes that the benefits to women of certain herbs during the childbearing year should not be denied. It must be remembered that herbs have medicinal properties and should not be used carelessly. Some should not be used in pregnancy under any circumstances, usually because they may cause miscarriage if taken in very large amounts, and a list of these follows.

Medicinal herbs contra-indicated in pregnancy

English name	Latin name
Angelica	Angelica archangelica
Autumn Crocus	Colchicum autumnale
Barberry	Berberis vulgaris
Black Cohosh*	Cimicifuga racemosa
Blood Root	Sanguinaria canadensis
Blue Cohosh*	Caulophyllum thalictroides
Broom	Sarothamnus scoparius
Cotton Root	Gossypium herbaceum
Fern (male)	Dryopteris felix-mas
Feverfew	Tanacetum parthenium
Golden Seal*	Hydrastis canadensis
Greater Celandine	Chelidonium majus
Juniper	Juniperus communis
Life Root	Senecio aureus
Lovage	Levisticum officinale
Marjoram	Origanum vulgare
Mistletoe	Viscum album
Mugwort	Artemisia vulgaris
Nutmeg*	Myristica officinalis
Penny Royal*	Mentha pulegium
Peruvian Bark	Cinchona officinalis

Pokeroot	*Phytolacca americana*
Rosemary	*Rosmarinus officinalis*
Rue	*Ruta graveolens*
Sage	*Salvia officinalis*
Sassafras	*Sassafras officinalis*
Sweet Flag	*Acorus calamus*
Tansy	*Tanacetum vulgare*
Thyme	*Thymus vulgaris*
Tree of Life	*Thuja arborescens*
Vervain	*Verbena officinalis*
Wormwood	*Artemisia absinthium*

* These herbs are safe to use in childbirth (see page 60).

Laxative herbs contra-indicated in pregnancy

Alder Buckthorn	*Rhamnus frangula*
Cascara	*Rhamnus purshiana*
Rhubarb	*Rheum sp.*
Senna	*Cassia angustifolia*
Yellow Dock	*Rumex crispus*

Culinary herbs contra-indicated in pregnancy

The following herbs are harmless in culinary doses but should not be taken in large quantities, i.e. more than as a flavouring for foods.

Celery Seed	Parsley
Cinnamon	Rosemary
Fennel	Sage
Fenugreek	Saffron
Oregano	

Essential or aromatherapy oils contra-indicated in pregnancy

The following herbal essential oils should not be used for massage in pregnancy or taken internally.

Aniseed	Juniper
Arnica	Nutmeg
Basil	Marjoram
Birch	Myrrh
Cedarwood	Oregano
Clove	Penny Royal
Cinnamon	Peppermint
Clary Sage	Rosemary
Cypress	Sage
Fennel	Thyme
Hyssop	Wintergreen
Jasmine	

Note: Lemon, Lemon Verbena and Lemon Balm essential oils may irritate, so do not use if you have sensitive skin.

Herbs for minor complaints of pregnancy

Many of the herbs for use in pregnancy and childbirth as prescribed by modern herbalists come to us from North American Indian women. The connection they saw between the earth, its fruits, creation and the mother is reflected in their wonderfully supportive system of healing the mother and preparing for birth.

After the well-being of the baby, the mother's health and welfare are of primary importance during pregnancy. Herbs that are appropriate for her individual physical and emotional needs are suggested in this section. An alphabetical listing of ailments follows, explaining symptoms and detailing their herbal treatment, with self-help and nutritional suggestions where appropriate. Although some of these complaints appear in Part Two: A–Z Directory of Other Conditions, their treatment during pregnancy is a special case.

Abdominal pain in pregnancy

Pain in the lower abdomen during early pregnancy may be caused by miscarriage or ectopic pregnancy (where the foetus is in the Fallopian tubes, and pain is sudden, sharp and severe), fibroid degeneration, kidney inflammation, appendicitis, or stretching of the uterine ligaments. If pain is accompanied by bleeding at any stage this should be treated as an emergency.

During late pregnancy pain may be caused by the onset of labour, placental separation, ruptured uterus, ruptured stomach rectus muscle, kidney inflammation, or appendicitis. All severe pain in later pregnancy should be treated as an emergency.

Stretching pains that occur as the ligaments supporting the uterus soften during pregnancy are nothing to worry about and may be soothed by a herbal tea and massage. Lower abdominal cramping is common in early pregnancy and is nothing serious in the absence of other symptoms above.

Herbal treatment
Infusion of Chamomile, Lemon Balm or Lime Blossom
Dose: Equal parts as a standard infusion, 1 cup three times a day. Any of these may be combined 50/50 with a decoction of Cramp Bark, dose as above.

In later pregnancy abdominal pain may be referred from the spine or pelvic joints (see BACK-ACHE). A warm bath with either Chamomile essential oil (2–3 drops) or 10ml tincture of Cramp Bark and 10ml tincture of Lobelia added will help.

Braxton Hicks contractions
These contractions, which are experienced as transitory tightenings of the uterus in later pregnancy (after twenty to twenty-four weeks), may be soothed by Chamomile, Rose and Lavender essential oils (1–2 drops each) in a carrier oil such as almond oil, massaged in gently in a clockwise circular motion.

False labour pains
These early pre-labour pains may be experienced in the last month of pregnancy. Use anti-spasmodic oils as above. Bergamot is another essential oil that may be used for massage in the last month.
Dose: Motherwort and Black Haw as a standard infusion, 1 cup as needed.

Bladder pain in pregnancy
Experienced as aching over the pubic bone area, this may be caused by cystitis. See Urinary problems in pregnancy (page 53).

Stomach pain in pregnancy
This may be caused by indigestion (see Heartburn in pregnancy, page 49). Acute pain may be due to gastroenteritis (food poisoning with diarrhoea and vomiting). In this case consult your practitioner.

Allergy in pregnancy
If you suffered from allergies before pregnancy these symptoms may well be aggravated, and the hormonal and metabolic changes of pregnancy may even create new allergies. Symptoms are commonly painful sinuses, red and itchy eyes, a blocked or running nose without a cold, wheezing, itching skin or rashes, digestive disturbances such as diarrhoea and constipation alternating, indigestion, severe wind or griping pains, or may appear as joint pains like arthritis or as swelling, or as persistent cystitis. If you start your pregnancy with any of these symptoms you should seek medical advice. It is not a good idea to treat allergy during pregnancy, by desensitizing for example, but you should definitely get help after the birth (see ALLERGY).

One way you can help yourself is by trying elimination of suspect foods from your diet one by one. (see Elimination diet, page 137). If you do this, make sure you get enough nutrition from other sources to replace eliminated foods. If there is a family history of allergy this is particularly important so as not to pass the sensitivity on to the baby. Foods that are common culprits here are wheat and dairy products; it is wise to eliminate both of these during pregnancy and breast-feeding.

If you know that you are sensitive to environmental allergens the best you can do is to avoid them where possible. In the cases of sensitivity to chemical residues in fruit and vegetables, it is best to avoid these completely by eating only organic vegetables where possible.

Hayfever is a common allergy, and herbal treatment of it would include the use of gentle anti-inflammatory herbs for the nasal passages, such as a standard infusion of Eyebright, Elderflower and Chamomile, and eye baths of Eyebright used daily.

Anaemia in pregnancy
Due to the increase in fluid in your body during pregnancy, a reduction in red blood cell levels takes place. If this is excessive, anaemia results. You may feel tireder than normal, breathless, irritable, and low in energy. In later pregnancy the growing baby's need for iron often causes mild anaemia. Treatment is necessary if haemoglobin falls below 10g/dl of blood. Below 5g/dl (35 per cent of normal) bed-rest is needed as well. Your blood is usually checked at sixteen and thirty weeks to prevent this occurrence. If you begin pregnancy low on iron stores because of heavy periods, you are more likely to develop anaemia. Levels of other minerals such as zinc, copper and cobalt, and Vitamins B_1, B_6 and folic acid also affect iron absorption (see Nutrition – vitamins and minerals, pages 128–37).

Nutrition
Before conception it is a good idea to take a multi-mineral such as those formulated by Cantassium for two to three months, to build up mineral stores. If you are diagnosed as anaemic, bear in mind that iron deficiency is not the only cause of anaemia in pregnancy, and natural sources are better absorbed than those from an inorganic source, which can cause constipation. A liquid tonic made from organic sources such as herbs and fruits can be bought at health food shops. Vitamin C aids absorption and should be taken in conjunction with a tonic. Foods that are naturally rich in iron are: watercress, parsley (consume in moderation), kelp, spinach, berry fruits, cocoa, alfalfa, brown rice, wholemeal bread, wheatgerm, free-range eggs and dairy produce. Avoid tea with meals as this

reduces absorption. A multi-vitamin and mineral tablet daily (including 400mcg daily of folic acid as recommended by the Department of Health) may improve deficiency.

Herbal treatment
The following are iron-rich: Burdock, Gentian, Raspberry Leaf. These can be ground finely and put into small capsules (see page 10) and two taken twice daily. Raspberry and Nettle tea are very high in minerals. It is also recommended that Raspberry Leaf tea be taken daily from month six onwards, in preparation for birth.

Anxiety during pregnancy
See Emotional problems during pregnancy, page 44.

Backache in pregnancy
This is so common in pregnancy that it is thought to be normal, but with good posture it can be avoided or alleviated. Often it is due to pre-existing structural imbalances that are exacerbated by the extra weight. It is often experienced as lower back pain or sacro-iliac pain and is due to the expansion of the pelvic joints and softening of the ligaments compounded by muscle weakness and poor posture. Pain may be felt in the buttocks or groin, or radiating into the thighs and down the legs. It is important to take medical advice, and physiotherapy or osteopathy may be needed to correct it.

Self-help
Stretching exercises and advice on improved posture may well help. Lessons in Alexander Technique are excellent for pregnancy and will help prepare for the birth. Swimming is excellent too, but avoid the breast-stroke if you need to hold your head above water as this puts too much strain on the lower back. Try yoga, including 'The Cat', an exercise specific for the lower back. Always wear flat shoes with good support. There are good books on the market recommending exercises for pregnancy.

Nutrition
Be sure you are getting enough calcium and magnesium (in green leafy vegetables, wheatgerm, dried figs and apricots, almonds and other nuts and seeds, and dairy products) and in Nettle tea. Drink plenty of liquid, especially water, to aid elimination from the kidneys and ease backache.

Herbal treatment
Back massage with herbal oils will provide relief and improve muscle tension. One or two of the following essential oils in a carrier oil are suggested: Bergamot, Chamomile, Geranium, Ginger, Lavender. 1–2 drops of each essential oil are added to the base oil which should be warmed first.

St John's Wort oil relieves pain and irritation of the nerve endings. Massage 20ml into the sacral area of the lower back to relieve irritation and pressure on nerve endings. If severe, a cold compress of St John's Wort herb applied to the back for several hours and renewed as it dries out will help (see pages 11–12). St John's Wort tincture taken internally, 20 drops every few hours, will provide pain relief.

Bleeding gums in pregnancy
This is caused by increased blood-flow and softening of the gums due to raised progesterone levels. Astringent and healing herbal mouthwashes will help, but remember to visit your dentist during pregnancy.

Herbal treatment
Combine tincture of Marigold (antiseptic and healing), with astringent tinctures of Agrimony, Blood Root or Bistort. Dilute one part tincture in eight parts warm water and swill the mouth for 2–3 minutes twice daily or more if needed. Diluted lemon juice is an alternative.

Candidiasis (thrush) in pregnancy
This is caused by the proliferation of a normally benign yeast, Candida albicans, on the mucous membranes of the vagina. Kept in check, it does not cause any problems, but with increased hormonal production in pregnancy it can cause thrush, a thick, white, cheesy discharge. Other symptoms are itching and soreness of the labia and vulva. Sometimes it is brought on by antibiotics used for urinary infections, as these destroy the ecobalance of the flora normally present, killing everything off and allowing the yeast to colonize.

Herbal treatment
Herbal douches or pessaries are not advised in pregnancy. Instead, you can soak clean folded cotton or a sanitary pad in a herbal infusion or diluted tincture (the latter is stronger) and wear next to the skin for two hours at a time, renewing it as it dries out.

Marigold and Sweet Violet or Golden Seal (tincture or infusion, equal parts) should be diluted one part to fifteen parts water with 1 drop of Tea Tree essential oil added. Marigold or Chamomile cream with Tea Tree oil added, 5 drops to 50g cream, is anti-fungal and soothing used locally. Apply two to three times daily.

Note: Essential oils are highly effective in small doses and can burn, so should always be less than 1 per cent of a dilution.

Self-help

Candida albicans thrives on yeast and sugar-containing foods, and clinical experience shows that avoidance of these can improve the condition. (See Anti-candida diet, page 139). It also responds to bio-cultures of lactobacillus that provide benign, 'good' bacteria to counter the 'bad'. These are found in natural live yoghurt and can also be bought as dairy-free freeze-dried capsules. Take 2 capsules three times daily, or eat one large tub of yoghurt. Some women find it helps to apply the yoghurt locally as well, although this is messy. Zinc and iron deficiency during pregnancy may predispose to thrush. In an attack take a dose of 15mg zinc and 25–50mg iron plus Vitamin C 250mg daily, two to three weeks. Continue for longer if thrush is recurrent.

Constipation in pregnancy

Because food moves more slowly through the digestive system, constipation in pregnancy is quite common, especially if there is a previous tendency towards it. If your diet is high in bulky fibre from wholefoods, fresh fruit and raw vegetables, it should not be a problem, however. This means cutting out white flour products such as bread, biscuits, cakes, pasta, pizzas, etc. Red meat slows the digestion down and may aggravate the problem. Check if iron supplementation is the culprit: large doses can cause constipation. It may also be a reaction to certain foods such as wheat and dairy products, so you could try eliminating these one at a time for two weeks, to see if the condition improves. (Make sure you are getting enough protein from other sources.)

Self-help

Alter your diet to include wholefoods and take plenty of fluids, particularly mineral water, between meals. Try iron-rich foods instead of iron supplements. Avoid straining when you pass a stool; try deep breathing instead. A squatting position supported by a pile of books on either side of the toilet is ideal. Nothing can replace a daily walk as a stimulant to a lazy bowel. Stimulant herbal laxatives such as senna should never be used in pregnancy.

Herbal treatment

The following herbs may be useful:

Dandelion Root: decoction, ½ cup three times daily, or tincture, 2.5ml three times daily.

Psyllium Husk: 1 teaspoon twice daily in a glass of water followed by another glass of water.

Beetroot fibre as a bulking agent (much more effective than bran).

Cloasma or melasma

This is a dark coloration that appears on the face during pregnancy due to hormonal factors. Foods rich in PABA, part of the Vitamin B complex, may help. The Common Daisy has a reputation for clearing this type of skin discoloration. It would need to be made into an infusion and dabbed on.

Cramps during pregnancy

Unfortunately many expectant mothers experience leg cramping, especially later on in their pregnancy. This may be due to the fact that as the baby grows it takes more calcium from the mother, as well as to the extra pressure of the baby's weight. It usually occurs in the calves of the legs or the feet, and is worse at night.

Self-help

Massaging vigorously helps, or try the following exercise: lean at arm's length with hands flat against a wall, feet flat on the floor about 1 metre away, putting a good pressure on the hands until the cramp goes.

Try to avoid calcium supplements as these are poorly absorbed. The following foods are high in calcium, in order of content: kelp, whitebait and sardines, Cheddar cheese, blackstrap molasses, parsley, dried figs, almonds, watercress, yoghurt, egg yolk, goat's milk and cow's milk. Kelp tablets are easy to take, you may need 6–9 a day. (See Suppliers, page 203.) Insufficient hydrochloric acid in the stomach may be a cause of poor absorption, if so ½ teaspoon of cider vinegar in water before meals may sort the problem out. Hydrochloric acid tablets are not recommended in pregnancy.

Herbal treatment

Cramp Bark decoction: 1 cup two to three times daily with 1 cup before bed. This is a specific remedy for this problem. Hawthorn Berry decoction may be added (equal parts).

Chamomile, Nettle, Borage, Oatstraw and Raspberry Leaf tea are high in calcium: 1 cup daily may prevent cramps. Alternatively they can be powdered and put into capsules and 2–6 taken daily.

Cystitis
See Urinary problems in pregnancy (page 53).

Depression
See Emotional problems during pregnancy, below.

Diabetes in pregnancy
This may be picked up on routine urine-testing during pregnancy. Women with pre-existing diabetes and those with pregnancy-related diabetes need careful monitoring during pregnancy and dietary control to avoid complications.

Emotional problems during pregnancy
Although it is the most natural thing in the world for a woman to be pregnant, it is a time of great change and she may find it difficult to cope with all the new feelings as they emerge, especially in the absence of an extended family and if supportive female family members such as her own mother are far away.

Anxiety
Because of the increase in hormonal activity in the early stages a pregnant woman may feel easily upset. Mood swings are common and any problems loom much larger. Even the happiest mother expecting a planned baby may find that doubts and uncertainties arise. These may be compounded by nausea and tiredness and you may wonder if you want the baby at all! Concern with the future may preoccupy your mind as you wonder how you will balance work and baby, and how well you or your partner will cope with all the changes a new family member will bring, especially if this is a first child.

Your diet may affect the way you feel. Cravings for sweet foods may lead to blood-sugar imbalances, hence mood swings and tiredness, so avoid sugary foods and sweet snacks between meals, especially if you tend to feel nauseous: have a sandwich, some nuts or fresh fruit (in moderation) instead.

These feelings should start to pass by the end of the third month as hormones stabilize and energy increases with the establishment of the pregnancy.

It helps to sort out any problems about work or finance well before the baby is due. Talk over fears and worries with your partner, a family friend, GP or midwife. Ante-natal classes provide a helpful forum for discussion with other parents; you will find you are not alone in these problems. Some hospitals provide pregnancy advisory groups and parenting classes. The National Childbirth Trust (see page 201) provides Bumps and Babies Groups in most areas.

Deep relaxation, meditation and affirmation are all skills worth learning at this time as well as giving yourself the time to indulge in ways that make you feel good. As your body reacts to the changes that are taking place deep emotions may surface, but this may be no bad thing, for as you create another life within, so you may be able to make positive changes in your own life.

Well-being, a feeling of calmness, content and acceptance often prevail in the second trimester. As you blossom, you look and feel marvellous.

Later on, as the birth approaches, fears and apprehensions connected with labour are common. Ante-natal classes providing information on the process and teaching relaxation methods to cope with the pain are essential.

Common fears are of something going wrong in labour, losing the baby, the baby having some kind of abnormality, being unable to feed or care for the baby, etc. As regards breast-feeding, an NCT counsellor will provide information and support.

Talking to a health care professional may ease your mind. The unknown is more frightening than the known. Tiredness and insomnia may contribute to worries, so try to get plenty of rest and sleep. (See also remedies for insomnia in pregnancy, page 49.) If anxiety or depression becomes severe, ask to see a counsellor or psychotherapist. It is not clear whether ante-natal and post-natal depression are linked. Some midwives think that ante-natal depression may actually work to a mother's advantage as it may help her if she needs to seek support for coping post-natally.

Herbal treatment
Infusions of any of the following, or two or three combined. All are relaxants and anxiolytics, given in order of strength; try the mildest ones first.

Caution: Valerian and Hops are the most potent and may cause drowsiness during the day. They should be avoided in the first trimester (three months) of pregnancy.

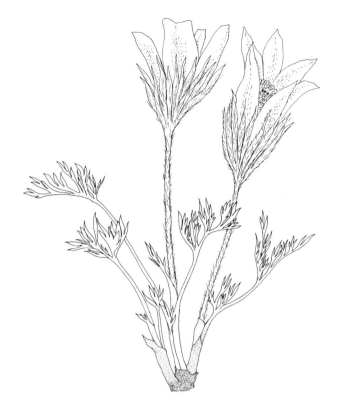

Pasque Flower *(Anemone vulgaris)*

Mild sedatives

Chamomile	2–8g	
Lime Flowers	2–4g	
Lemon Balm	2–4g	} per cup
Passion Flower	½–1g	
Motherwort	2–4g	

1 cup three times daily and 1 at bedtime, or tinctures, 2ml or 40 drops, twice daily.

Stronger sedatives

Valerian	½–1g	
Hops	½–1g	} per cup

1 cup three times daily, or tincture, 1ml or 20 drops, twice daily.

Oats *(Avena)*, tincture 2.5ml three times daily.

Caution: Do not take Hops if you are depressed (see Depression below).

Restlessness and irritability

Cowslip is excellent for the restlessness of late pregnancy. Skullcap strengthens the nerves and is effective for nervous tension.

Try Cowslip: tincture 2ml; infusion 2g. Skullcap: tincture, 2ml; infusion 1–2g. Both twice daily. Take half the dose if combining them.

Depression

Any of the following are a good general tonic and lift mood by nourishing the nervous system.

Lemon Balm: tincture, 2ml; infusion 2–4g. Nettles: tincture, 2ml; infusion, 1–3g. Oats: tincture, 2ml. Lavender: tincture, 2ml; infusion, 2–4g. They work well combined, in which case take quarter of the dose of each, three times daily.

Note: There are many proprietary herbal tablets for stress and anxiety on the market, some of which may be too strong for use in pregnancy. Check their ingredients carefully, and take half the recommended dose. If in any doubt or if the condition does not improve, consult a medical herbalist.

Dr Bach's flower remedies

These are excellent for treating emotional upheaval. They are homoeopathic remedies made by a special process of either sun-warmed infusion of flowers, or boiling. There are thirty-eight remedies, each one specific to a particular emotion. You need to choose one or more whose negative aspect most corresponds with your mood. Taking them will produce the positive (opposite) aspect. The remedies are completely safe to take at any stage in pregnancy.

The Bach flower remedies help increase self-confidence in ability to cope with the whole process of pregnancy and birth. Careful selection as needed can highlight the emotionally fulfilling aspects of pregnancy and anticipation of approaching motherhood.

Those that women have found particularly helpful during pregnancy are: Aspen, Cherry Plum, Elm, Mimulus, Mustard, Olive, Rock Rose, Star of Bethlehem, Walnut, White Chestnut, Wild Oat, and Rescue Remedy (the last is a combination for shock and overwhelming emotion, particularly good in labour).

Dose: Choose up to six remedies, and put 2 drops of each in a 30 ml bottle of spring water. Dosage for Rescue Remedy is 4 drops in spring water. Take 4 drops, four times daily.

See pages 174–5 for a full list and indications of the remedies.

If you are unsure which remedy to choose, consult a practitioner, or the Dr Bach centre (see page 203).

Fluid retention (oedema) in pregnancy

Oedema is common in late pregnancy, manifesting in slight puffiness of hands and feet as the increased fluids in the body enter the soft tissues, and can be quite uncomfortable. Towards the end of pregnancy the fluid levels in the body rise to prevent dehydration during labour. Excessive weight gain, warm weather and being on your feet a lot makes it worse. Resting usually gives relief, especially with the feet up. Drinking less is not a solution and may deprive the baby of needed fluid. Oedema may cause carpal tunnel syndrome with the swelling pressing on a nerve, causing pain in the wrist and hand. See Pre-eclampsia (page 51) if general swelling is accompanied by headache and a general unwellness.

Herbal treatment

Externally: Aromatherapy massage is very effective in providing relief, using essential oils of Lavender, Lemon, Chamomile, Geranium: 1 drop of each in 50ml base oil. It is necessary to massage in long smooth movements along the limbs towards the heart. Massage is of most benefit if a partner or friend can do this for you, although it will also work if you do it yourself. Some good books on massage, including massage in pregnancy, are available.

Internally: Cleavers, Horsetail, Couchgrass, Dandelion Leaf; 1–4g of each per cup, 1 cup infusion three to four times daily. Making up a thermos flask and sipping it throughout the day is an alternative. This is a gentle diuretic that will remove excess fluid.

Haemorrhoids (piles) during pregnancy

These fleshy protuberances that balloon out from the anus form small nodules that can be very sore and itchy and may bleed. Constipation (see page 45) and straining to pass a motion aggravate them. They usually occur in later pregnancy, or after the birth, but are reversible.

Caution: Commercial preparations for haemorrhoids contain mercury and local anaesthetics that should be avoided in pregnancy.

Self-help

Try not to strain when passing a motion; ideally use a squatting position. You could try this with your feet on books either side of the toilet. Exhaling deeply through the mouth is more effective and less damaging than straining. Follow recommendations for varicose veins in pregnancy (see page 54) but use ice-packs instead of hot and cold showers.

Herbal treatment

Externally: Cold compresses, made with herbal infusions on lint, gauze or cotton, are ideal to apply to the area (see page 12 for directions). Choose from either Witch Hazel, Plantain or Oak Bark (for astringency) and Comfrey, Mullein or Marshmallow (for soothing), and add Marigold for healing. In addition, either Pilewort or Witch Hazel ointment is specific, and should be applied after washing morning and night and after each bowel movement. Witch Hazel tincture or powder can be added to a cream base. As an emergency measure, distilled Witch Hazel is available from any chemist, although it is not as good as tincture of Witch Hazel. Proprietary brands of Pilewort and Witch Hazel ointments are available over the counter (see page 203).

At night, sitz baths (see pages 12–13) are an alternative to compresses. Simply make 1–1½ litres of infusion as above and sit in the bath or bowl for 20 minutes at a time. The infusion can be reheated and used several times.

Heartburn (indigestion) of pregnancy

During pregnancy the 'valve' between the gullet and the stomach is softened and becomes lax. Gastric acid may regurgitate upwards, causing irritation and a burning sensation behind the breast-bone. This is very common, occurring in 50 per cent of women, and is usually worse on lying down, at night and when overtired.

Self-help

Self-help measures can be very effective. It is best to eat small meals frequently and not to eat late at night. Chewing food thoroughly will help, as well as avoiding spicy, greasy, fatty or acidic foods that obviously irritate the problem. Do not drink any fluid with meals but have a drink half an hour afterwards. Taking a herbal digestive tea such as Peppermint (no more than 3 cups daily), Lemon Balm or Lemon Verbena after meals is particularly helpful. If you still find it a problem, careful food combining may be the answer (see page 144). Starches (carbohydrates) are not taken at the same meal as proteins but at separate meals, and vegetables may be combined with either of them. This causes less acid to be produced and eases digestion.

Herbal treatment

- Tincture of Peppermint and Meadowsweet: 2.5ml of each, diluted in water. Take as needed.
- Infusion of Peppermint and Meadowsweet: 2–4g Peppermint and 4–6g Meadowsweet per cup, three times daily.
- Slippery Elm powder or tablets: 2–4 tablets three times daily before meals; can be sucked or chewed for greater effect. To make a soothing drink, heat a cup of milk and water mixed and add 2g powder, stirring well. Good before bed.
- Charcoal tablets: 2–6 daily.
- Papaya enzyme tablets or pineapple bromelain tablets may also help. Chew 2–4 with a meal. All the above tablets are available as proprietary brands over the counter.

Caution: Some 'natural' digestive aids contain hydrochloric acid; avoid in pregnancy.

Insomnia in pregnancy

This is very common, due to difficulty in getting comfortable in bed, or because of heartburn which is worse when lying down. Some women are disturbed by having to get up to pass water several times a night, or the baby may be moving about. Mental excitement or anxiety can keep you awake. If this is the case, regular practice of meditation can relax you and aid sleep. A quiet mind often means a quiet body too. If you worry about not sleeping, this can set up a vicious circle, with sleep refusing to come. Avoiding beverages containing caffeine is essential if you find sleeping a problem. Other causes of insomnia in pregnancy may be food too late at night, or watching television late at night, especially if the content is disturbing. Overtiredness or lack of exercise will not help either.

Herbal treatment

Gentle sedatives: herbal teas are excellent in pregnancy. Taken during the day as well as in the evening, these will help to relax you at night. Combine any of the following to your own taste, for a pleasant-tasting tea: Lime Flowers, Passion Flower, Skullcap, Chamomile, Lemon Balm, Orange Blossom, Rose Petals.
Infusion: 2–4g of each per cup, 1 cup three times daily, and 1–2 cups before bed. Sweeten with organic honey to taste, as this also has a reputation for aiding sleep.
Stronger sedatives: Valerian and Hops have a 'hypnotic' effect; they can make you feel drowsy and a little spaced out, but are good when feeling desperately tired and not sleeping, if taken before going to bed. Decoction of Valerian: 1g per cup, sweetened; tincture: 3ml diluted. Infusion of Hops: 1–2g per cup, sweetened; tincture: 1–2ml diluted.

They are sometimes combined with Passiflora as proprietary tablets, and available over the counter, but half the recommended dose should be taken.

Caution: Do not take Valerian in the first trimester (three months) of pregnancy.

Oat tincture (Avena) is a safe insomnia remedy even in the first month of pregnancy: 1–3ml before bed.

Herbal bath oils: Essential oils of Chamomile, Lavender, Orange Blossom, Rose Geranium, or Otto of Rose, if you want to really treat yourself. Add 2–3 drops to a warm bath of any one or combine them, 1 drop each.

A massage with these oils, diluted 1 drop each

to 50ml of a carrier oil, is wonderful if you have a willing partner.

Relaxation techniques

Try a standard relaxation of muscle tension and release throughout the body, starting at the toes and going through all the muscles – calf, thigh, tummy, etc., clenching hard and letting go, all the way to your head. Deep regular breathing (feel your abdomen rise with each in-breath), is helpful if you can get into the habit.

Sufficient pillows under your bump and lower back will help you to get comfortable as the recommended position is on your side. You can buy a specially shaped 'Preggy Pillow' to support your bump. You should not lie on your back as this compresses the major blood vessels, returning blood to the heart. It is not difficult to learn to sleep on your side even if you are naturally a back sleeper, as this is the only comfortable position during pregnancy.

High blood pressure (hypertension) of pregnancy

If your blood pressure rises abnormally high after the normal slight fall in early pregnancy, there are a number of natural self-help measures you can follow, in conjunction with any treatment you are being given. Blood pressure should be compared with pre-pregnancy levels. A blood pressure of between 110/90 and 145/90 is considered normal in pregnancy, but above this, especially if the lower figure rises, is considered cause for concern. Danger signs are swelling of the hands and face, visual disturbance and headache (see Pre-eclampsia, page 51). As hypertension is a potentially serious condition, follow your doctor's advice.

Self-help

A vegetarian diet has been shown to lower blood pressure if it is based on 75 per cent fresh fruit and vegetables (especially raw, in salads). Onions, garlic and leeks are particularly good. A minimum of dairy products, with most of the protein in the diet coming from vegetable sources, like pulses, is combined with grains to give a complete protein. No caffeine beverages should be drunk. Eat fresh garlic if you can, added to salads, or take freeze-dried fresh garlic, in capsules two to three times a day. Citrus fruits, all high in Vitamin C, will strengthen blood vessels, or take a Vitamin C supplement. (See Healthy whole food diet, page 126.)

It is very important to get plenty of rest and sleep, and to reduce stress levels. Make sure you do not put on too much weight, and take plenty of exercise.

Herbal treatment

Note: None of the following is a substitute for a doctor's prescription.

Skullcap or Wood Betony as relaxants for associated tension and anxiety may be all that is needed. Try a tincture, 2.5ml twice daily of each, or see Emotional problems of pregnancy (page 46).

To lower blood pressure: Infusion of Hawthorn Berry and Leaf, 1–2g per cup, three times daily. Infusion of Lime Flowers, 2–4g per cup, three times daily. The two may be combined 50/50. Decoction of Cramp Bark, 2–4g per cup may be added to Hawthorn Berry and Lime Flowers in proportion of 2:1. This dilates the arteries, lowering blood pressure.

Dandelion Leaf as a natural diuretic will help, particularly if there is fluid retention; 4–10g per cup three times daily. Other herbal diuretics are Cornsilk, Cleavers, Yarrow, Horsetail, Couchgrass.

Morning sickness (nausea of pregnancy)

Nausea with or without vomiting is common in early pregnancy, and is often the first sign. It can happen at any time of day, several times if you are unlucky. Tiredness may accompany the nausea, or just feeling generally off-colour. The nausea is thought to be caused by chemical by-products of increased hormonal activity in pregnancy building up, creating a general toxicity in the body.

Self-help

You may feel liverish, and walking a mile a day may help sort this out. Nausea may also be the result of low blood sugar, especially if it is an early morning problem and is relieved by eating. Increased levels of progesterone may activate the vomiting centre in the brain. Pressure from the uterus in the late stages of pregnancy may also cause nausea. It will help to get up slowly in the morning and have a cup of herbal tea with a few dry, plain biscuits. (Ask someone else to bring it; you will not benefit if you start running around!) As a wide range of herbs are useful, a consultation with a medical herbalist is worthwhile. However, you will probably find some of the following will work for you. It may be that one will be effective for a time, then appear to stop working, in which case you should try another. Alternating the herbs on a daily basis may be more successful for some women. Nausea may be nature's way of getting you to rest in early pregnancy, when it is so important, so if all else fails this may be what you are needing most!

Herbal treatment

- Ginger is excellent, but it needs to be dried or crystallized, not fresh. It usually works right away but the effect decreases as time goes on. Tincture of dried ginger: 20 drops in a little water every hour, for up to five hours. Infusion of ginger powder: 1g per cup of hot water.
- Black Horehound is an anti-emetic. Tincture: 1–2ml three times daily. Infusion: 2–4g per cup three times daily.
- Spearmint Leaves may be added to improve the taste. They are anti-nauseant as well. Mix 50/50 with the above.
- Roman Chamomile: Tincture: 20 drops every hour, up to six doses, until you get relief. *Caution:* It may cause vomiting if taken in excess.
- Dandelion: Tincture: 20 drops three times daily. For liver congestion, 'bitters' are effective. *Caution:* Some bitters are not to be taken in pregnancy: see Herbs contra-indicated in pregnancy (pages 41–2).

Supplements

Deficiency of Vitamin B_6 has been suggested as a cause of nausea. Supplement with 10–20mg daily (best as part of a B complex supplement).

Consult your GP if vomiting is excessive or prolonged, when it is known as hyperemesis.

Placenta praevia

If the placenta implants low down in the uterus early in pregnancy it may obstruct the opening of the uterus later on. Fortunately, this is rare, and usually the placenta moves upwards as the uterus expands. Signs that all is not well include bleeding in late pregnancy as the baby presses on the placenta. This may be slight at first, becoming profuse quite quickly, and will be painless and bright red. It is a medical emergency, so get help quickly. Hospital rest is the only course of action and the baby may have to be delivered by caesarian section.

It is not advisable to try to treat yourself.

Pre-eclampsia

This is suspected when two or more of the following symptoms present: high blood pressure,

oedema, and protein in the urine. Blood pressure rises should be compared with early pregnancy levels, since an individual rise of 20mm mercury diastolic could indicate pre-eclampsia. Headache, visual disturbance and epigastric pain are signs of impending eclampsia (see Eclampsia below). Seek medical help urgently.

Preventing pre-eclampsia

Eat plenty of protein (60–80g) daily. There is 25g protein in ⅓ cup of milk, or 4 eggs or, 2 cups of cooked beans, or 50g nuts, or 100g fish, meat or cheese. Do not limit salt intake but be sensible about the amount you eat. Lack of adequate salt may cause pre-eclampsia.

Orthodox treatment of pre-eclampsia involves potassium supplements. Increase potassium levels naturally by eating foods rich in this mineral, such as bananas, unpeeled potatoes, chicory, raw beetroot. Dandelion Leaf is an excellent remedy as it affects the liver and kidneys, and is also high in potassium. Eat foods high in calcium: dairy foods – goat's milk, yoghurt and cheese being preferable to cow's – nuts, dried fruit, and green leafy vegetables. Molasses and kelp are good dietary supplements. Herbs rich in calcium include Alfalfa, Raspberry Leaf and Nettles. Adequate calorie intake is essential. RDA is 2400 (as much as for a labouring man).

Caution: Improperly managed pre-eclampsia may be fatal. If you suffer from it, use dietary measures only in consultation with your doctor or midwife.

Eclampsia

Swelling of body tissues, high blood pressure and protein in the urine together are all signs of a dangerous condition that can cause convulsions and ultimately the death of the baby from lack of oxygen. It is a medical emergency. A caesarian section may be necessary to save both mother and baby. Generally you would feel very unwell before this stage and would get help before the eclampsia became full-blown. The usual course of treatment is anti-hypertensives and bed-rest. Dietary measures and relaxation techniques such as yoga and meditation are a good idea once the condition has stabilized, to keep blood pressure down.

Polyhydramnios

Excess amniotic fluid around the baby may lead to hard swelling of the abdomen with symptoms of breathlessness and heartburn caused by the pressure. Fortunately this is very rare, but it is sometimes diagnosed at ante-natal checks. It is most often caused by twins, and there is a predisposition with diabetes. Some authorities believe bed-rest may possibly make pre-term labour more likely. Polyhydramnios does not harm the baby although it may possibly be associated with certain foetal abnormalities. The baby has more room to move and may present in a breech or other awkward position during labour, therefore careful monitoring is required.

Stretch marks

Stretch marks or striae around the growing abdomen and across the breasts are so common that they are thought to be normal: they are caused by the skin stretching quickly, with resulting damage to its collagen fibres. Unfortunately the marks are permanent, although they do fade eventually. They can be simply prevented, however. Skin will stretch an enormous amount naturally, but if well oiled every day in pregnancy will remain supple to the end, and no unsightly marks will remain. In the author's experience, every woman who has followed this advice has had no marks. If you have already developed some, try massaging a very little Vitamin E oil into the red marks every night. A healthy wholefood diet containing plenty of vitamins and minerals, particularly Vitamin E and zinc, is thought to help prevent skin damage (see pages 128–37 for food sources).

Herbal treatment

Use Wheatgerm Oil for prevention or combine wheatgerm and almond oil 50/50 if the smell of pure wheatgerm oil puts you off, add Lavender essential oil 1 per cent (20 drops to 100ml carrier oil). Massage once a day into abdomen, breasts and thighs, preferably after a warm bath. Try Marigold infused in oil too, which can be bought ready-made or is easy to make at home. Apply as above.

Tiredness during pregnancy

Tiredness is very common between weeks six to fifteen and twenty-six to forty. Hormonal changes are the usual cause, although the discomforts of later pregnancy and insomnia can compound the lack of energy.

Self-help

Poor nutrition is linked to fatigue, which is why first-class diet is so important (see page 39).

Sugary foods can cause blood-sugar swings which increase tiredness. Lack of energy may be an indicator that essential minerals or more protein are needed. If you are very exhausted, see your practitioner as this may be a sign of Anaemia (see page 43), especially if you are breathless. Good sleep is essential. Moderate exercise encourages sleep and gives more energy. A brisk hour's walk every day during pregnancy is a good habit. Meditation practice may increase levels of well-being as well as relaxing you. Rest is very important, and often you will find your body is directing you to this, especially in late pregnancy when you should rest as much as you need to. For some women, just carrying the baby and supplying it with nutrients takes all their energy. Anything on top of this can be stressful, so try not to overcommit yourself. A nap in the afternoon will help. Don't leave it too late to leave work if you are tired as you need to rest to build up stamina for the birth and for looking after the baby. It is recommended to reserve use of herbs for tiredness in later pregnancy.

Herbal treatment

- Proprietary herbal iron tonics, such as Floradix, available over the counter, which is a combination of iron-rich herbs and vitamins, is particularly recommended for fatigue. Follow directions for dosages, usually 10ml two to three times daily. It can be taken in early pregnancy and consists of concentrated iron-rich fruit and vegetables.
- Siberian Ginseng is an excellent tonic for women, available over the counter as an elixir or syrup. Avoid Panax Ginseng (usually called Korean or Chinese, sometimes – erroneously – American Ginseng) as this is too stimulating and can cause raised blood pressure in pregnancy as well as containing undesirable hormones for pregnant women.
- 'Thymoleptic' or supportive remedies like Oats, St John's Wort, Borage, Betony and Alfalfa raise the spirits and promote a general feeling of well-being.

As infusions, 2–4g of any of the above per cup, three times daily.

Formula for tiredness in pregnancy

St John's Wort	2 parts
Betony	1 part
Alfalfa	1 part
Borage	1 part

Total: 100ml/g a week.
Dose: tincture 5ml three times daily, or infusion of dried herb, 1 cup three times daily.

- Infusion of Nettles and Raspberry Leaf is full of minerals and may be taken daily instead of other beverages such as ordinary tea. It is especially recommended for the last month of pregnancy: 2–4g of each per cup, one to three times daily.
- Bitter liver tonics such as Dandelion, Burdock, Milk Thistle or Blessed Thistle can be taken occasionally as a boost to energy: 1–2g root as decoction. Either ½ cup of infusion twice daily for a week or 20 drops of tincture in water two to three times daily.

For tiredness during last four to six weeks of pregnancy
Raspberry Leaf: as a tea twice daily.
Squaw Vine: 20–30 drops twice daily.
These are also considered excellent as preparation for birth.

Supplements
Vitamin B complex: 25–50mg once daily.
A multi-mineral may also be appropriate as you may lack essential trace elements, especially in late pregnancy.
(See pages 128–37 for food sources of above.)
Queen Bee Royal Jelly, although not herbal, is recommended as some women have found it of great benefit for increasing energy in pregnancy. It is available as proprietary brand capsules over the counter. Chinese sources are considered to be superior.

Urinary problems in pregnancy
Urinary cystitis in pregnancy is often caused by bacterial infection ascending the urethra to the bladder and causing inflammation. There is often a niggling problem with increased frequency of passing water, which may be painful, and a sensation of aching around the pubic area. It is common in pregnancy due to laxity of the smooth muscle around the urinary outlet, allowing bacteria or inflammation to ascend more easily. In pregnancy cystitis can quickly develop into a kidney infection with vomiting and backache as the first symptoms. An attack can trigger preterm labour or mimic it, so treat this as an emergency.
Another cause of cystitis is an acid or, more unusually, alkaline urine. Have urinary pH tested or do it yourself. The pH or acidity/alkalinity of the body as reflected in the urine is important: it should be 7 or 7.5 but can become acid if it drops to 5, as the body tries to rid itself of excess acidity, which is usually the case with cystitis. The urine is alkaline when the body cannot rid itself of acidity, but the problem is the same.

Self-help
To correct acidity, get some exercise every day in the fresh air, especially if you have a sedentary job, and practise breathing deeply. Drink plenty of water as it is important to keep up fluid intake.
Avoid acid-producing foods such as meat, white flour and white sugar, which may aggravate (see Alkaline diet, page 142). When you have an attack, fast on vegetable juices and barley water, not fruit juices.
Pelvic-floor exercises will help as they tone up the muscles around the urinary exit (see Abdominal and pelvic exercises, page 195).
Other helpful measures include those that are common sense at any time. Wear cotton underwear and leave off tights. Always wipe yourself from front to back, wash as soon as possible after making love, do not use perfumed soap or vaginal sprays.

Herbal treatment
Based on herbs with a gentle anti-microbial action combined with those that have a soothing and anti-acid action. Note: Some of the herbs used to treat cystitis in Part Two: A–Z Directory of Other Conditions are contra-indicated in pregnancy.
If the pH is alkaline, initial treatment is to acidify the urine. Cranberry juice is best, 1 cup three to four times daily. Available in cartons or bottled in major supermarkets.
Combine from the following:

- *Anti-microbials*: Horsetail as decoction (30g to ½ litre cold water, left to stand for two to three hours then heated), 3–4 cups daily. Tincture (2–3ml), three times daily. Substitutes are Couchgrass or Cornsilk; follow the same directions.
- *Demulcent*: Marshmallow Root to soothe sore tissues (30g to ½ litre cold water, made as above), 3–4 cups daily.

- *Anti-acids:* Birch Leaf or Meadowsweet herb can be added to the above if the urine is very acid. They are mild, alkaline diuretics, good if there is intense burning with an urge to pass water but very little produced. Make as above.
- Essential oil of Lavender, diluted 1 per cent in a carrier oil, massaged into the abdomen just above the pubis, will help.

If the problem is an acute one it should clear up in two to five days. If the cystitis has become a chronic problem, the treatment may need to be carried on for two to three weeks, in which case take only 2 cups a day. If it does not clear or if there is blood in the urine, see your doctor. Have your urine checked in any case to make sure the bacterial infection has gone.

Supplements
Vitamin C in high doses can clear up urine infections. Take up to 1–3g daily for a few days only. Build up the dose gradually, and if it causes a runny stool, drop the dose back to a comfortable level. For long-term use, take 50mg maximum daily during pregnancy. Be careful as Vitamin C can sometimes cause acid urine and discomfort: look for a gentle form such as calcium ascorbate, preferably slow-release, or natural C from Acerola cherries.

Stress incontinence in pregnancy
In late pregnancy, as the hormones relax the muscles at the outlet of the bladder and the baby presses on it, a little urine may be leaked, usually when you laugh or cough. It is nothing to worry about, although you may need to visit the toilet often. Pelvic-control muscle exercises help (see Abdominal and pelvic exercises, page 195), and you should continue with these after the birth.

Varicose veins in pregnancy
The extra volume of blood in the body stretches the walls of the veins, and the pressure of the uterus on the veins returning blood from the legs causes them to balloon out, becoming tender and sensitive. The first sign is often heavy and aching legs, especially at the end of the day, usually towards the end of the term. Subsequent pregnancies are more susceptible to varicose veins. A family history may predispose you to them; if this is the case, take extra care. The veins of the labia may also become varicosed (vulval varicosities), as may the anus (see Haemorrhoids, page 48).

See also VARICOSE VEINS for herbal treatment.

Self-help
The best medicine is preventive. Take enough rest and do not stand too long if you can help it. It may be necessary to give up work sooner than planned, especially if it involves standing most of the day, for example.

Lying with the legs up during the day as frequently as possible, wearing support stockings and improving circulation by stretching exercises all help. One exercise is to lie flat on your back with legs raised high and spread against a wall, and the back supported on the floor, for ten minutes at a time.

Alternate hot and cold shower treatments directed at the legs – a burst of as hot water as bearable, followed by a longer burst of cold, repeated several times, will tone up the smooth muscles of the veins, opening and closing them. Five minutes of this treatment twice a day will improve the condition. Exercises that help are brisk walking and swimming, especially a kicking stroke, but avoid breast-stroke with head out of the water because this puts a strain on the lower back.

For more information on exercises see Janet Balaskas, *Active Birth* and Elizabeth Noble, *Essential Exercises for the Childbearing Year.*

5 Childbirth and Post-natal Care

'Birth, natural birth . . . surely the greatest event in a woman's life.'
Juliette De Bairaclai-Levy, Herbalist

Attitudes towards childbirth

As this truly momentous event in a woman's life approaches, whether or not it is her first child, it calls to the deepest part of her, and she feels all her resources and strength called upon.

Our Western culture largely determines mental attitudes towards childbirth; this is clear from observations of other cultures where different attitudes prevail. Herbal medicine has been used in childbirth since time immemorial, and still is in many parts of the world, so it may be of interest to look briefly at this. Herbs were also once in widespread use in Great Britain by 'wise women' who attended at childbirth. In fact some of these have been taken up by the orthodox medical profession.

Some cultures saw birth as a challenge, with the mother proving herself by going alone into the bush to labour and deliver. It is more common, however, for a great deal of emotional and physical support to be provided; often the whole female side of the family will be present. A traditional midwife may play a part, providing massage and herbs as required. Although in some cultures a labouring woman may be isolated and attended only by women, in others she traditionally has her male partner as her main support, as in Indonesia. If not actually present at the birth, the father may have an assigned role, usually to protect the sanctity and safety of the birthplace and take part in any religious ceremony. This is all powerful 'medicine' for the expectant mother. She feels that the family and the whole community are involved and supporting her efforts, and indeed they are all concerned that everything should go well for their prospective new member, for their survival depends on it. In affluent Western culture the setting may be very different but the need for security and support by the woman in labour is the same.

The instinctual or primeval urge to labour lies below the level of conscious thought within the lower brain and it is this level that needs to be accessed by the mother during birth if the natural processes are to be set in progression for all to go well. Just as animals seek out a calm, safe place where they will be uninterrupted in giving birth, so women in labour, if they are allowed, will do the same. This may not be easy in a high-tech hospital environment unless sensitive provision has been made. A woman in labour also needs attendants she knows and trusts and protection from emotional disturbance.

Choice of care in childbirth

Questions you may want to ask yourself when making your choice are: Where do I want to receive most of my ante-natal care? Who do I want to see for most of my ante-natal care? Where do I want to give birth? Who do I want to help me deliver the baby? Remember, you don't have to be rushed into a decision about your care, you should have time to talk to different birth-care providers, and to go away and think about it. If you change your mind later on and would prefer a different maternity package, you can change your booking. In England the Maternity Charter (1994) specifically states that women should be able to choose the type of maternity care, place of birth and attendants at the birth, and should be treated with consideration at all times.

Hospital birth
You may be offered shared ante-natal care between your GP and the hospital you choose. You will be registered with a hospital consultant and your baby will be delivered in the hospital maternity

unit, usually by a midwife unless there are complications. You may visit the maternity units of local hospitals, when you should ask to speak to the supervisor of midwives. However, there are other choices.

GP units

If your GP is qualified to do so, she or he may provide ante-natal care and deliver your baby in the unit. (If your GP does not hold this qualification you may receive care from a different GP for the duration of just your pregnancy, although a familiar GP provides a continuity of care that is reassuring for many mothers.) Most of the care in GP units is provided by midwives. Unfortunately they are becoming rarer as local health authorities close them down.

Domino scheme

An abbreviation for 'Domiciliary In and Out' this is on offer in many areas. Midwives in small teams provide women with continuity of care throughout the ante-natal period, during birth and postnatally, referring to an obstetrician should any complications develop. The mother returns home from hospital with her baby shortly after the birth but always has the option of a longer stay if she so wishes or if there are complications. She will be able to consult her GP as usual.

Most GPs are unwilling to provide care during delivery and midwives are universally acknowledged to be the experts in normal pregnancy and childbirth. Approximately 75 per cent of babies in the UK are delivered by midwives. Check with your local midwives that continuity of care will remain even if your pregnancy becomes complicated. In some areas this can be arranged for all aspects of your care, a big advantage because fragmentation of your care can be particularly distressing if problems have developed and if for instance you have an unexpected caesarian or forceps delivery. Recent reports show that low-risk women do better and have a lower rate of intervention with midwifery care only.

Home birth

This is becoming more popular again in spite of the trend towards more obstetrical care. You will need to approach the supervisor of midwives at your local maternity unit, stating you intend to have a home birth and asking her to supply a midwife to attend you. It is not your responsibility to provide GP cover for the midwife, but the Health

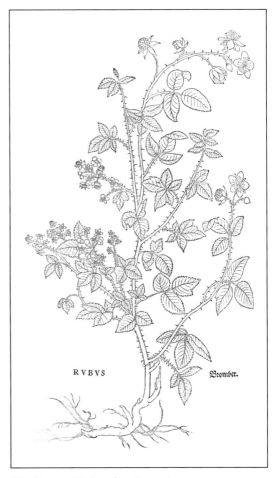

Blackberry (*Rubus fructicosus*)

Authority's. Your own GP may not be keen for you to have a home confinement, especially if he or she has no experience in this area. However, you can look around for a GP who is amenable. It is as well to bear in mind that most doctors are not happy about first births at home, but it is your right to choose. Recent statistics show that home deliveries are no more dangerous than hospital deliveries in most cases and for low-risk women are actually safer. In Holland 40 per cent of babies are delivered at home. For many women the comfort of home surroundings allows for greater relaxation and a non-medicalized birth.

If you need further help on deciding, refer to leaflets on home birth from the National Childbirth Trust (NCT) and Association for Improvements in Maternity Services (AIMS), to make an informed choice (see page 201).

Herbal preparation for childbirth

Herbal 'partus preparators' (childbirth preparations) have been used from time immemorial in all cultures, and have an excellent record, providing a type of care that is not available in modern orthodox medicine with its emphasis on treatment of disease or complications rather than prevention of them.

Herbs used by North American Indian women before childbirth included most notably Squaw Vine, Blue Cohosh, Black Cohosh, Birth Root, Cramp Bark and False Unicorn Root. These are mentioned for interest only and should be prescribed at the correct time and in the correct dosages by a medical herbalist.

Other 'partus preparators' from the European tradition include Raspberry Leaf, Lady's Mantle, Red Clover, St John's Wort, Blessed Thistle, Hawthorn, Motherwort, Goat's Rue, Nettle and Fennel. Raspberry Leaf is probably the best known, having a long history of use by midwives in this country. It is a superb preparation, toning and strengthening the uterus and at the same time making it more flexible for labour. However, it should be taken only in the last three months of pregnancy as it has been known to overstimulate the uterus. If this is the case, and you find Braxton Hicks contractions (see page 43) increased, cut back the dosage and the problem should settle down.

Preparation herbs are generally safe if taken only in the last six weeks; however, if in any doubt, it is best to take advice.

Caution: You may be tempted to use some of the remedies contra-indicated in pregnancy (see pages 41–2) to stimulate the onset of labour if you are two weeks or more overdue and induction is imminent, but *do not do so*, as this may be dangerous. Consult an experienced medical herbalist for advice.

The process of labour

Pre-labour
Pre-labour contractions can start and stop over a period of several hours, or even days, as if the uterus is getting ready. They are not as painful as those of real labour; if you are in any doubt, they are probably not the real thing.

Irregular contractions coming between ten- and thirty-minute intervals and not increasing in power and frequency are usually practice contractions. The contractions of true labour come regularly and increasingly quickly, building up to a peak of intensity and then subsiding. There is then a trough of quiet until the next contraction starts. Towards the end of labour, they reach a pitch of intensity as the uterus reaches the climax of its work. It has to enable the cervix to open, by pulling it upward and dilating it, and to propel the baby down the birth canal for delivery. It does this by contracting and relaxing several opposing sets of muscles, which must work in harmony.

Simple and useful advice to stimulate labour is intercourse and nipple stimulation; the prostaglandins and oxytoxin produced are powerful labour hormones.

Imminent labour
The signs of the beginning of true labour may include some or all of the following, not necessarily in the order given.

The show
This is a clear or slightly bloodstained mucus from the loss of the plug that closes the cervix during pregnancy. It may take place over several days or all at once. Labour can start anything from a few hours to several days later.

Loss of waters
The amniotic sac surrounding the baby releases its fluid which is clear and almost odourless. It may be just a leak from the forewaters in front of the baby's head, or the whole sac may burst, releasing a lot of water, in which case labour should start within forty-eight hours otherwise there is a danger of the unprotected baby becoming infected. In this situation induction of labour may be suggested. Breaking of the waters often happens at night. For instance, bending over to attend to a toddler may cause it, so in late pregnancy try not to bend; squat or kneel instead.

Bowel changes
The bowel may need to empty itself completely in several movements to prepare for birth.

Regular and painful contractions
The first contractions resemble intense period pains, often in the lower back. They reach a powerful level and come regularly at intervals of between two and ten minutes.

First stage

The cervix has first to efface or 'thin out' before it can open, and the longest part of the first stage is concerned with this and the first 4–5cm of dilation. Intervals between contractions are between five and ten minutes at the beginning, usually closing to two to three minutes or less towards the end. You are normally advised to go into hospital when contractions are coming five minutes apart, or to call the midwife if you are having a home birth.

The first stage may take anything from six to eighteen hours in a first labour, and an average of six hours in a second. If you would like to have a check from a midwife at any stage either at home or in hospital, telephone the hospital to arrange it. Variations in length of labour can depend on many factors including the position of the baby's head. A well-fitting, well-flexed head usually means a quicker labour.

Every woman pregnant for the first time wants to know what the birth will be like. It is impossible to give a very satisfactory answer, as every woman experiences it differently. Pain is subjective, but it is best to be prepared for an intensity of pain or sensation you have not experienced before. Some women describe it as resembling severe menstrual cramps, others say it is more of an energy rush. There is no doubt, however, that once labour has started you will be completely taken over by it. Natural endorphins (pain-killing hormones) are released as nature's way of making it bearable. It should be bearable; if it is not, this may be an indication that something is wrong. Breathing techniques learnt in ante-natal classes help, as you control the pain by breathing in with it and releasing it with your outbreath. Painkillers are available, of course, if you need them, as is TENS (transcutaneous electrical nerve stimulation) which electrically inhibits pain receptors in the area and stimulates the body's pain-killing chemicals. Some women manage quite well with just gas and air (Entonox). Herbal remedies can be taken if you have organized these yourself beforehand, and so can homoeopathic potencies of herbs which may be easier to take.

Plenty of support is essential. Building up good relations with the midwives on call may help you most: seeing a friendly face in labour is immensely reassuring. As previously mentioned, you can request continuity of midwifery care throughout pregnancy and birth, and postnatally. If this is not possible, however, try to have present in addition to your partner a female friend or relative with whom you get on well and who ideally has attended some ante-natal preparation with you, as the labour may be long and your partner needs support too. Having a partner who knows what is happening and who can remind you to relax and go with the contractions, is of course invaluable for many women.

Women have different methods of coping. Some adopt and maintain a certain position, others walk about; some need to express their pain and effort vocally, others are controlled; some retire into their own world whereas others want lots of support and sympathy. Either way you must do what is right for you. Taking each contraction as it comes, not thinking too far ahead, and above all staying in control help. Many women report that consciousness is altered during labour, with a correspondingly different perception of pain and of time; it sometimes sounds worse than it actually is! Focusing on the purpose of bringing forth your child gives it bearability that other forms of pain do not have.

Active birth

There is no doubt that remaining upright during early labour is the most advantageous position, helping gravity and the descent of the baby, and so if you plan to do nothing else, at least aim for this. You may feel that walking around is not for you and makes the pain worse, in which case ask your attendants to support you upright, or sit on the edge of the bed. All-fours or forward-leaning are extremely useful positions for second stage and delivery. It is possible to remain upright even on a delivery table by supported squatting, for example, or kneeling.

The worst possible position for both mother and baby is lying flat, which increases the work of the uterus as it has to work against gravity. This position has been used in the past for the convenience of the medical attendants, but you should encounter a more sympathetic attitude today.

Massage and water baths in labour

Massage is very helpful for some women, providing pain relief and relaxation. Firm massage of the lower back with circular movements over the sacrum with the thumbs and palms of the hands is especially good. Some even recommend the use of a wooden rolling pin. Massage of the legs and feet helps blood return to the uterine area and is soothing as well. Any area that aches will benefit from massage. Some women experience intense pain in the inner thighs, and find upward stroking or inner-thigh kneading and buttock shaking effective in releasing tension and helping 'open up' for the birth. As with other prenatal exercises, it is good to practise this beforehand with a partner so that you are both comfortable about doing it.

Immersion in warm water helps, and water baths are becoming a popular option for some women following Leboyer's technique. Some hospitals which do not have a birthing pool allow the use of one if you can supply it. However, unless they specialize in the technique, they are unlikely to deliver your baby in the water.

Transition stage

When energy flags towards the end of the first stage herbal remedies will help (see Herbal birth plan, page 61). Fluids such as fruit juices during the first stage will keep up blood-sugar levels. Nausea and vomiting can occur, in which case water will keep you from dehydrating. However, there is no reason why you should not be able to have snacks if you feel like them, as it is possible to neutralize acid stomach contents rapidly if necessary, and inhalation during anaesthesia can be prevented.

The transition stage marks the end of the first and the start of the second stage, when the cervix is nearly full open and before contractions change rhythm for the second stage and delivery of the baby. Contractions may be coming very fast and this may be experienced as a period of irritability or despair by some women, when everything seems too much. There may also be an interval of quiescence at the end of transition and before the second stage starts, when nothing is happening. This rest period before the beginning of the end should be respected as such. Known by midwives as 'Rest and Be Thankful', this stage may last for anything from a few minutes to two hours.

Second stage

The contractions become expulsive and of a bearing-down nature, often giving an uncontrollable urge to push, though sometimes this may not be felt at all. You will be urged to push, however, once the cervix is fully dilated. The second stage may vary from only a few minutes in a second labour to up to two hours or more in a first. The baby's head will be descending through the pelvic canal and women sometimes instinctively feel the top of the head as it 'crowns' at the vaginal entrance.

The baby's head emerges, the mother gives another push, and the body is born as the shoulders clear the entrance. Unless there are problems (with foetal distress, for example), the baby can be delivered up on to the mother's tummy, where the airways can be cleared of mucus. Alternatively, you may like the midwife to deliver the baby and leave him or her in front of you to pick up for yourself, if no suction is needed and the room is warm enough. Episiotomy (in which an incision is made to prevent the perineum tearing as the baby is born) should not be routinely necessary if the perineum is supple enough and the birth is proceeding normally (see Herbal birth plan, page 61, for oils to massage the perineum). The baby's head can be guided out carefully to prevent tearing. Midwives say that tears heal better than cuts, but a very bad tear may take a long time to heal (see After the birth, page 62, for herbs to expedite healing).

Third stage

The cord should not be clamped until it has stopped pulsating, otherwise the baby will be deprived of some of its blood supply. Very soon after the baby is born, the uterus contracts to separate the placenta from the wall and push it out. The placenta is usually delivered in twenty minutes to an hour if left to expel itself. If the newborn baby suckles at the breast, hormones that stimulate the process are released. If you want a completely natural birth (see below) check that the midwife understands about a 'physiological third stage', otherwise an injection of Syntometrine may be given to contract the uterus artificially and prevent haemorrhage. If bleeding is not excessive, however, this should not be routinely used, and there is no need to pull on the cord to hurry up the placenta.

The initial examination of the baby by the delivering midwife should be done in front of you. Both mother and father should have the opportunity to welcome their newborn, and the baby to cuddle up to the mother and suckle. These first moments of bonding are now known to be extremely important. If the mother needs stitches these can be done while she holds her baby. Afterwards it is lovely for parents and baby to be left alone, so that the three of them can get to know each other and share the new experience which is such a personal one.

You will probably be exhausted, but full of triumph and joy as well, or you may need to sleep and let the experience sink in. Food and drink are very welcome at this time. Usually you will be given a wash, or may take a shower if you feel like it, followed by a well-earned sleep, or at least peace and quiet for a few hours. Your baby should remain with you unless there are complications and the infant needs special care. Should this be the case, in some units you can accompany your baby.

For more information on a natural third stage see Sally Inch's book, *Birthrights* and leaflets from AIMS and NCT (see pages 201 and 205).

Natural childbirth

By definition this is a birth that takes its natural course, with no intervention on the part of the attendants, who allow the time-honoured process to go at its own pace. In order for all the natural processes to work as they should, mind and body must work together in harmony. If this balance is upset, distress and complications can set in. Intervention is very likely in these circumstances as contractions may become inefficient and labour prolonged. If the birth is not proceeding well, she may require assistance which could prove life-saving.

Advocates of natural childbirth are often concerned at increasingly routine medical intervention in childbirth, based on the assumption that what is necessary in some cases must be good for all. Doctors are relying more and more on foetal monitoring machines to assess the progress of labour, and it is as well to be aware that you may be offered procedures such as artificial rupture of membranes (ARM) or augmentation of labour by intravenous Syntocinon to hurry things along. There is some debate as to whether continuous foetal monitoring is an appropriate substitute for an attendant midwife's skill. It also means that the woman is unable to move around when attached to the machine. If you do not want routine intervention it is as well to be prepared with a birth plan of your own, and to know all the eventualities so that you and your partner can make informed decisions if necessary.

There is a real danger that the human approach is being lost in modern obstetrics and traditional ways of supporting women in labour ignored in favour of a more high-tech approach across the board. However, some maternity hospitals are trying to be more user-friendly nowadays by providing information and a more homely atmosphere.

There should be more encouragement for women to be actively involved in decisions affecting themselves and their babies. If this is not apparent and you want a natural birth, it may be wise to choose another hospital.

Contact AIMS or NCT or other childbirth organizations for support (see page 201). The Association of Radical Midwives is also useful for support and mothers are encouraged to attend meetings.

Use of herbs in childbirth

Probably the most important factors for an easy labour are fitness of the muscles used in childbirth, general stamina, breathing techniques, and a relaxed state of mind, all subjects taught in antenatal classes (see page 37). Most significantly, these classes teach that knowledge of the process taking place breaks the cycle of fear–tension–pain.

Herbs can be taken to relieve the pain of childbirth to some extent, but work better to increase the effectiveness of contractions, thus lessening pain and shortening the length of labour. Do not expect them to match the strength of orthodox pain relief like morphine, however. Ideally a medical herbalist should be consulted with a view to drawing up a herbal birth plan (see below). Some herbalists will also attend at a birth (contact the National Institute of Medical Herbalists, see page 202).

As well as the herbal remedies which act on the uterine muscles (see page 57), herbal essential oils can be easily and effectively massaged in or inhaled during childbirth. Herbs can also be used during the physiological or natural third stage of labour, to facilitate delivery of the placenta and prevent post-partum haemorrhage.

Herbal birth plan

The birth plan includes herbs that may be recommended by a medical herbalist to facilitate the process of labour which you can have available during the birth in case you wish to try the more gentle herbs before stronger painkilling drugs. The individual situation must of course be judged at the time by yourself and your attendant midwife. The author usually supplies a herbal birth kit with instructions, put together after consultation with the expectant mother and her partner. You may want to make your own along these lines. In the author's experience, there has never been any problem with hospital staff about the use of the herbal remedies if they are consulted beforehand, but it is best to mention them in your hospital birth plan. Herbs are easier to use at home, of course, and they seem to come into their own in the home environment.

Herbs for the first stage
• Chamomile tea to drink at the onset of contractions and throughout if possible when thirsty.
• Squaw Vine and Raspberry Leaf infusion, 50/50, 30g to ½ litre water for each, sweetened with honey, as labour becomes established. Aim to drink 1 cup an hour, for as long as you can. Squaw Vine is known for its ability to open the dilating cervix and Raspberry Leaf to facilitate contractions. Some women become nauseous and unable to stomach anything during labour; if this is the case take tincture of Squaw Vine and tincture of Raspberry Leaf, 4 drops of each in a teaspoon of water, or under the tongue.
    Herbal remedies can gently speed up or slow down contractions in the first stage in the case of under- or over-activity of the uterus. Black Cohosh and Blue Cohosh are effective herbs, but do consult an expert before taking them. The aim is to promote regularity and effectiveness of contractions.
• Anti-spasmodic remedies: Cramp Bark or Black Haw will help ease painful contractions. A 1-litre decoction of 50/50 of the herb would need to be made beforehand, kept warm and sipped frequently.
• Analgesics such as Valerian. Tincture, 2–5 mls hourly as needed, up to ten hours.
• Sedatives: Californian Poppy, Skullcap and Motherwort. Tincture, 2–5 mls hourly as needed, up to ten hours.
    Unlike the allopathic drugs, herbal remedies are calming without sedating, enabling you to remain fully aware of the birth process.

Herbs for the second stage
The intensity of the second stage makes it unlikely that you will want to take anything, unless contractions are becoming ineffective in which case frequent sips of Raspberry Leaf infusion will be invaluable. You will find it is enough to keep on top of the pushing contractions, and if you do this successfully then hopefully pain relief will not be needed; endorphins are high at this point. Bear in mind that the end is near, that the birth of your own personal miracle, your child, is imminent. You may like your partner or midwife to help with local applications to your abdomen and perineum of warm or cold flannels soaked in diluted essential oils as well as to mop your brow.

Local applications
• *Relaxing:* Containing essential oils of Chamomile, Lavender and Rose, 1–2 drops to 50ml drops of almond oil. This can also be used for a firm lower back massage in a carrier oil, or applied to the perineum, on a warm compress well diluted with water, as it is analgesic and soothing. (This is also good for helping stretchiness of the perineum if applied regularly for a month before the birth and even during it.) Cold compresses of Lavender and Rose Geranium on the wrists and forehead are reviving.
• *Stimulating:* Containing essential oils of Rosemary, Ginger, Penny Royal, or Clary Sage, 1 drop as above for massage. These can also be diluted in water and applied as a warm compress above the pubic hair. (Do not apply this formula to the sensitive perineum.)
• Oils can be heated in an oil vaporizer for inhalation. As well as Chamomile and Lavender for relaxation, Ylang Ylang or Jasmine are good as they are uplifting.
To take
• Panax Ginseng (Korean Ginseng): A sterling herbal remedy if the second stage is long and you are exhausted. Available as tablets, tincture, capsules or as an elixir in individual glass phials; 1 tablet/capsule as needed or 5ml of elixir or tincture.
• Composition Essence (a mixture of stimulating herbs available from Potter's Herbal Supplies) can be taken in drops, 5 at a time, diluted.
• Ginger can be used in any form, such as drops of tincture, as a tea, or fresh chopped added to tea, crystallized or as oil in capsules.
• Dr Bach's Rescue Remedy (see page 175) may prove invaluable for exhaustion and overwhelming emotions. If it cannot be taken, the lips can be moistened with it.

Herbs for the third stage
Herbs used in the third stage are best prescribed for you by a medical herbalist as they are quite

strong in their action and will help deliver the placenta quickly and stop bleeding if necessary.

It is necessary to prepare all remedies beforehand ready to take. For example, make a flask of the herbal tea when the first signs start, and remember to take one with you if you are going into hospital. You should have someone with you who knows how to dispense the remedies, as this will be difficult to do this yourself once you are in labour. Partners also appreciate having something helpful to do for you, such as massaging, preparing oils, making teas, etc. instead of waiting around for hours feeling helpless.

After the birth

Healing the perineum
- Marigold (often called Calendula in the shops) tincture diluted on cotton compresses applied to the perineum will heal any tears or an episiotomy quickly, dilute one part to thirteen parts water, renew as they dry. If too sore to touch, just pour very dilute tincture, 5ml to 500ml, over the stitches while sitting on the toilet.
- Marigold cream applied in addition, twice daily after a week, will help heal scar tissue.
- Witch Hazel or St John's Wort in addition for bruising. Dilute tinctures as above.

Note: If there is much swelling and bruising, try soaking sanitary pads in the diluted tincture and freezing them. A pad can then be worn next to your skin until it thaws out, to be replaced by another. These are more comfortable than frozen peas, which are sometimes recommended.

Recovery after birth
As you will be very tired initially, rest is the most important factor in recovery. The old-fashioned 'lying-in' was very sensible, but today a woman is often under pressure to get up and back to work in the home, before her body has recovered. You need longer than a week in hospital to get back on your feet. Most women are glad to get home, but ideally you should have two weeks' total rest and then take it easy for a month. You may have had intervention or even surgery; you will be learning to breast-feed if this is your first baby, and you will be surviving on much less sleep than you require. It may be difficult to organize, but try to get some help, especially if you have other children. This is just the practical side of things and does not include getting used to the demanding new person in your life, wonderful as the baby may be, or overcoming any trauma associated with the birth itself.

Treatment
Supportive herbal remedies would include those for ANXIETY, tension and insomnia in pregnancy (see pages 46–7). For tonic herbs to aid recovery, see Exhaustion after childbirth (below) and for herbs to enhance milk production, see Breast-feeding (below).

After-pains
Herbal anti-spasmodic drops are a very useful remedy to help the uterus contract to its pre-pregnancy position and to alleviate discomfort. They can be bought ready-made from suppliers (see page 203), 10–20 drops in a little water taken just before breast-feeding, as the pains are felt most when the baby feeds. They are also good for recovery if the birth has been a traumatic one.

Other remedies for after-pains are:

Black Cohosh   1 cup decoction (1–2g) 3 times daily
Cramp Bark   1 cup decoction (3–4g) 3 times daily

or a mixture of half of each. Either can also be taken as a tincture, 2ml three to four times daily. As the remedies may also reach the baby in your milk it is necessary to keep to small doses during lactation.

Anaemia after childbirth
Anaemia is quite common depending on the amount of blood lost during birth. It will be picked up at the post-natal six-weekly check, but if you are very exhausted and pale, take professional advice before that. See Anaemia in pregnancy (page 43).

Exhaustion after childbirth
Tonic herbs: Damiana and Ginseng are powerful remedies and good for exhaustion. Ginseng comes in many forms – Korean is most effective: also try either Codonopsis or Siberian Ginseng for a more gentle remedy – and can be taken as tea, elixir, capsules or tablets, 1 three times daily, or tincture, 5–10ml once or twice daily. Damiana can be taken as tea, 2–3g per cup, three times daily, or tincture. If breast-feeding, cut back the dose if it makes the baby restless or sleepless.

Oats provide a more gentle tonic, 2.5ml fluid extract or 5ml tincture, three to four times daily. Or St John's Wort, 4ml tincture three times daily, or as tea, 2–4g per cup three times daily.

Proprietary brands of Damiana and Ginseng are available over the counter.

Supplements

Continue to take pregnancy multi-minerals and take Vitamin B complex, 25–30mg once daily.

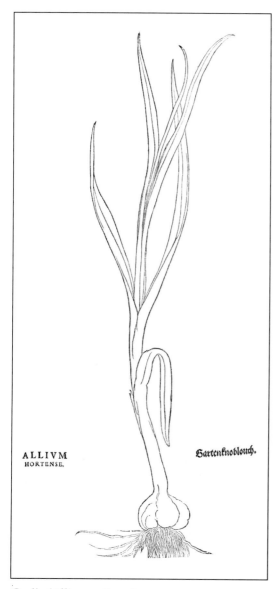

ALLIVM HORTENSE. *Gartenfnoblouch.*

Garlic (*Allium sativum*)

Vitamin A, D and E drops for breast-feeding mother and baby are available in pharmacies.

Post-partum injuries

Certain areas may have sustained bruising or even damage during birth. Changes in the position of the uterus and cervical problems will usually be picked up at the six-week medical check after the birth. Bladder problems such as frequency of passing water or leaking are common to start with (see urinary incontinence, pages 186–7). Injury to the pelvic bones are not uncommon and are best treated by an osteopath or chiropractor, who can put them right if out of alignment.

Breast-feeding

Breast milk is ideal for babies, as it contains certain trace elements, amino acids and essential fatty acids that are not found in modified cow's milk formulas: in fact a total of over 200 substances are found in breast milk. Mother's milk provides not only the correct nutrition but, through the antibodies it carries, immunity for the baby against early infections, and it may also prevent allergies, if there is a family history of these. Furthermore, breast milk is much cheaper and easier, as it is always available.

Although there is a knack to breast-feeding that needs to be learnt, there is no reason why most women should not be able to do it. Perhaps the most important factors are support and good advice at the outset. You should ideally put your baby to the breast as early as possible, preferably immediately after delivery. If the correct setting is provided at this initial stage, nature will take its course, but a good midwife will spend time showing a new mother and baby how to 'latch on'. The first milk (colostrum) is scant but very rich and will give the baby a taste for milk, as well as being full of important antibodies.

There are few contra-indications to breast-feeding, except for example if the baby has to be in intensive care, although as previously mentioned mothers may accompany their babies in some hospitals. If your baby is ill it is particularly important to try to establish breast-feeding to provide extra immunity. Breast milk is also easier to digest than formula milk. It should be possible to express some milk, by means of a breast pump. If no pump is available at the hospital, the NCT have a breast pump hire scheme, and there should be an agent in your area. See also Engorged breasts (below).

Breast size does not affect a mother's ability to produce milk. The hormone prolactin is produced in abundance after delivery and is stimulated further by the baby's sucking to activate the milk-producing cells in the breast. The nerve endings in the nipple also transmit a message to the pituitary gland to send oxytocin to the breast and to activate the 'let-down' reflex, so that the milk enters the nipples. It is a beautifully regulated process whereby the baby gets the right amount of milk, providing feeding is allowed on request.

The experience of breast-feeding is a richly emotional one for mother and child, both of them experiencing satisfaction, pleasure and comfort. However, the delicate balance of milk production depends on interaction of baby and mother, so if the latter is anxious, in pain or in some other way upset, this can interfere with the let-down of milk. Furthermore, it is not unusual for it to take as long as three to four weeks to get established properly. This is why it is so important to have a supportive environment from midwives, partner and family. It is well worth persisting if you want to feed your baby yourself, and do remember that you can get help. Breast-feeding counsellors trained by the NCT and the La Leche League provide support and information for women wishing to breast-feed (see page 201).

If you cannot breast-feed *do not* feel bad about it. With the right attitude and love the experience of bottle-feeding can also be very satisfying for a baby. There are some very positive aspects to it, one being that both the mother and her partner can share the feeding. Women back at work sometimes find that combining bottle and breast can also work well.

Use of herbs during breast-feeding
Herbs have a long history of supporting the breast-feeding mother. Drinking certain herbal teas ensures plentiful milk in which the benefits are passed on to the baby. Chamomile tea drunk by the mother will relax her baby and help them both to sleep. Careful selection of the right herbs is necessary as you would not want your milk to taste unpleasant or cause diarrhoea in the baby. Teas are best but small amounts of tincture will do no harm. Generally medical herbalists prefer not to treat mothers for any chronic illnesses during breast-feeding, but to wait until later. Tea and coffee are not recommended during lactation as they are far too stimulating for the baby. Plenty of water and herbal teas, particularly those mentioned below, are most beneficial.

Herbs to enhance lactation
Infusion of either one or several of the following: Fennel, Dill, Caraway, or Aniseed, 1–2g per cup. This makes a pleasant drink several times a day and the carminative effect will also help prevent colic in the baby.

Supplements during lactation
Lactating women need increased amounts of the following (see pages 128–37 for food sources):
Vitamin C: not more than 500mg daily.
Vitamin A as beta-carotene: not more than 2500 IUs daily. (Vitamin A as retinol is best avoided during breast-feeding as in pregnancy, see page 00.)
Vitamin D: 400 IUs daily.
Vitamin B: Vitamin B_1, B_2, B_3, B_{12}, folic acid as B complex: 20–25mg daily.
Vitamin E: cold-pressed vegetable seed oils such as safflower added to the diet are the best sources: 1 tablespoon daily.

Good sources of calcium are very important as are other minerals – magnesium, zinc, selenium, copper, and manganese – to build healthy bones. Food sources are best but you could supplement with a multi-mineral such as the Cantassium minerals for pregnancy.

Problems with breast-feeding
Insufficient milk
If milk supply is inadequate it may be that you are not getting enough rest and sleep, good enough nutrition, or are under stress of some sort. Try to get more sleep, if necessary in the day when your baby sleeps. Ask for help from your doctor or health visitor; breast-feeding counsellors are able to provide support and information. Often it is only a temporary problem.

Herbal treatment
The following remedies may help, all of which are tolerated perfectly well by a baby.

- Borage (Starflower): 3–4g per cup, or tincture 5ml. Or can be taken as oil of Borage (Starflower oil) in 500mg capsules, 1 three times daily, or Evening Primrose oil in 500mg capsules 2 three times daily, for the essential fatty acids necessary to build up milk supplies.

- Goat's Rue: 1–2g per cup, or tincture 2ml.
- Saw Palmetto: 1g per cup decoction, or tincture 2ml.
- Milk Thistle: 1.5–3g per cup, or tincture 4ml.
- Nettles: 2–4g per cup, or tincture 5ml.

Dose: Infusion/decoction of dried herb or tincture three times daily, half dose if combining all.

(See also Herbs to enhance lactation, above.)

Failure of milk supply

Take Chaste Berry as a decoction, 1g per cup, or tincture 1ml three times daily for up to one month. Can also be bought as proprietary tablets.

Engorged breasts

The milk may come in suddenly and the breasts become over-full, hot and painful due to the increased blood flow and excess fluid in the breast tissue. If this happens it may be difficult for the baby to suck as he cannot get a grip on the swollen nipple. It may be necessary to express some milk. This is done more easily if you apply hot compresses with flannels to get the milk to flow. Add 1 drop essential oil of Rose Geranium, Lavender or Chamomile to a basin of warm water. One reason for engorgement is that the baby is not feeding often enough – another reason for feeding on request, which benefits both mother and baby.

Note: Wash the oil off thoroughly before feeding.

Herbal treatment

An ancient and effective treatment is to apply a chilled bruised cabbage leaf to the breast inside the bra, replacing as necessary for up to twenty-four hours. This has a guaranteed anti-inflammatory effect.

Another remedy is Echinacea, 10 drops of tincture or 2 tablets every four hours.

Mastitis

If engorgement is not resolved, a painful inflammation of the breast tissue may result, usually because of a blocked duct. The breast may feel lumpy and there may be a tender red patch. Continue breast-feeding if possible, massaging the lumps towards the nipple as you do so. If you have a temperature and feel flu-like, it is a consequence of milk leaking into surrounding tissue within the breast. Contact a breast-feeding counsellor. Occasionally, if the treatment fails to resolve the problem, antibiotics may be necessary.

Herbal treatment

Follow instructions for Engorged breasts (above), plus herbal poultices applied for relief of inflammation.

- Marshmallow Root and Chamomile Flowers, powdered: take equal parts and mix to a poultice consistency. Apply on a dressing. Repeat as often as necessary, covering with cloths or plastic film to keep warm. If powdered herbs are not available, use a cloth wrung out in an infusion.
- Comfrey is also good. Use fresh mucilage from the root or leaf if possible, otherwise dried, which will need to be soaked overnight and pressed out. Saturate a dressing with comfrey, then apply to the breast after rubbing some olive oil into the skin to prevent sticking. Cover with plastic and leave until dry, then reapply. Comfrey ointment can also be used, but is not as effective.
- Applications of hot compresses of essential oils of Rose Geranium, Lavender or Chamomile, 1 drop diluted in water. Thyme oil may be added for its anti-bacterial effect.

If the condition does not resolve or recurs, you may have infective mastitis, in which case contact your midwife, health visitor or doctor.

Note: Wash off the application thoroughly before feeding.

Sore nipples

These may be caused by sensitivity to the baby's sucking and are the commonest reason for giving up breast-feeding.

Correct positioning at the breast is essential to ensure that the baby is latching on to the areola (the pigmented area surrounding the nipple beneath which lie the milk ducts) in order to obtain the milk and avoid damaging the nipple. Help in positioning from a midwife or breast-feeding counsellor may be needed in the early days.

In addition the following may help:

- Breast milk left to dry on the nipple.
- Marigold or Chamomile ointment. Apply after every feed.
- Witch Hazel tincture dabbed on without dilution. Be sure to wash off before feeding.

The NCT offer the following advice:

- Get really comfortable before feeding; use relaxation techniques, listen to music, think about milk flowing, have a warm drink.

- Expose breasts to the air as much as possible.
- Check that your feeding position is not causing the problem. Hold the baby close to you tummy to tummy, on his or her side, with head and neck in a straight line. To ensure a good feeding position bring the baby to the breast, not the other way round, and make sure s/he does not have to turn his or her head to reach the breast.
- Try to avoid leaving the baby until ravenous before feeding, then s/he will be more gentle on your nipple.
- Seek advice, as skilled help with positioning may be all you need.

Cracked nipples

These can be very sore but usually heal quickly. You may need to express milk from the affected side and feed from the other breast in the meantime. Seek advice from a midwife, health visitor or breast-feeding counsellor for skilled help with positioning.

CANDIDIASIS or thrush may be the cause of persistent cracked or sore nipples or deep breast pain. Check the baby's mouth for white spots which unlike milk curds do not rub off easily, see pages 139–41 for foods to avoid, and seek help from your doctor.

Herbal treatment

- Comfrey or Marigold ointment applied frequently.
- Diluted essential oil of Chamomile, 1 per cent in wheatgerm oil massaged in several times a day.
- Breast milk massaged in.

Nutrition and weight gain

Nutrition needs to be very good while breast-feeding. Extra Vitamins A, C and D are needed, especially in the winter. Sufficient protein is required, ideally 50g daily. You may crave sugar because glucose makes up a large proportion of mother's milk, but avoid snacking on sweets and biscuits, instead, eat a sandwich containing some protein to keep blood-sugar levels balanced. Obviously you need to drink plenty of liquid while breast-feeding.

Some women eat more than they need for themselves and their baby during pregnancy and find that they are still considerably overweight after the birth. However, during breast-feeding many women lose this.

Post-natal depression

This is a growing problem, almost exclusive to the Western world, and may be due as much to cultural and environmental factors as to the drop in hormone levels after the birth. Three to four days after the birth it is usual to experience the baby blues as the result of the sudden fall in oestrogen levels, and women often feel weepy and unaccountably sad at this time. However, these feelings normally pass within a few days.

Post-natal depression may be triggered by a difficult birth where there has been medical intervention such as a caesarian section, or immediate separation from the baby after birth. It is more likely in women who have previously experienced post-natal depression. If they lack family and community support, women may feel isolated and unable to cope with the demands of a new baby or to adjust to life-style changes. Coming to terms with combining working and looking after a child is particularly difficult for some women. Many women and their partners suffer from sleep deprivation with a new baby and this contributes to post-natal depression.

Symptoms vary greatly in severity from a general feeling of exhaustion and depression while still coping, to being so badly affected as to be unable to look after the baby. Other symptoms are lack of appetite and feelings of anger towards the baby when it cries, followed by terrible guilt. The depression may last for a few weeks or for up to a year following the birth and may recur with adverse circumstances. Baby blues can also affect women when they wean their babies, a grieving at ending the nursing relationship.

Self-help

If symptoms are fairly mild you can help yourself. Ensure that you get enough sleep. Try to sleep during the day when the baby does, if your night's sleep is very broken. Arrange regular breaks away from the baby: getting out of the house for even a short while helps. Develop coping strategies. Talk to other mothers, join an NCT Bumps and Babies group (see page 201). Take a holiday away from it all – but do not leave the baby behind! – to help you start enjoying being together again.

In severe cases of post-natal depression, mental symptoms may also include acute anxiety, panic attacks, hallucination, phobias and, more rarely, violent or psychotic behaviour, in which case professional help is imperative for the safety of mother and baby.

Herbal treatment
Treatment includes boosting the nervous system with general and nerve tonics and anti-depressants to start with, while addressing the hormonal imbalance. Add sedative herbs as needed:

Anti-depressants: Borage, Siberian Ginseng, Rosemary, Damiana.

Nerve tonics: St John's Wort, Damiana, Vervain, Oat, Prickly Ash.

Hormonal Herbs: Chaste Berry, Sarsaparilla.

Sedatives: Passion Flower, Lemon Balm, Skullcap.

A helpful combination you could try is as follows:

Formula for post-natal depression
Chaste Berry   25 per cent
Oats   25 per cent
St John's Wort   25 per cent
Borage   25 per cent
Dose: 100 ml/g a week. Tincture 5ml three times daily, or dried as decoction of Chaste Berry to which add other herbs as infusion, 1 cup three times daily.

Borage is specific for post-natal depression and can also be taken in capsules as oil of Borage (Starflower oil), 500mg three to four times daily, instead of tea. It is a useful addition to any post-natal depression formula.

In addition, Dr Bach's Flower Remedies (see under EMOTIONAL PROBLEMS) are excellent, especially Walnut for a time of transition, Mustard for this particular type of depression and Sweet Chestnut if the cause is of greater depth, leading to despair. See pages 174–5.

Essential oils of Jasmine, Clary Sage and Ylang, Ylang are specific for post-natal depression. Use 1 drop in the bath, or evaporate in an essential oil burner, and dab on wrists diluted in carrier oil 1 per cent.

Further information and advice are available from the Association of Post-natal Illness (page 201).

6   Weight Problems and Dieting

'In anorexia, bulimia and compulsive eating, what we see are women trying to change the shape of their lives by trying to change the shape of their bodies'

– Louise Eichenbaum and Susie Orbach.

Why diet?

Dieting has as much to do with mastering the female form as with any health consideration. It has always been desirable to emphasize the difference between the male and female form, and in this century this has been in terms of thinness; gone is the admiration for the Rubenesque figure. In the past, binding some parts of their bodies and padding others have been common practice among women. Decades of corset control have been replaced by dieting. The slimming craze dates back to the 1960s when Women's Liberation threw out the corset and the bra, but for most women it has brought slavery to food instead of liberation. The ideal is to have no flesh to support.

Women today are targeted by magazine slimming articles showing young, thin models who themselves have to diet to achieve this 'natural' look, or whose pictures are touched up to improve their looks. There is great pressure on young girls to conform, and patterns of restricted eating are often set at a very young age, but most of these dieters do not get any thinner, they just become obsessed with food. To a greater or lesser extent, this may lead to eating disorders (see Anorexia nervosa and Bulimia nervosa, pages 78 and 81).

Many of the myths surrounding thinness equate it not only with attractiveness, but also with success and self-control. Interestingly, these are primarily male attributes rather than female nurturing qualities. By denying a fuller figure the natural characteristics of femininity are also denied. Many women are not in fact overweight but just feel fat; if life is not going well it is their figures that are at fault.

For some women, control over life becomes synonymous with control over the body, and a pattern of over-eating then under-eating is established that is hard to break. Their lives become ruled by dietary considerations. Real weight gain may then start to be a problem.

Obesity

Excessive weight gain is a major problem in affluent Western societies and there tends to be a higher prevalence of obesity in women than in men. About one in seven adults in the UK is at least 20 per cent overweight, and in the USA the figure is even higher. The definition of obesity is the presence of a greater proportion of fat cells than normal, or an increase in the size of fat cells (see below). Not all heavy people, for example heavyweight boxers, are obese.

The determination of normal or excess weight used here is based on actuarial figures used by life insurance companies to give estimates of mortality caused by obesity. Ideal weight is expressed as the proportion of weight to height and abnormalities fall either side of this. The commonest formula is the Body Mass Index method (BMI) which is arrived at by dividing the weight in kilograms by the height in metres squared. The normal range for women is 20–25; obesity starts at 27–30 and gross obesity is calculated at 40+. Mild obesity is taken as being 20 per cent above the upper end of normal range of weight for height, and overweight at 10 per cent above. Severe obesity is rare and would be 100 per cent above ideal weight for height (see chart, opposite). Most obese women in the UK and the USA fall into the mild obesity category.

The main factors governing the development of obesity are primarily genetic: because of an inherited predisposition, the regulatory point may be set

Weight table for women

Which group are you in?

To find out whether you are underweight or normal weight, overweight, or obese, first find your height, then run your finger across to your present weight.

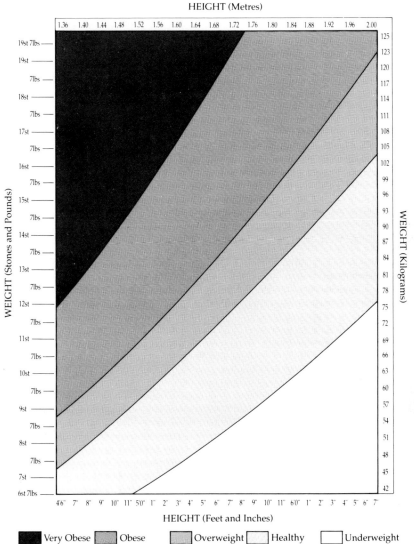

HEIGHT (Metres)

WEIGHT (Stones and Pounds)

WEIGHT (Kilograms)

HEIGHT (Feet and Inches)

■ Very Obese   ▨ Obese   ▨ Overweight   □ Healthy   □ Underweight

at the wrong rate in early childhood. Secondly, there are social factors: for various reasons obesity is much higher in lower socioeconomic classes, perhaps because better-off middle-class women have more time and money to devote to their figures, and their knowledge of nutrition may also be better. (It is interesting to note how social factors operate in different cultures, for example in some developing countries being overweight is considered desirable as it indicates wealth, and fatter women are considered to be more feminine.) Third come hormonal and metabolic factors, and fourth, psychological factors.

Problems associated with obesity

1 Increased mortality.
2 Specific medical disorders: hypertension, late-onset diabetes.
3 Degenerative diseases: atherosclerosis, high cholesterol levels and coronary heart disease.
4 Associated disorders: there is a direct correlation with gallstones, and increased incidence of gout, hiatus hernia, and VARICOSE VEINS. Gynaecological problems such as loss of periods (see page 23) and infertility (see page 33) are common, as are complications in pregnancy. Development of osteoarthritis of weight-bearing joints is likely (see pages 155–7). Excess weight worsens many chronic problems because of the extra strain on the body it imposes, and this is especially true of heart and respiratory disease.
5 Greater risk under anaesthetic and during surgery.
6 Greater risk of accidents and injuries.
7 Social and psychological problems, which include embarrassment about appearance resulting in unhappiness on social occasions, and failure to attract the opposite sex and difficulties within marriage. Lack of participation in sport is common, and getting no exercise only makes the problem worse. Self-imposed social isolation as the result of obesity may lead to depression.

Metabolic reasons for weight gain

Excessive weight gain consists of a relative increase in the number of fat cells and the quantity of fat they contain. Fat is stored underneath the skin and around various internal organs. When fat is stored as protein, lean body mass increases as well. Women have more subcutaneous fat than men to start with. Weight gain is caused mainly by an intake of food in excess of that required for the body's energy needs. There are other reasons as well – genetic, hormonal, psychological and social – which will be discussed below. The allocation of energy from food is decided largely hormonally by the endocrine glands. The body also has reserves of energy stored as glycogen, found in the liver and muscles, enough for no more than two to three days without food.

Basal Metabolic Rate (BMR)

The normal energy needs of the body consist of a basal level; this covers the needs of the myriad vital functions of the body at rest, including temperature maintenance. Extra energy is needed to burn up food when it is eaten, and for physical activity, and these are not included in BMR. The rate is measured at rest, twelve to eighteen hours after the last meal.

BMR is calculated as output in kilocalories per kilogram of weight. The 'average' female of average weight/height between the ages of eighteen and sixty has a BMR of 24 kilocalories per kilogram, that is, 1350 kilocalories per day. To give an idea of what this means, we need 1 kcal per minute to maintain life, another 0.5 kcal when asleep, 6 kcal when sitting and thinking and 9 kcal during exercise.

Different people have different rates, however, and individual BMR is very variable, which may go some way towards explaining why some women never get fat and others get fat easily. Many overweight women suffering from metabolic problems really do eat very little.

Factors affecting BMR

1 Eating food and digesting it raises BMR, the amount being proportional to calories eaten (protein does this by 20–30 per cent and fats and carbohydrate by 5 per cent over a 24–hour period).
2 Vigorous exercise raises BMR, and regular strenuous work or exercise raises it permanently.
3 Hormonal action: in women this falls faster than men and is affected by factors such as menstruation – BMR rises pre-menstrually and falls after menstruation, and is raised during pregnancy and lowered in lactation. Hormones from thyroid and adrenals directly affect it.
4 In the short term, BMR is raised by excitement and lowered in depression. Acute illnesses raise BMR but it falls during starvation.
5 In the long term it falls with age, and varies with climate and diet.

Because stores of fat are less metabolically active, those who have more fat tend to have a lower BMR. Interestingly, it has recently been discovered that some normal healthy people function perfectly well at basal levels much lower than previously thought, with important implications for weight gain.

The other index that is important in predicting weight gain is the amount of energy used every day. This can be done via an equation showing:

Estimated Average Energy Requirement (EAR):
EAR = BMR × PAL (Physical Activity Level) = 1.4

which is average for a sedentary worker with very little physical activity – only 20 per cent of all daily energy needs are for maintaining life.

Age 19–49 = 8.10 (1940) kcals per day
50–70 = 8.00 (1900) kcals per day
75+ = 7.61 (1810) kcals per day
(Multiply by PAL of 1.6 for moderate activity and 1.8 for strenuous activity.)
If you take BMR of the average woman
in kcal = 1350
kcal used in digestion of 2000 calories
at 10 per cent = 200
Energy used to maintain life = 350
Total = 1900

Using this calculation you can see that any extra intake above 2000 kilocalories if not burnt up by exercise will have to be stored by the body, usually as fat.

The thermogenic response, whereby any extra calories are lost as heat created by the body, tends to happen more within the physically fit and normal weight range.

Unfortunately, the majority of women in the West lead a fairly sedentary life and their basal metabolic activity contributes the largest proportion (around 70 per cent) of all their energy needs. This does not leave much margin for error when food consumption rises.

It is obvious where the preoccupation with calorie-counting encouraged by most weight-loss diets originates, but that is not the whole story by any means. BMR is lowered in both obesity and starvation, and this is why most dieting to lose weight is unsuccessful in the long term. As food intake is reduced, so correspondingly is BMR, in order to conserve energy. Thus, food eaten after dieting has a greater capacity to turn to fat.

The best way to increase BMR is regular, vigorous exercise, and the best way to maintain weight loss is through a sensible and nutritionally sound, not necessarily restricted diet. Only these two approaches in combination can help in the long term.

Genetic reasons for weight gain

In some overweight women normal BMR may be well below average and is probably associated with an abnormal thermogenic response – extra calories are not lost as heat. These women may just be more efficient at metabolizing their food. They need little energy for daily activities and so need little food: if they take more they will inevitably put on weight. They do not usually show any signs of being hypothyroid in spite of their slow metabolism. Often there is a family history of being overweight and the woman may have been so since childhood. Repeated dieting will be disastrous for these women as the body's 'thermostat' sets the basal rate ever lower following each attempt. However, environmental factors also play a part in obesity, and not all those genetically disposed to obesity need to remain overweight.

Hormonal reasons for weight gain

Disorders of the appetite control centre in the hypothalamus in the brain are the main cause of overeating. The hunger and satiety mechanisms may be faulty because of an hereditary disorder, but more often because of faulty and irregular patterns of diet and negative emotions. As a result, incorrect signals are sent between the two centres and the digestive system.

Lower thyroid hormone levels can lead to hypothyroidism: you should get your thyroid level checked if you are exhausted, develop constipation, become very sensitive to temperature and your hair gets in poor condition. Excessive levels of corticosteroid hormones from the adrenal glands lead to increased production of glucose and more fat being laid down. Other hormonal changes include those following childbirth (this often coincides with less exercise, although not less work!) and the menopause – the familiar 'middle-age spread'.

Psychological factors in weight gain

Psychological factors play a major part in many cases of excessive weight gain. Over-eating can reflect a woman's psychological state. Unmet emotional needs may be satisfied orally, in the way that a baby's needs are satisfied. 'Comfort eating' is well recognized as a reaction to stress, and usually reverses when the stress is relieved. Dieting can become addictive, however, with a woman being convinced that if only she can be thinner, life will be better. Feelings of boredom, frustration or rebellion may also relate back to childhood experiences with feeding. Indulgence in food, especially sugary food, can be used as an escape and becomes literally addictive. Depression is often associated with over-eating. Bingeing and overeating lead to ANXIETY, and Bulimia nervosa (see page 81) may develop. Anorexia nervosa (see page 78), an excessive preoccupation with weight gain followed by severe weight loss, is most common in adolescent girls following personality or family conflicts.

Social factors in weight gain

There are many reasons for simple obesity/overweight problems apart from metabolic or hormonal factors. Some social factors include the following:

Over-eating

All of us over-eat at some time, for example on holiday or at Christmas, when we are also taking it easy and not burning the extra calories off, and in many people this results in weight-gain, although this can usually be reversed quickly.

Persistent over-eating is a problem that appears to be connected with underestimation of food intake. Some women report that they are eating less than they are, and when they get down to analysing it are in for a surprise.

Faulty nutrition

Poor nutritional condition is caused by junk food diets and/or lack of money and lack of education on nutritional matters. A poor diet often tends to consist of foods such as fats, sugars and unrefined carbohydrates – white bread, cakes, biscuits, chips, etc. Fried foods may feature prominently in the diet. Alcohol consumption is often high. The need for extra carbohydrate snacks between meals is created by the poor nutritional value of food consumed. It is significant that the greatest proportion of the overweight falls into this category, which is also often the lowest socioeconomic group.

Social eating

A lifestyle which includes professional or social commitments such as business lunches, receptions, conferences, cocktail parties, etc. often involves irregular, or infrequent and too large meals. There are more women executives and senior members of the professions than ever before, with a tendency to over-eat rich gourmet food and over-consume alcohol.

Poor eating habits

Eating the main meal late at night, continual snacking and eating very fast without chewing properly all hinder efficient digestion. The habit of TV meals means that people are distracted by the programmes they are watching from an awareness of what and how much they are consuming. Television advertisements for tempting foods encourage repeated sorties to the kitchen. Food needs to be eaten, as the Buddhists say, mindfully, and with respect for the body. A proper mealtime, quietly sitting down, is essential for it to work at its best. This said, it is by no means the case that all overweight women have poor eating habits.

Changing eating patterns

Eating out frequently is becoming more common, as are takeaway meals high in saturated fats and refined carbohydrates. Women consume more alcohol than they used to; social drinking is on the increase and so is drinking alone.

Food advertising

Women are often persuaded to buy foods that look delicious but are processed, full of sugar and fat and lacking in vitamins. Chocolate and other confectionery have huge sales in the UK. Despite government health reports of the harm done by fats and sugar, they continue to be omnipresent and marketing even sometimes presents them as good and wholesome; in the case of refined sugar there is no basis at all for this.

Lack of exercise

Exercise is decreasing, with an estimated 30 per cent of adults taking regular exercise, and only a proportion of these doing enough to influence their health beneficially. Of the older generation – age sixty and over – some take a little but a large proportion (50 per cent) take none.

Why dieting often fails

This is mainly the result of the body adapting to dieting in order to compensate for the lack of energy input. How it does this depends to some extent on the severity and length of the diet and individual health and constitution.

Basal rate is generally higher in the obese because of increased lean body mass, the body's attempt to correct the situation by laying down less fat. During dieting the body attempts to correct the situation as it sees it, that is, to conserve resources because it is starving (for example, on a restricted diet of fewer than 1000 kilocalories a day for over a week). The tissues it chooses to sacrifice are those it sees as metabolically least useful; in the case of the sedentary overweight woman, unfortunately this is not fat, but lean mass or protein. The body seeks to retain tissue that is most active, and, particularly in someone who diets a lot, this will be fat.

The body cannot be expected to know what you want it to lose; it has several reserves, including blood glucose, as well as glycogen stores to convert to glucose, fat and protein. As the lean mass falls, so does the basal rate. A lower calorie intake when dieting leads to a progressively smaller weight loss at each attempt. To counteract this during dieting you would have to take strenuous exercise. This is why most diets do not work.

Initial weight loss is due to loss of glycogen (and water) which is a readily accessible source of energy – up to seven pounds may be lost in a short time. As glycogen is essential to the body, all of it has to be regained after the diet.

Another way the body adapts to less food intake is to slow down physically, to conserve energy. Although you may not notice this, you will probably rest and sit around more when dieting, which makes it even more difficult to lose the desired weight.

Dishearteningly, those who are very fit and active and relatively slim, and who therefore have a larger proportion of their body mass as lean muscle or protein, lose body fat naturally as part of their weight loss, their metabolic rate does not fall and they do not have problems afterwards.

Exercise

We take far less daily exercise than our ancestors, who as hunter nomads are supposed to have walked forty miles a day! A few thousand years is a short time in evolutionary history and our bodies have not adapted to the kind of affluent Western life-style where few people take any exercise that actually benefits their health. To compensate, it is necessary to do aerobic exercise, literally to aerate your tissues. Oxygen is vital for good metabolism, which is sluggish without it. It is necessary to work at exercising until you are breathless, which means that new oxygen is burning energy stores and aerating your whole system beneficially. The lymph and blood systems will also be stimulated to pump better, removing any waste products from the tissues.

Pulse check

A pulse check is one method to show if you are achieving the right results by exercise. To do this safely, subtract your age from 200 (for example, age 26: $200 - 26 = 174$ beats per minute). When your pulse reaches a count of 174 (or whatever your own particular figure was) during exercise, keep working out at the same pace for ten to fifteen minutes. Always warm up first and do not stop suddenly; march or walk yourself down to your normal pulse rate. To be really beneficial, exercise needs to be taken at least three times a week, even for only fifteen minutes; it is frequency that is important. Regular exercise raises metabolic rate permanently. You can attend an aerobics class and exercise to music; cycling, jogging, and swimming performed enthusiastically are also forms of aerobic exercise. Jogging and running should be on a soft surface, not on tarmac or pavement. A mini-trampoline or personal bouncer is a good investment but do not use this if you have a prolapsed womb.

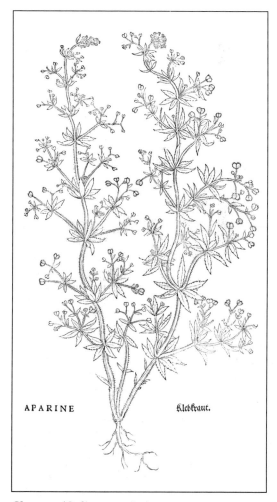

Cleavers (*Galium aparine*)

Popular methods of weight reduction

There seem to be as many diets on the market as there are women wanting to lose weight. Novel diet plans constantly fill new books and range from reasonable to downright dangerous in their efforts to persuade diet addicts to try yet again. It seems that a successful and easy way of losing weight is the modern version of the Holy Grail.

If you look at the medical facts, there are only two possible methods of reducing weight, which can be combined. One is moderating, reducing or strictly controlling food intake, and the other is increasing energy output by physical activity. The suggestion that certain foods burn up calories faster than others has not been proved, nor has the existence of 'brown fat' cells that supposedly burn up energy at a greater rate.

It seems surprising that authors of diet books are so ill-informed about metabolism. Most diets fail because they do not take into account what they do to the dieter's body and, worse, leave her feeling it is all due to a lack of will-power. It is not surprising that so many women, not understanding why they don't succeed, become obsessed with dieting.

There are several schools of thought among advocates of dieting to lose weight. The main ones are outlined here.

Restricted food intake

Moderation in food consumption is really a myth as a method of weight loss unless the dieter is only just above target weight, or has gained weight very recently. It is not easy to achieve moderation, which is why it most often fails to work as it is not usually maintained for long enough. For habitual dieters basal metabolic rate is the other factor; as this decreases with lower intake, it becomes necessary to eat less and less as time goes by to produce even a small loss, which is even more difficult to stick at.

Calorie-controlled or restricted diets

These consist of diets ranging from 800 to 1500 kilocalories a day. Unless a wide range of foods is eaten, vitamins and minerals are likely to be in short supply. Diets of fewer than 1000 kilocalories a day will cause depletion of essential micronutrients unless supplements are taken. Conventional reducing diets of 1200–1500 kilocalories produce a slow weight loss. The energy deficit is so small and any weight loss after the initial loss so slow, however, that women usually abandon them. Women generally feel that their lack of will-power has led to their failure, not realizing they are up against impossible odds. There may be an apparent success initially on a very restricted intake but the returns are diminishing, especially on returning to the diet previously eaten. It is easy to get obsessed with continual calorie-counting which is not always that accurate.

Very low-calorie diets

Diets below 500 calories a day are definitely not to be recommended. Loss of essential nutrients is certain unless special ready-made food supplements are used in conjunction, and the immediate health risks, to the heart for example, are unacceptable. Many over-the-counter, get-slim-quick diets use mixed vitamin and mineral powders combined with protein, but although they may work initially, this is all too often not the case in the long term. The benefit of these prepackaged diet formulas of 400–700 kilocalories is questionable considering their substantial cost.

'Starvation' diets for the obese are sometimes performed in hospital, and weight loss is often impressive, but dangerous complications can arise. The metabolic effect comes into play and in most cases, unless the operation is followed by a continuous strict dietary regime, all the weight is regained over time. The usual tendency is to overeat afterwards to compensate. In one study done in the 1920s of people in good health following a very restricted diet over a six-month period, they all ate ravenously for a while when they stopped the regime, due to uncontrollable hunger. This may be the body's attempt to provide for the possibility of future periods of starvation. It is significant that most of the sample, although of normal weight before, tended to become overweight after the study.

Appetite-suppressant drugs

Although these have shown moderate results in initial weight loss, when they are stopped the situation is reversed and combines with a return to previous eating patterns to undo it all. Prescription-only amphetamines and similar drugs have been used in the past, but because of their side-effects, not least addiction, they tend to be prescribed less now. They should always be a last resort, for essential short-term weight loss before surgery, for example.

Carbohydrate- and fat-exclusion diets

Low-carbohydrate diets have been among the most popular for weight loss, limiting or excluding bread and other bakery products, pasta, rice, potatoes and of course sugar. Unfortunately these diets drain the body of glycogen in the initial stages without touching the fat stores at all. As the glycogen levels fall, so do blood-sugar levels (HYPOGLYCAEMIA), and dieters commonly experience symptoms of dizziness, shakiness and weakness. As low glycogen levels stimulate the hunger response in an attempt to get some fast-burning carbohydrate into the body to raise blood sugar, ravenous hunger results. Low carbohydrate is replaced either with high protein and/or higher fat content, which is not a good idea. This is the case with many commercial low-calorie foods. High-protein diets for any length of time carry their own risks and are not recommended: for example, high-protein lean meat is not actually low in fat just because the fat is trimmed off. Fat contains twice the calories of carbohydrate. It is not sensible to cut out all fats, as essential fatty acids are vital to normal metabolism, but a fat-reduction diet is very appropriate to weight loss.

Instead of calorie-counting, it does make sense to consider which foods are fattening and which are not; be vigilant against those that are calorie-rich, in particular fatty foods (most fat in the diet comes from fatty meat, butter and margarine, milk, cheese, cooking fats and oils, cream-rich dishes and pastries and biscuits). Alcoholic drinks, particularly spirits, are calorie-rich.

With persistence, some weight will eventually be lost on a moderate exclusion diet but loss will only be maintained if moderation is maintained.

Balancing diet following dietary recommendations

Government reports recommend that for health reasons:

- Fat be reduced to half present levels of intake, and saturated fats (butter, cheese, cream, milk, cooking fats) be no more than 10 per cent of the diet. The diet should contain essential fatty acids, as found in vegetable seed and nut oils.
- Sugar be reduced to half present levels of consumption.
- Carbohydrate be increased by half and consist of slow energy-releasing unrefined carbohydrate – cereals, potatoes, beans, lentils, etc. – rather than refined products. Unrefined carbohydrate is the best source of energy and should form 50 per cent of the diet.
- Dietary fibre be increased to Dietary Reference Value (DRV) of 40g.
- Protein: DRV is 45g a day for women, much less than is eaten at present.

(See also pages 123–5.)

General hints for choosing and cooking food

- Avoid frying and roasting food. Grill or bake preferably, or use very little oil – 2–3 teaspoons at a time. Olive oil is best. Use special cooking pans that require no fat for frying.
- Reduce or cut out red meat. If you eat it, cut off all fat.
- Cut down on chips and fat-roasted potatoes; save them for a once-weekly treat. Dry-roast or boil potatoes.
- Use more vegetable protein in your meals, such as pulses, ideally combined with rice, preferably brown. Tofu from soya is a good substitute protein. Aim at having two to three vegetarian main meals a week, even if you are a meat-eater.
- Replace full-fat cheese with low-fat and cream with yoghurt or fromage frais. (Eat no more than 100g of cheese a week.)
- Eat bread containing unrefined flour and use wholemeal flour and unrefined brown sugar (in moderation) in cooking.

High-fibre diet

A diet high in natural fibre, from skins of fresh fruit and vegetables, for example, and unrefined carbohydrate from grains, combined with a moderation of intake and avoidance of foods known to be calorie-rich, has shown the best success rates for long-term weight loss.

Fibre is important for a regular bowel movement, and in studies of people following high-fibre diets, is shown to be preventive of bowel disease. Among other things, it creates a wholesome micro-climate of bacteria in the bowel and reduces food-transit time, so less toxicity is produced. Naturopaths suggest that fat harbours toxins to a greater degree than other tissues, and the more of it there is the more difficult it is for the body to metabolize normally, hence fat stores are created. (See Healthy wholefood diet and Biogenic diet, pages 126 and 139.)

Note: Addition of wheat bran to the daily diet is not

the answer; natural fibre is less irritating, much bulkier and therefore more healthy for the colon. Beetroot fibre, available powdered in capsules, is a more acceptable dietary addition.

Behaviour modification

Behavioural therapy is used to try to modify behaviour patterns leading to obesity. The theory is that women respond with hunger to inappropriate 'food cues' such as time of day, emotional appeal and other psychological associations. They will be advised to *stop dieting*, to eat what they want at meal-times. Treatment focuses on changing habits like ready availability of food, particularly high-calorie snacks, and slowing down the rate of eating. Rewards for goals reached and self-monitoring methods are used, including detailed record-keeping and nutrition education. The therapy takes time, especially if life-long habits need to be changed, but is moderately successful. Cognitive therapy has recently been used to overcome self-defeating attitudes. As an alternative, counselling may provide individual women with insight into their problems, to help break the pattern of inappropriate eating responses.

Self-help

In the long term, the following will help you lose weight without dieting.

1 Develop self-awareness to help you break out of the negative cycle of under-eating and over-eating. Recognize the pattern: eating for comfort – guilt and self-criticism – dieting – then rebelling and bingeing. Accept that you may have psychological needs that are not met, and find ways of fulfilling them without resorting to food.
2 Realize that dieting does not resolve psychological issues, and get help if you need it. Control over life through dieting is an illusion: in fact dieting leads to loss of control over eating.
3 Become aware of your appetite and the amount and type of food you eat. Keeping a food diary helps some women. You could also note your emotions at the time.
4 You may need help to get back in touch with physiological hunger and establish new eating habits. Don't be afraid to ask for referral to a therapist – support is so important.
5 Any moderation in food intake needs to be sensible and accompanied by an increased amount of vigorous exercise, to lose weight and to keep it off.

6. Balance your diet rather than restricting calories. Remember that most of us eat more than the government-recommended amounts of fat, starch and protein, and far less dietary fibre. Judicious food-combining is helpful for the improved digestion of food (see Food combining diet, page 144). This is particularly good if food intolerance has been a cause of weight fluctuation.

Keeping weight off

Establish new eating habits.

1 Stop dieting!
2 Eat a regular balanced meal three times a day, with the most substantial at midday, to avoid the hypoglycaemic response. It may be necessary to eat small meals often at first. It is very important to keep blood-sugar levels balanced for weight control – if you suspect you have a blood-sugar problem see Hypoglycaemic diet (page 143).
3 Avoid stimulants, including coffee, sugar, tea, chocolate, cigarettes and alcohol. Over-use of these indicates an underlying blood-sugar imbalance. This is usually connected with stress, so lifestyle changes may be appropriate.
4 If persistent over-eating has been the main problem in weight gain, eating small meals is often recommended to bring a disordered appetite-centre in the brain back into line, but take advice.
5 Eat slowly and chew well. The satiety response that lets you know you are full occurs twenty to thirty minutes after starting eating.
6 Try to eat in a calm environment, out of the office for example, or away from the rest of the family for a while if necessary. Reschedule your day if business interferes with eating, and avoid long business lunches where possible.
7 Get some support from your doctor, counsellor, self-help group, etc. Women often find that associations like Weight Watchers work for them because they provide motivation and encouragement.
8 Taking control again over eating will empower you. When you feel good about yourself and the way you look people respond to you positively, increasing your confidence further.

Herbs to aid weight loss

Although herbal remedies can play a valuable part in weight loss, they have been abused by over-the-counter herbal weight-loss preparations consisting mainly of strong herbal laxatives and diuretics. These merely encourage a greater weight loss of water than usual on a diet, often through diarrhoea.

The only way to lose weight permanently is to raise the metabolic rate and take more exercise, as described on page 73.

You can also raise your metabolism by making your body more efficient at converting food into energy if you use herbs to stimulate the thyroid gland gently and improve a sluggish digestion.

To remove toxicity from tissues see Colon cleansing (page 146). This is not a short-term measure, however; any significant improvement will take place over four to six months.

Liver-cleansing is important for improving digestion and removing toxicity. See Liver diet (page 148), which should be followed for four to six weeks initially.

It is also important to pay attention to lymph-system cleansing to stimulate the lymph glands that remove metabolic breakdown products. Really vigorous exercise such as running, or daily jumping on a bouncer, stimulates the flow of lymph. Lymph is pumped around the body better, ridding it of excess fat build-up. Local treatment includes skin-brushing daily with a natural bristle brush purpose-made to encourage tiny lymph vessels under the skin to work well.

Liver herbs: Dandelion Root, Burdock, Barberry, Oregon Grape, Black Root, Golden Seal. These herbs need to be taken in conjunction with a High-fibre diet (see page 75) to be effective.

Gall-bladder herbs to aid fat breakdown: Blue Flag, Fringe-Tree, Boldo.

Lymph-cleansing herbs: Cleavers, Cone Flower (Echinacea), Poke Root, Chickweed, Burdock, Blue Flag, Ribwort Plantain, Fennel.

Metabolism–enhancing herbs: Bladderwrack, Cola, Cayenne, Astralagus, Atractylodes, Liquorice, Ginger.

Dose: 2–3ml tincture twice daily of one of each group (with exception of Cayenne which should be taken in very small doses, ¼ml daily). Decoction/ infusion: ½–1 teaspoon dried root, 1 teaspoon dried leaf per cup twice daily. Individual combinations are best; for example, if there is a lot of mucus or fluid retention use more lymph-cleansing herbs. The following is a helpful formula you could try for two to three months.

Formula for weight loss

Atractylodes	20 per cent
Cleavers	20 per cent
Burdock	20 per cent
Boldo	20 per cent
Oregon Grape	10 per cent
Cola	10 per cent

Total: 100ml/g a week. Dose: tincture, 5ml three times daily, or decoction/infusion of dried herb in equal parts, 1 cup three times daily.

- In addition a tea of Fennel Seed and Cleavers, 1 teaspoon per cup three times a day, with the above formula.
- Spirulina, an algae that is very nutritious and provides essential nutrients that aid fat breakdown, as well as giving the feeling of being satiated; 1 tablespoon in water or juice before meals.
- Bladderwrack or Kelp, 5ml tincture or 5g dried herb as decoction three times daily. As powder, add to food. Rich in iodine, it stimulates the thyroid.

Bladderwrack is considered the main active herb for weight loss, and usually shows results over two to three months in conjunction with other measures suggested. Due to its very strong taste, it is more palatable as tablets. These can be purchased over the counter, in which case 2–3, three times daily, for up to four months.

Some proprietary tablets made by long-established herbal manufacturers such as Potter's Herbal Supplies or Gerard House (see page 203) will contain the above constituents: check labels.

Vitamin and mineral supplements

These aid conversion of glucose to energy. Try for a month initially with other measures. Do not take long-term without the advice of a practitioner.

- Vitamin C: 1–3g daily.
- Chromium (GTF) (part of glucose tolerance factor for blood sugar balance): 100mcg daily.
- Zinc (involved in numerous enzyme reactions in digestion and the energy production cycle): 15mg daily.
- Vitamin B_3 (part of GTF) and B_6 (production of hormones including insulin for blood-sugar control): 100mg of each daily.
- Co-enzyme Q10, an essential co-factor in cell energy production, thought to metabolize food more quickly: 30–60mg daily.

- Also helpful: digestive enzymes – natural enzymes, Papain and Bromelain: 250–500mg with a meal.

Eating disorders

Three types of eating disorder are recognized: Compulsive eating, Anorexia nervosa, and Bulimia nervosa.

Compulsive eating

In this disorder, very large quantities of food are eaten during a binge. As no steps are taken to eliminate it, considerable weight gain is inevitable, leading eventually to obesity. The causes are generally those that relate to Bulimia nervosa (see below).

Self-help

See measures under Obesity above (page 68).

Herbal treatment

See herbs for emotional problems under Anorexia nervosa and Bulimia nervosa below.

Anorexia nervosa

In 1992 the Royal College of Psychiatry estimated the number of secondary-schoolgirls in the UK with anorexia as being around 10,000, and that 1 in 500 girls and young women between the ages of fifteen and twenty-five suffer from this condition, with about 100 dying from it every year. 40–50 per cent of anorexics go on to develop the sister syndrome Bulimia nervosa (see below).

'Anorexic' is a medical term which literally means 'loss of appetite'. 'Nervosa' simply means nervous, that is, to do with upset of the nervous system. The fact is that far from losing her appetite the anorexic will undoubtedly feel hungry much of the time, but denies this hunger.

Although Anorexia nervosa is often described as 'the slimmer's disease', the condition is not just a case of over-dieting and slimming. An anorexic is approximately 25 per cent below her normal body-weight. She usually weighs between 5½ and 6½ stone. Age of onset is usually between eleven and thirty-five years, although the condition may persist into later life. Only one in 10 sufferers is male.

Symptoms of anorexia

There are a number of warning signs. If some, or all, of these symptoms apply to you, then there is a strong indication that you are likely to become anorexic:

- Loss of weight: 1–2 stones or more.
- Fear of being overweight.
- Strictly limiting the amount you eat, counting calories or weighing all your food compulsively. Obsessively writing down the amounts you have eaten in a diary.
- Constantly thinking about food.
- Avoiding meals and pretending that you have already eaten.
- Making yourself sick, or taking laxatives after food.
- Weighing yourself at least once, or more often, every day.
- Exercising as much as possible, in an attempt to burn off calories and lose more weight.
- Emotional problems: isolation, withdrawal from people, unhappiness, depression, mood swings, insomnia or agoraphobia.

Five or more of the above are an indication; for a diagnosis of anorexia, the following in addition must be present:

- Periods have ceased (amenorrhoea) for at least three months.
- Lanugo (unusual body hair) is present, and head hair is dry/brittle and thin.
- Severe constipation.
- Abdominal pain, dizzy spells and a swollen stomach.
- Bad circulation, skin cold and dry, possibly discoloured.
- Tiredness and weakness.
- Suicidal feelings.

Anorexia is not a disease and is reversible if sufferers start eating normally again. Rather, it is a psychological disorder with a complex causation.

Causes of anorexia

Social: Cultural and social pressures on women in the Western world to be slim, as portrayed in the media, leads to their dissatisfaction with their own bodies.

Psychological: A need for control – power over weight may perhaps be the only power some women feel they have in life; by obsessively focusing on it problems and emotional confusion can be ignored. Anorexia is a way of coping.

Ironically, although anorexics often refuse help, this is often an attempt to draw attention to their plight.

A fear of growing up, of puberty, of adulthood with all its pressures, decision-making and responsibilities is partly to blame. Low self-esteem is invariably reported by anorexics.

A fear of being sexually attractive may be a root cause, possibly as a result of having been sexually abused. Consciously or unconsciously a woman may attempt to desexualize her body as a defence strategy.

For girls at home, parental strife, marital break-up, separation and divorce are all precipitating causes. High parental expectations, whether real or imagined, are perceived as a threat to be coped with. Many anorexics are perfectionists and fear failure; consequently they become workaholics. Stressful events such as a bereavement, leaving home, examinations or unhappiness at work may play a part.

Obsession with weight loss may escalate into anorexia if the original weight goal is superseded by another, lower one, and so on. Loss of judgement is common; an anorexic will view her body as fat when there has been great loss of weight and she is actually emaciated and fragile.

Treatment and recovery

It is important to recognize that the first crucial step towards recovery is both acknowledging and accepting that something is wrong. Confide in a close family member or friend. Give them permission to help. Ask for support in contacting a doctor, a health visitor, therapist or self-help group. It is crucial that there are people who will understand and offer support and help in the early stages.

Sources of help

General practitioners and hospital treatment

Unfortunately doctors may belittle the problem, or suggest that all that is needed is dietary advice. If this happens, you should look for a doctor who is prepared to understand the depth of the problem and support you. Before you go to the doctor, it may help to write a brief account of what has been happening. Make it clear that you cannot manage to solve this problem on your own if that is indeed the case. You may need to see a counsellor or psychologist as well as a nutritionist.

Once your condition is diagnosed, you will be expected to stop losing weight. If you continue to lose weight, people may step in and take charge of your life. If you are a child you can be put into hospital against your will, if your parents request this, even if you are over the age of sixteen. You must realize that people are not against you; they care and do not want you to die.

Inpatient hospital treatment consists of response-reward behavioural techniques and/or drugs. As a patient you may have things taken away from you and you may be restricted to bed-rest; you earn privileges by weight gain. Some patients have described this as inhumane. Their families, who are usually feeling guilt-ridden, may be excluded, and their feelings and needs not met. Many girls leave 'fattened up' but still with a very low body-image and anorexic thoughts and feelings. Relapse statistics are high.

Note: In most cases, people with anorexia can be helped without being taken into hospital.

Therapy

Some GPs can refer you to a counsellor or to a hospital as either an outpatient or an inpatient. As an outpatient, it is important that you continue to see your GP as well as having counselling. Some hospitals have special adolescent units and family therapy departments. Most hospitals have psychology departments.

If you are under sixteen, it is likely that you will be referred to a Child and Adolescent Psychiatry Service for treatment. Alternatively, you may be referred to a paediatrician and/or dietician. If possible, the options should be discussed with your GP. If you are given a choice you should consider counselling seriously because this will help you to talk about the problems you are experiencing, and, more importantly, will help you to identify what the problems actually are. You will also need help with the physical problems of eating.

Cognitive/behavioural therapy is the method commonly used by psychologists (based on learning new patterns of behaviour); treatment should be client-centred and focused on the individual's needs. A system of short-term goals and rewards set between the therapist and the client as well as exploration of physical and emotional needs, family relationships, etc. is important. You may be encouraged to write a 'Feelings and Food' diary, so that you can monitor both your progress and your feelings associated with food. This is useful, especially during the initial stages of recovery, and can be dropped later when it is no longer needed. Relaxation techniques and stress management are essential. A major part of therapy involves re-appraising attitudes to food – rather than seeing it as 'good food' or 'bad food', the sufferer learns that a balanced intake needs to incorporate both, and fear of food needs to be replaced with acceptance and enjoyment.

Self-help

Remember that recovery is gradual, set realistic short-term goals (with a therapist), focus on what you have achieved and do not look back. As you gain weight some of the old fears will return, but this is only temporary and will pass when you begin to get better. Therapy should help you cope. It will be necessary to learn how to recognize proper feelings of hunger and fullness, and this will take time. It will also be necessary to keep to diet sheets given by a dietician, or other therapist, at first, until you can depend on recognizing these feelings. You should try to eat the agreed amount. Do not in any event skip a meal. Occasional binge-ing, usually of refined, sugary carbohydrate 'for-bidden' foods, is normal and you should try not to panic if this happens. Carbohydrate foods should be eaten three times a day to prevent this craving.

Ask for the support of family and friends, make some decisions about mealtimes with them and stick to them.

Herbal treatment

It is essential that this is taken in conjunction with counselling and nutritional advice.

Herbal treatment focuses on returning digestive function to normal, building up the bodily strength again and supporting the emotional side. In the early stages a herbalist would concentrate on bitter herbs to stimulate digestion and its reflex action on the whole body. (The recommended herbs are shown in italics.)

Liver herbs: Barberry is specific for this problem, and should be taken in addition to bitters. Dose: tincture, 2–3ml three times daily. An equally effective alternative is Burdock, 8ml twice daily.

Bitters: Angelica Root, Centaury, Wormwood, Gentian, to stimulate and normalize appetite. Dose: tincture, 10 drops of one of these, three times daily. A proprietary formulation called Swedish Bitters is available over the counter or from suppliers. Take as directed.

Anti-nauseant herbs: German Chamomile, Black Horehound, Spearmint. Dose: tincture, 5ml in water as needed.

For anxiety: Skullcap, Californian Poppy, Valerian, Passion Flower, Wild Lettuce. Dose: 5ml tincture of one, or combine two or three together, in which case half of dose, three times daily. Alternatively, as infusion in equal parts, 1 cup three times daily of Skullcap, Rose Petals, Lime Flowers and Passion Flower.

For agitation and nervousness: Hops (not if depressed). Dose: tincture, 1–2ml three times daily.

General tonics for debility and convalescence: *Oats,* Alfalfa, Siberian Ginseng. Dose: 5ml of one three times daily.

Sprouted Alfalfa may be eaten fresh in a salad, or can be bought as tablets, in which case 2–3, three times daily with food. Dr Reckeweg's Alfalfa tonic is particularly recom-mended (available from various suppliers, see page 203). Dose: 1 dessertspoon three times daily.

Nutrition

It is suggested that severe depletion of the mineral zinc, essential to normal adolescent development in girls, may account for many cases of anorexia nervosa. The symptoms of extreme zinc deficiency are the same as of anorexia. Certainly becoming anorexic will itself deplete the body of many essen-tial micronutrients, which need to be replaced. A mineral test is very important to assess the degree of mineral loss, especially in long-term anorexics. (For interim use a simple zinc tester is available from Larkhall Laboratories; see page 203.) It is best to take professional advice on zinc supplementa-tion as intake affects uptake of other important minerals.

Supplements

Vitamin B complex: 50–100mg daily.
Vitamin C: 500–1500mg daily or more, up to bowel tolerance levels.
Calcium: 500–1000mg daily.
Magnesium: 250–500mg daily.
Zinc: 50mg daily, or more under supervision, following a professional zinc test.
Iron: as natural iron tonic, from vegetable and herbal sources, such as Floradix, 1 dessertspoon three times daily.

Associations offering advice and support
See under Eating Disorders, page 201.

Bulimia nervosa

Bulimia is an eating disorder characterized by recurrent uncontrollable bouts of over-eating in a short period of time followed by self-induced vomiting and/or laxative abuse and/or starvation to get rid of or counter the food intake.

A variety of other names have been coined to describe the condition, such as the 'binge–purge cycle' and the 'dietary chaos syndrome'. Essentially, there are two subgroups of bulimics: normal-weight bulimics and anorexic bulimics. Some may be overweight; some sufferers are slightly overweight before they develop bulimia, and some become overweight as a consequence of this behaviour.

In recent years, bulimia has been recognized as a condition separate from anorexia nervosa, although 40–50 per cent of anorexics become bulimic. Although there are similarities between the two conditions, such as attitudes concerning control of food intake and the overwhelming fear of weight gain, each disorder has its distinguishing features.

Symptoms of bulimia

If some or all of the following apply to you, then you may be bulimic:

- Irresistible desire to eat.
- Abnormally large amounts eaten in a short time.
- Consumption of high-calorific food during a binge, usually refined, sugary carbohydrate.
- Hiding eating during a binge.
- Termination of such eating episodes because of abdominal pain or self-induced vomiting.
- Repeated attempts to lose weight by severely restrictive diets, self-induced vomiting or use of laxatives.
- Frequent weight fluctuations greater than 10 pounds due to alternating binges and fasts.
- A clearly abnormal eating pattern.
- Depression and self-disgust following eating binges.
- Absence of a diagnosis of anorexia nervosa or any other known physical cause.

Causes of bulimia
Physical

- A biological predisposition to obesity (see Obesity, page 68).
- Pre-menstrual carbohydrate, sweets and chocolate craving.
- Intolerance or hypersensitivity to certain foods.

Psychological

- Certain tendencies: usually depression and alcohol or drug dependency.
- Emotional difficulties: many women sublimate emotional conflicts by eating. Food is used as a source of comfort, to counteract boredom and loneliness, and to express negative emotions like depression and anger, blocking out painful thoughts which cannot be acknowledged so that the food issue replaces them and becomes 'the problem' instead.

Social

- Pressures on women to diet. Fatness is associated with greed, indulgence, loss of control and other negative qualities. A common belief is that being slim and beautiful will lead to being successful, loved and happy.
- Conflicting messages about food through advertising. Some is portrayed as slimming and 'good' for you, and some is very fattening and 'bad' but very desirable.
- Women have so many conflicting roles to play: the daughter, the sexy wife or partner, the caring mother, the successful career woman, etc. These different roles have conflicting body images attached.
- Eating together is sociable, feeding ourselves and each other shows we care – it is a way of nurturing. It is easy to see how this can get out of hand.

Onset of bulimia

Binge-eating usually starts between the ages of fifteen and twenty-four. It may start for any of the reasons above, but the main one is usually the desire to be slim.

It may follow a phase of anorexia nervosa, or be the result of feelings of self-dislike, particularly about size and weight. A major stressful event may precipitate it. Bulimia is not uncommon in women who feel isolated at home as housewives and mothers of young children, experiencing all sorts of frustrations and resentment.

Characteristics of bulimic behaviour

Sufferers who rely on fasting as a means of weight control tend to go through bingeing phases which may last for some days followed by several days of starvation to 'counteract the damage'. Others who practise self-induced vomiting and other forms of purging will often complete the binge/purge cycle within a couple of hours. They will abuse laxatives and slimming and diuretic (water-reducing) tablets; often appetite-suppressant drugs such as amphetamines are obtained under false pretences. Excessive exercising is common.

Bulimia sufferers believe that purging after a binge stops weight gain. However, laxative abuse does not work because all food is absorbed into the small gut before it can reach the large bowel. Self-induced vomiting is not as effective as might be thought either. Binges are usually on fast foods high in sugar and refined carbohydrates. These start to be digested almost as soon as they enter the mouth, quickly leave the stomach and are rapidly absorbed. Binges can last from half an hour to two hours and it is impossible to retrieve everything eaten.

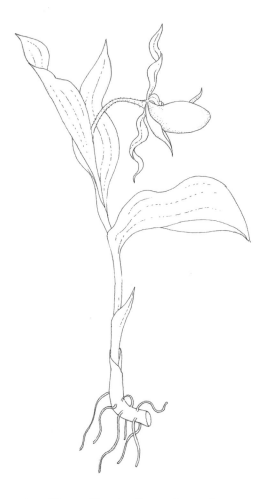

Lady's Slipper (*Cypripedium pubescens*)

Long-term effects of bulimia
Mental and emotional
Obsessional behaviour patterns are habit-forming so that sufferers may consider that even a normal meal or a small over-indulgence warrants a 'clear-out'. When relief at having disposed of the food wears off, feelings of guilt, shame, self-disgust, humiliation and depression set in. These feelings can be so strong that the desire to binge, ironically, is sometimes re-activated within a few hours. Bulimics may have to lie and even steal to satisfy and hide their habit. They may have severe mood swings and be aggressive towards family and friends.

Bulimic behaviour may be a revolt against society or family. By doing what other people would regard as disgusting – being sick, eating out of rubbish bins and other behaviour considered anti-social – women are making their protest.

Physical
The severity of symptoms will vary depending on how long bulimia has been practised; on the body's capacity to tolerate and counterbalance the chemical disturbance; on the frequency of episodes, and the quality of nutrition that is absorbed in between times.

The effects of bingeing are abdominal distension and pain; swelling of the hands, legs and feet; swelling of the salivary glands around the face and jaw-line. The effects of vomiting are hypoglycaemia (low blood-sugar); chemical imbalance (progressive loss of potassium and sodium); predisposition to dental decay and gum disease as a result of bingeing on sugary foods; bleeding from the upper intestinal tract (forced vomiting may be traumatic enough to cause injury to the throat and oesophagus); lack of protein causing fluid retention in the body tissues (oedema) including puffy face and ankles.

Sufferers who practise laxative abuse feel ill and chronically tired out as a result of chemical imbalances which can be life-threatening if very severe. Chronic diarrhoea causes dehydration and a loss of body salts and minerals which may result in loss of muscle strength and heart irritability. Also, large amounts of laxatives may cause loss of bowel tone and secondary constipation which can propel sufferers into greater abuse.

Amphetamines affect the central nervous system and mimic the effects of adrenaline, increasing energy levels, heightening mood, reducing surroundings awareness, concentration, appetite and physical coordination. When the effects have worn off, the sufferer feels confused and irritable, and has a hangover. Alcohol has similar effects, leading to further problems. Stress and tension, together with chemical imbalances, may cause irregularity or cessation of periods.

Treatment and recovery

The most important step is to recognize that bulimia is a problem. Although knowing this eating behaviour is not normal, some women come to regard it as a way of life. It may be years before they seek help because they feel that the bulimia is disgusting and they are afraid of rejection. The longer they use it as a coping strategy, trapped in the vicious circle, the harder it becomes to break free, and the more frightening the prospect of change. The sufferer has to really want to give it up.

Seeking a lasting recovery from bulimia needs perseverance and courage. It involves being willing to try ways of coping with the emotional difficulties that cause the bingeing. Different approaches work for different women.

Sources of help

General practitioners and hospitals
Confiding in a GP is often the first step; take notes with you of your feelings and experiences and questions you need to ask. If the GP is not sympathetic you have the right to change to another without giving an explanation.

You may be hospitalized or, more likely, seen as an outpatient, so that the chaotic eating pattern can be tackled within an everyday setting. Some in-patient programmes are strictly behavioural and involve response-reward techniques. Couple and family therapy is important in the sufferer's recovery so that the family/spouse is involved rather than isolated. So often the family feel that they are the guilty party, and hospitals can sometimes offer a carers' support group.

Therapy
A relationship needs to be built up with a counsellor or psychologist. The areas explored will include past history, relationships with family, friends and sexual partners and feelings and motives underlying bulimic behaviour. Help will include developing a more relaxed attitude to food and weight, stopping the use of dangerous methods of losing weight, stabilizing weight at a 'natural' set point, identifying triggering factors, and devising more positive ways of reacting to life's stresses rather than using bulimia as a coping strategy.

A therapist should listen intently and with empathy while at the same time retaining objectivity and detachment, and should provide an accepting, trusting, supporting rapport. With the therapist you can explore your strengths and weaknesses and develop self-awareness and a clearer understanding of the problem. Behavioural therapy may be used; the idea is to unlearn an unwanted pattern of behaviour by appropriate guidance and practical assignments, perhaps in the form of short-term weekly goals being given to help regain control over eating. This can be valuable to sufferers who have developed a conditioned response (bingeing) to stressful situations and emotions. Having become aware of the triggering factors, new reactions to them can be learnt.

Often sufferers are afraid to give up bulimic behaviour because they fear change. Relying on food to get themselves from one day to the next, some sufferers lose all ability to solve their problems.

Depression can be a big barrier and it is not unusual for sufferers to feel worse before they feel better. Women may suddenly find for the first time in months or even years that they have capacity to feel. Many hidden negative emotions which have been repressed for so long will begin to surface, and they may need help to resolve these.

Group therapy

Benefits include a sense of belonging and the realization that there are others in the same position. As a result of lending support to each other, members come to realize that they are valuable individuals. These factors improve sense of self-worth and restore shattered self-confidence as well as easing feelings of isolation.

Orthodox drugs

Certain anti-depressants are used in managing food cravings and depression. These drugs are for patients prone to endogenous depression (as a result of a chemical or hormonal reaction) rather than the more common type of 'reactive' depression caused by life events such as bereavement, rejection, work problems, etc. There are herbal alternatives: see Anorexia nervosa (page 78) for sedatives and nervines. Other alternative therapies, such as hypnotherapy, acupuncture and homoeopathy may also help.

Bulimia and weight gain

Giving up the relentless pursuit of weight loss and focusing on behavioural change usually causes a tremendous amount of anxiety. A bulimic presented with a normal diet plan will believe that this will cause her to get fat.

Studies have shown that we all have our own weight 'set point' which is on the whole at an equilibrium. When dieting ceases, after a while weight usually stabilizes to an acceptable level, even when eating three meals a day.

When vomiting and laxative abuse cease, sufferers may experience an uncomfortable sensation of fullness and bloating. Their stomach and ankles may swell. This is temporary and is due to re-hydration. When a normal diet and eating pattern is established, and the tone of the intestinal muscles has returned, the symptoms should subside.

If you have been maintaining an exceptionally low weight for your age, height and bone structure, by long periods of fasting and/or vomiting directly after meals, you are bound to gain weight when you stop doing this. You may become heavier than you would like, but need to accept that nature did not intend you to be thin. Therapy will help you appreciate a new you.

Self-help

- Try to give up dieting.
- Avoid thinking in terms of 'good', 'bad' and 'forbidden' food.
- Do not weigh yourself every day.
- Avoid getting really hungry. Have three meals a day with perhaps a small mid-morning and mid-afternoon snack as well.
- Eat with family or friends if possible at conventional meal-times and do not skip meals.
- Meals should be well balanced and contain all the essential nutrients and a variety of tastes and textures; follow the dietary advice you are given. A small amount of fat, especially essential fatty acids found in vegetable oils, is needed for tissue repair and energy. Important vitamins must be included: B complex with extra B_5 and B_{12} is recommended, as is Vitamin A. Carbohydrate should be included in each of the three daily meals, with lunch and dinner being a combination of carbohydrate, protein, salad or vegetables.
- At mealtimes: try to slow down the rate of eating by finishing a mouthful before starting another and resting between mouthfuls. Practise leaving something now and then. Help yourself to smaller portions. Concentrate on eating; never do anything else, like watching television, during a meal. Avoid drinking with food; instead, have a drink twenty minutes afterwards.
- Limit the amount of food available in the house. Practise shopping in small quantities and always make a shopping list.
- Spend time every day in deep relaxation, positive visualization, meditation or yoga. Try to live day-by-day, setting realistic goals. Remember, the odd relapse will not put you back to the beginning.
- Understanding that bulimia masks a diversity of interwoven problems helps the sufferer to look beyond the food and weight issues to a new self-awareness.

Herbal treatment

It is essential that this is taken in conjunction with counselling and nutritional advice.

See Herbal treatment for anorexia (page 80). Choose from all those herbs mentioned for emotional problems. Bitters and herbs to stimulate appetite are not appropriate.

Anti-nauseants should be taken before food: German Chamomile, Black Horehound, Spearmint, Dose: as tincture, 5–10ml of each.

Anti-emetics: Ginger root, dried as decoction or as tincture, 1ml in water; or as powder, a pinch in tea, after food if necessary. You can take every hour if you wish.

Hepatics or liver herbs to detoxify are important: Barberry, Dandelion and Milk Thistle for regeneration of liver cells. Total: 100mg a week. Dose: tincture, 2–5ml three times daily, or infusion/decoction of dried herb in equal parts, 1 cup three times daily. Take for 2 months.

Tonics: As for Anorexia nervosa (see page 80).

Dr Bach's Flower Remedies: Crab Apple is specific. See page 174 for a comprehensive list of Dr Bach's remedies.

Supplements

Follow guide-lines for vitamin supplementation for Anorexia nervosa (see page 80), but take professional advice on mineral supplements. A mineral analysis test is recommended before proceeding, as mineral levels are likely to be abnormal.

Associations offering advice and support

See under Eating Disorders, page 201.

7   Menopause

How Changing Woman Stays Young

When Changing Woman gets to be a certain old age she goes walking towards the East. After a while she sees herself in the distance looking like a young girl walking towards her. They both walk until they come together and after that there is only one – she is like a young girl again.

– Apache Indian

Menopause – the word derives from the Greek, meaning month and cessation – is part of nature's plan for the end of woman's fertility. It happens naturally between the ages of forty-five and sixty, when periods stop, although it can occur earlier. The average age of onset of menopause in the UK is fifty. It is also known in medical terms as the 'climacteric', meaning critical period, and is sometimes referred to as the fifth climacteric. The climacteric is a transitional period beginning before the menopause and continuing after it and may last for anything between a few months and several years. An established menopause is defined as six months without a period.

According to survey, the age of menopause in Western society is coming down four to five years on the previous generation, although it is not known why. Suggestions are that postponing the childbearing years, a first pregnancy after forty, taking hormones (the contraceptive pill, fertility drugs, treatments for PMT, etc.) and surgical sterilization may throw the female system out of balance. Smoking is associated with premature menopause. An artificial menopause is caused by total hysterectomy, with the ovaries removed, which can happen at any age. It is also caused by radiation damage or by cytotoxic drugs used to treat cancer. It leads to an immediate menopause in most cases, and symptoms are likely to be more severe than in a natural menopause.

Attitudes towards menopause

The cultural context in which menopause is experienced can affect the physical and mental/emotional symptoms. It is seen as the end of the so-called 'curse', but instead of being a liberation it is largely perceived in society as yet another women's problem, this time 'the change'. In medical terms it is increasingly being seen as a deficiency disease. It is disturbing that every physical milestone in a woman's life is regarded as a 'disease', and this says something about the way that half our society is regarded.

The perceived importance of femininity in its narrowest sense, as opposed to personal, mental and other more subtle female qualities, adds stress to this period of transition. It devalues men as well as women, by attaching esteem only to that which is youthful. Older or traditional cultures, on the other hand, often revere the wisdom that comes with the years.

Certainly perceptions of menopausal symptoms vary greatly between cultures. It is significant that in studies carried out in traditional cultures such as the Japanese and Arab, psychological menopausal symptoms do not seem to be a problem, although this may be changing in modern Japan. It seemed to be the case where the older woman traditionally had a special role to play; perhaps being able to leave purdah is a significantly greater event.

Social strata are indicators of how successfully women will cope with the climacteric. Well-educated, well-off women, usually middle-class, may fare better possibly due in part to greater availability of information. In less well-off groups stereotypes of menopausal women may be unquestioned and low expectations reinforced by men and by other women.

It is not only men, however, who are negative about menopause. The novelist Fay Weldon, quoted in Gail Sheehy's *The Silent Passage – Menopause*, said that the very word is used by men 'to describe you as being horrible, miserable and unattractive . . . in using it [women] are inviting a definition that is diminishing to them'. Unfortunately women in their forties are often unsympathetic too and may avoid or ignore the fact that friends are going through it. It does not help that many women apparently say nothing about their experience of menopause to anyone outside the family. As Germaine Greer points out, the woman of a certain age becomes 'invisible', whereas she previously used sexuality as a means, consciously or not, to gain goals. If this is important to her, the rejection compounds the sense of loss of status.

To some women, on the other hand, the menopause comes as a welcome relief, bringing freedom from menstruation, contraception, and sometimes unwanted attentions from men. They feel it is a liberation; they can be themselves at last. Interestingly, Arab women appear to experience it only as a relief. Could this be because their position in the family and society is already determined and being post-menopause makes no difference? Some Western women also describe the post-menopausal years as the best time of their lives, however, full of energy and a sense of new direction.

It is the lack of a positive attitude that denies women a potentially rewarding experience. When children have grown up, what better time to branch out in all the directions that have been previously closed by other commitments? This is the ideal time to explore and develop other aspects of femininity. Menopause also forms a natural break for reflection on the rest of your life, it is literally a pause in time, heralding the third age of woman – a more inward phase, after the hurly-burly of childbearing and rearing.

Imagine the scenario where a woman can welcome a new era and recognize the end of fertility without regret. Her time for childbearing is over and she has fulfilled her part in nature's plan. She may sadly have lost children, or she may have chosen to remain childless. If she has been reluctantly childless then now surely is the time to let that go. This does not mean denial, indeed a period of mourning may be appropriate as the past is released. Help may be needed to let it go. It is taking time to recognize these periods that is important.

A new perspective is needed, not just for women but for men too. People are living longer than ever before. The Third Age is defined as being between fifty and seventy-five. There are 14 million Third Agers in Great Britain today, and if the trend continues this will be the largest group in society by the year 2020. Evolutionary history has not favoured women after the menopause; only 150 years ago average life expectation was just forty-five. Nowadays women still have a third of their lives to go at menopause. A strategy for better health after age fifty is imperative, and this is also a time for fulfilment of dreams, old passions and desires not satisfied, and projects uncompleted. Time to enjoy life!

If attitude is so important at menopause, what can be done to encourage a positive approach? Where do we focus our energies? And how should younger women prepare for it to make it a good experience? It becomes obvious that it is necessary to educate each other, and to raise awareness of these issues in society generally. Older women need to find their own place physically, psychologically, socially and spiritually, but they will have to help themselves. Fortunately there are signs that menopausal women are coming out of the closet; Germaine Greer and Gail Sheehy among others have encouraged a vanguard of women writers and other women to speak out.

Many women approaching menopause are so busy as workers, wives, mothers and carers of elderly parents that they do not think about their own health, and in this way are still caught up in the attitude of the previous generation to menopause. However, our mothers and grandmothers did not know about HRT, the risk of osteoporosis, breast cancer, cancer of the womb or heart disease, or expect to live so long, so they did not have the same choices to make.

In order to adopt a natural approach to menopause, a plan of action is needed, a blueprint for a healthy body and mind, so if you are one of those women who experience unpleasant symptoms, there is no need to take hormone replacement therapy (see page 99) at the first hot flush. An account of how the passage of the menopause takes place and of some of the changes that may happen during it follows.

Hormonal changes in menopause

Before menopause, changes in the hormone balance have been going on for some time. Symptoms may have been noticed for anything up to ten years before periods stop. Hot flushes may occur around period time, emotional lability may become noticeable, tiredness is quite common. Often, menstruation does not end suddenly. In the pre-menopausal stage (before bleeding stops), irregularity is common, with periods coming less frequently although they may also come more frequently. They may also be heavier, with flooding, or alternatively may become very scanty. As menopause approaches the relationship between the pituitary gland and the ovaries is upset, with FSH (follicle stimulating hormone) and LH (luteinizing hormone) levels much higher as the body tries to stimulate the ovaries to produce more. In turn there is decreased production of the hormones oestrogen and progesterone.

As the ovaries decrease production, a type of oestrogen is produced by the adrenal glands which can replace up to 75 per cent of the pre-menopausal levels, in some women right up until the seventies. Other women, due to poor health, unfortunately produce much less. It is also produced in small amounts from body fat, so thin women run the risk of producing less. A small amount of progesterone is produced, as well as testosterone. The amounts of oestrogen present in the body after menopause vary. Hormones adjust gradually in a natural menopause and it is this time of transition that is often uncomfortable. Also, it may not be obvious that menopause has happened until it is over, as any period could be the last.

Symptoms of menopause

According to surveys, 16–30 per cent of menopausal women experience no uncomfortable symptoms at all, and of those who do only 10 per cent have symptoms that are bad enough to need treatment. However, a much larger proportion of women than this are currently taking HRT supplementation. This raises big questions, and it is wise to examine the evidence for and against.

The constellation of symptoms associated with menopause are wide-ranging and it is difficult to find a consensus of medical opinion. However, a number of categories of symptoms may be defined as follows: few women experience all of these and severity is variable.

Vasomotor

Vasomotor changes in the small blood capillaries cause sudden hot sensations and flushing, especially of the face and neck, often followed by a chill or perspiration as the heat fades. It is usually worse if the weather is hot or if you get upset about it. For some women hot flushes are intense and difficult to cope with, and can cause embarrassment, but the truth is that other people rarely notice. Not all women experience night sweats but these can become a real problem if you suffer insomnia as a result.

Depending on which surveys you look at, the figures for women who experience flushes vary between 60 and 75 per cent. What is not shown, however, is that severity is very variable. The flushes may be very quick, in which case they are often called flashes, or prolonged. Some women report them occurring for several times a week for up to a year, or at worst several times a day for up to five years.

What causes flushes is not clear, as there is no direct tie between low oestrogen level and dysfunction of the skin. There does appear to be a flushing band where this occurs, since above a certain oestrogen level, that is, pre-menopause, flushing does not happen, and at a lower level post-menopause it does not occur. There is a correlation with poor adrenal gland function. Interestingly, flushing is not seen as a problem in all cultures. There is not even a word for it in Japanese! Interestingly, naturopathically it is suggested that there may be a connection with diet, and it is significant that the traditional Japanese diet is high in essential fatty acids from fish.

Genital

Due to the drying effect of the slow-down of oestrogen production on the mucous membrane of the vagina, intercourse may be difficult or painful. Prolapse of the womb or bladder is possible if tone and elasticity of these are poor. Infections, itching and vaginal discharge are more common. Bladder stress incontinence may be a problem as loss of tone occurs here. Pelvic floor exercises are effective to alleviate these problems (see page 195).

Emotional and mental

Depression and anxiety are possible, when the transition is taking place, due to hormone levels fluctuating. Weariness and episodes of the blues can occur, but this is usually temporary. Exaggerated feelings may be due as much to negative outlook as hormonal depletion. (Judgmental labels such as 'menopausal neurosis' do not help.) Other symptoms such as nervousness, irritability, anger, excitability, panic attacks, weepiness, lack of concentration, forgetfulness and fear of nervous break-down are reported. These form part of the climacteric syndrome classification used by doctors. It is important to distinguish between the effect of ageing that is common to both sexes, and the effect of menopause on women.

Demineralization of bone

This leads to brittle bones and Osteoporosis (see page 93).

Hypothyroidism

Due to reduced production of the hormone thyroxine, metabolism is slowed down, leading to weight gain, constipation and other symptoms. If severe, supplementation with the drug thyroxine is the orthodox treatment.

Poor skin and hair condition

Thinning and drying of skin and poor hair condition may occur.

Transitional problems

Anaemia and other blood deficiencies, heavy bleeding (menorrhagia), PMT, breast swelling and tenderness (because of water retention), loss of libido, headache, backache, joint pains, rheumatism and menopausal acne are reported by some women. Tiredness or exhaustion for a while is not uncommon.

Nutrition in menopause

It is obvious that women entering menopause need to maximize their input in every way, especially dietary, for a good level of hormone production to be maintained. There are plenty of foods and herbs that promote production of hormone precursors to help build hormones and facilitate the process of new oestrogen production. Support for the adrenal glands is particularly important; exhausted adrenals are not able to produce the hormones needed. For good adrenal function, Vitamin B complex and minerals including chromium are required. Less stress and more rest are imperative. A poorly functioning liver from years of dietary indiscretion will not help matters (see page 148). Dietary insufficiency is known to be related to hormone imbalance, and those experiencing premenstrual difficulties due to dietary problems have been shown to be more likely to suffer menopausal discomfort. Hot flushes may be related

to a low blood-sugar problem, or may even be an allergic problem aggravated by hormonal swings.

One school of thought suggests that without a monthly period less elimination of toxins takes place and so what we eat becomes even more important. It is necessary to build up a good supply of minerals, particularly calcium, magnesium, and selenium. Changes in the parathyroid hormones means that metabolism of calcium is no longer efficient and it may be leached from the bones. Studies have shown that increased intake of these minerals slows down the loss of mineral density in the bones and there are less bone fractures in those taking them. Moderate exercise is even more important now; cycling and brisk walking, which have been shown to preserve bone mineral density, are particularly good.

Oestrogenic foods

Hormones are made in our bodies from the food we eat; plant hormones are contained in these foods. A list of those most beneficial for menopause follows.

Seeds: Almost any sort, for example sesame seeds, pumpkin seeds, sunflower seeds, including sprouted seeds such as alfalfa, fenugreek, mung bean, lentil. Add to salads.

Wholegrains: Preferably organic – oats, wheat, rye, millet, buckwheat etc. These should be soaked, then cooked whole. Add to salads or serve instead of rice.

Fresh fruits: Bananas, avocados, papayas, mangoes.

Dried fruits: Prunes, dates, figs, raisins (all high in calcium).

Honey: Also bee pollen and Royal Jelly.

Culinary herbs: chervil, chives, garlic, ginger, nutmeg, horseradish, sage, parsley, rosemary, seaweed (kelp). Watercress, nettles and all dark green leafy vegetables are rich in minerals.

Cold-pressed oils: Safflower is especially high in essential fatty acids. Use for cooking and adding to food.

Nut oils such as walnut and hazelnut, natural sources of Vitamin E, are essential for healthy skin and hair and are tasty in salad dressings.

Women from countries where naturally grown vegetables, seeds and fruits feature abundantly in the diet do not suffer from menopausal symptoms in the same way as those on Western diets, which tend to be high in protein but depleted in minerals.

We eat far more protein than is necessary. Foods to avoid or cut down considerably include meat in particular: if you do eat it, eat only organically reared meat, to avoid artificial hormones that can imbalance the hormones.

Also beware of sugar, coffee, chocolate, alcohol, and any foods with chemical additives. Limit dairy products to occasional eggs and milk as traces of hormones are present in milk from dairy herds. Eggs are in any case best eaten in small quantities. Natural yoghurt is the most beneficial form of dairy produce.

Herbal treatment of menopausal symptoms

Plant hormones

Up to 5000 plants are known to contain phytosterols or hormones, and many of these contain phytoestrogens. New research suggests that hundreds contain phytoprogesterones (natural progesterone). Many of these plants feature in our diet, (see Oestrogenic foods above). Nature seems to have packaged these in such a way as to produce a natural beneficial balance of oestrogen and progesterone in the same way as in the human female, which would eliminate the hazards of pure oestrogen replacement. Certainly it would explain the actions of the herbs used to best effect for hormonal problems by generations of herbal practitioners who have always believed that they contain hormonal precursors or forerunners of the female hormones, enabling us to produce our own from them.

Plants containing phytosterols do not have the same direct action as synthetic hormones or work as quickly, but they provide lasting improvement that does not reverse when they are stopped. In the case of Wild Yam, its plant sterols provided diosgenin, the base for the contraceptive pill (see page 7).

An American doctor, John Lee, author of *Natural Progesterone: The Roles of a Remarkable Hormone*, suggests that lack of progesterone rather than of oestrogen is to blame for the symptoms of menopause and proposes that natural progesterone made from plant sterols is the answer. Synthetic progesterone has been designed to be absorbed orally, so he claims that natural progesterone needs to be applied externally. He recommends a progesterone preparation made from Wild Yams called Pro-gest, widely used in America. This is a vast and exciting field of research waiting to be explored further.

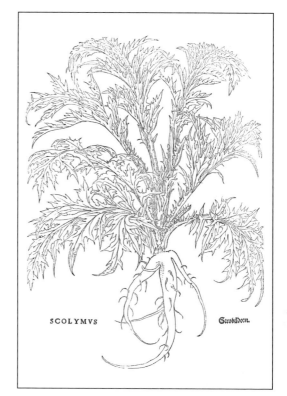

Milk Thistle (*Carduus marianus*)

Herbs known to contain phytosterols, include: Sage, Wild Yam, False Unicorn Root, Red Clover, Lady's Mantle, Motherwort, Astralagus, Chaste Berry, Sarsaparilla, Saw Palmetto, Vervain, Black Cohosh, Liquorice and Borage.

An alphabetical listing of ailments in menopause follows, explaining symptoms and detailing their herbal treatment with self-help and nutritional suggestions where appropriate. If you cannot find an ailment that is bothering you here, look in the A–Z Directory of Other Conditions at the end of the guide (page 151).

Abdominal pain
See page 151.

Anaemia
For treatment see Anaemia in pregnancy (page 43).

Anxiety and mood swings
These are very upsetting for some menopausal women and may continue for some time, possibly alternating with feelings of depression (see below).

Irritability and weepiness are common, and may be greeted unsympathetically by other family members. Moods may lift as quickly as they come and the see-saw of these emotions is difficult to handle. It helps to bear in mind that this is a temporary phenomenon.

Herbal treatment
- Gentle relaxants and sedatives: try Skullcap, Motherwort, Californian Poppy.
- Dr Bach's Flower Remedies: Walnut for times of transition and Impatiens for irritability are excellent. Scleranthus is very helpful for instability. For a full list see Dr Bach's Flower Remedies, under EMOTIONAL PROBLEMS.

If PMS (see page 16) has been a problem previously, it is not uncommon for a constellation of these symptoms to carry on into menopause, and possibly worsen.

Emotional problems of menopause
Depression
Depression is usually characterized by feelings of powerlessness and low self-esteem, which are coincidentally common to women going through the passage of menopause. Symptoms of hormonally related or endogenous depression include insomnia, early-morning wakening, poor appetite and sometimes loss of weight.

There is no evidence to show that long-term depression is linked with low oestrogen levels, and in fact it is probable that other life changes around the time of cessation of childbearing are strong factors in this type of reactive depression. This view may be confirmed by looking at the experiences of women in other cultures.

Different studies show the numbers of women experiencing depression fluctuating widely, between 21 and 78 per cent. One researcher found one in ten women affected. Factors affecting development of menopausal depression are variable. It was reported that women with depressive tendencies previously were more likely to suffer from depression at menopause, as were those that already had a considerable amount of responsibility at work as well as in the home. Having no time to themselves was a major factor. However, those who worked outside the home were less likely to become depressed, unless their work was very stressful.

Evidence that low oestrogen levels and depression may coincide just prior to menopause or just after (in other words for a short time only) due to surges and falls in oestrogen levels is backed up by women who report that this was a transitory phase, and some counselling at the time was all that was needed to sort out the problem areas.

However, it is suggested that use of the contraceptive pill or HRT can actually cause depression as both maintain artificially high blood levels of oestrogen, so that ordinary symptoms are made worse when these fall slightly.

Another contributory factor to depression is that some women may have a very heavy family commitment at this stage in life, not only as wives and mothers but often as carers for elderly parents. Unfortunately for such women, as parents live longer, the caring mother role turns into a caring daughter role, and if there is no break in between she has cause to be depressed.

On the positive side, not only are herbs for the body important but also food for the soul – love and appreciation. Those in happy established relationships that feed these needs are more likely to be positive about menopause. Those in stressed relationships are more likely to have problems. If a relationship with a partner is not affirming for you, now is an opportunity to work out why. Take heart – it is not uncommon for couples to grow closer after this time, nor is it unknown for a woman to start a new passionate affair after the menopause!

In some cases, if the approach of menopause is denied, it can be a source of panic and consequently severe symptoms when it starts, rather like an unexpected menarche for a young girl.

When depression is severe there may be a case for treatment, but not necessarily with HRT.

Herbal treatment
Depression is often a physical as well as psychological problem, reflected in poor energy. It may be necessary to use herbs to boost energy before others to treat the depression itself.

- False Unicorn Root is the chosen remedy to rebalance hormone levels. To this add one of the following herbs:
- Saw Palmetto, Rosemary or Damiana to raise energy. However, do *not* use these if there is over-agitation or anxiety as well as depression, as they will overstimulate. A gentle agent to use in this case would be Oats. (Natural plant-based iron tonics and vitamins may also help.)
- Vervain, St John's Wort, Motherwort, Lemon

Balm, after improvement is perceived. These often work best as individual simples of 50–100ml tincture a week for up to three months.

Otherwise try the following formula for a month.

Formula for menopausal depression

Tincture of Motherwort	25 per cent
Skullcap	25 per cent
False Unicorn	25 per cent
Vervain	25 per cent

Dosage: 100ml/g per week. Take 5ml three times daily, or as infusion/decoction of dried herb in equal parts, 1 cup three times daily. It is sometimes appropriate to add some bitters such as Gentian or Wormwood (a very small amount, i.e. 5 per cent of the total) as these have a beneficial tonic effect.

Note: Hops are not recommended in depression.

Dr Bach's Flower Remedies (see under EMOTIONAL PROBLEMS) are highly recommended for depression (particularly Mustard for gloom that descends for no apparent reason), and for anxiety and other emotional upsets at this time.

Fluid retention or oedema

As a result of hormonal fluctuation, aldosterone, the hormone which regulates water retention, often functions poorly. The symptoms are similar to those of PMS (see page 16). Some women find that they are bloated, with fluid retention in the abdominal area, the face and sometimes the hands and feet as well. This is the major component of weight gain in menopause.

Herbal treatment

- Aromatherapy massage is very effective in providing relief, using the following essential oils: Lavender, Fennel, Thyme, Chamomile, Geranium. 1 drop of each in 50ml base oil. It is necessary to massage along the limbs upwards towards the heart. It is of most benefit if a partner or friend can do this for you, although you can massage your legs yourself.
- Atractylodes or Siberian Ginseng for bloating.
- Fennel Seed and Dandelion Leaf infusion (60g to 1 litre), 1 cup three to four times daily. (Making up a thermos flask and sipping it throughout the day is an alternative.) This is a gentle diuretic that will remove excess fluid.

Otherwise try the following formula for a month.

Formula for fluid retention

Cleavers	40 mg
Horsetail	30 mg
Couchgrass	30 mg

(Quantity for 2 litres, make as above, 1 cup three times daily.)

Self-help

Nutritional measures include avoiding salt, as this retains water, sugar and caffeine. Drink plenty of water as it helps to flush out the kidneys. Vitamins and mineral supplements that may help include magnesium, Vitamin E, Evening Primrose oil and Vitamin B_6. An organic, wholefood diet with plenty of unrefined carbohydrate will help, as this removes toxic by-products from the tissues that retain water (see page 126).

Heavy bleeding (menopausal menorrhagia)

Flooding is not a normal symptom of menopause and should be reported to your doctor if severe (i.e. if it is difficult to soak up the flow with sanitary towels) or continues for a long time. Other causes of heavy or prolonged flow include *uterine fibroids*. The usual orthodox treatment is a surgical scrape or D & C, which usually only works for a while until the uterine walls thicken again with excess build-up of endometrium, and more heavy bleeding results. A hysterectomy may be recommended if this is not successful.

Herbal treatment

Herbs always provide relief but are not a cure in all cases. The following herbs will work to stem the flow of blood, if only on a temporary basis.

Formula for menopausal bleeding

Tincture of Birth Root	20 per cent
Greater Periwinkle	20 per cent
Cramp Bark	20 per cent
False Unicorn Root	20 per cent
Shepherd's Purse	20 per cent

Dose: take 5ml every hour for five or six hours until bleeding stops, then take five times for one day, decreasing to 5ml three times daily for a week. Fresh tincture of Shepherd's Purse, if you can get it, works best. In an emergency, take 1ml under the tongue frequently until help arrives.

It is necessary to look at the wider context and consider hormone-balancing herbs and herbs to normalize menstruation. These include Chaste Berry, True Unicorn Root, Golden Seal, Black Haw. The advice of a medical herbalist is invaluable.

Self-help

Treating the liver and reviewing your diet may be beneficial. (As a guideline, avoid heavy and mucus-forming foods such as dairy products and meat, especially if the blood is very dark in colour, as this may indicate stagnation due to dietary factors.)

Rest as much as possible when the flow is heavy, with your feet up. Try cold compresses over the lower abdomen at the same time; add a drop of anti-spasmodic essential oil such as Chamomile or Bergamot to lessen bleeding. Alternatively, try cold-water sitz baths for ten minutes at a time (see page 12 for directions).

See also Pre-menstrual and Menstrual problems, pages 18 and 21.

Supplements

Iron from natural sources (not inorganic, or ferrous sulphate), or herbal iron tonics, at least 6mg daily.
Multi-mineral: 1 daily.
Vitamin C with bioflavonoids: 500mg.
Vitamin B complex: 50mg.
Rutin tablets: 2–4 per day.

Post-menopausal bleeding

Caution: If bleeding recurs after menstruation has ceased for at least six months you must have a complete medical check-up as there are other causes such as FIBROIDS, vaginitis (see page 97), endometritis. Withdrawal of oestrogen therapy can also cause bleeding. More serious causes are cancers of the uterus, cervix, or ovary.

Hot flushes

Although these are the symptoms most complained of by women in menopause, they vary greatly in the amount of distress they cause (see above). Treatment with herbs works well in most cases. You may need to take quite high doses to begin with, and cut down later.

Herbal treatment

Herbal formulas to treat flushes and sweating are usually based on oestrogen- and progesterone-promoting herbs, in order of importance: Sage, Wild Yam, Chaste Berry, False Unicorn Root, Red Clover, Lady's Mantle, Motherwort and Astralagus. Supportive herbs for the adrenals, such as Liquorice and Borage, are important. Other herbs would be used as needed in individual cases.

You may find the following formula helpful.

Formula for menopausal hot flushes

Tincture of Sage	25 per cent
Wild Yam	25 per cent
False Unicorn Root	25 per cent
Lady's Mantle	25 per cent

Dosage: Total 100–150ml tincture a week. Take 5ml three to five times daily, depending on severity, and 10ml before bed if severe at night. If symptoms do not abate within a few days make a new remedy, increasing the amount of Sage to 50ml. The herbs can also be powdered, in equal parts, and put in size 00 capsules: the dose is 2, three or four times a day, and 2–4 before bed, depending on severity.

- Infusion of Sage, drunk cold, is effective if sipped frequently during the day, but does taste very strong. (It will help symptomatically but will not provide the hormone-rebalancing effect of the combined formulas.) Alternatively, essential oil of Sage, 2–3 drops, can be added to a glass of warm water and sipped. (Check the purity of any oil with your supplier before taking it internally.)
- Other herbs used for hot flushes: Raspberry, Vervain, Hops, Black Cohosh, Sarsaparilla, Pasque Flower, Mugwort. Hops are bitter and may be taken in capsules or pills. To balance a formula combine several herbs. Although these herbs have an oestrogenic action they are equally progestogenic and it is suggested that this last action may be one that brings relief in many menopausal symptoms.
- Chinese herbs include Schizandra (to prevent sweating and aid sleep), Rehmannia (for night sweats) and Dang Gui or Chinese Angelica (as a hormonal balancer), in equal parts. To this formula add Toasted Chinese Liquorice, which makes it more palatable and gentle on the stomach as well as giving the adrenal glands a boost. For centuries in China women have taken Dang Gui for menopausal problems.
- Evening Primrose oil and oil of Borage (Starflower oil) have a reputation for relieving hot flushes in high doses. Take up to 1000mg two or three times a day or EPA from fish oils. Try also Vitamin E: maximum dose 100mg or 300–600 IUs daily.

Caution: No one taking anti-coagulant drugs for thrombosis should take Vitamin E. Do not take Liquorice or Panax Ginseng if you have high blood pressure.

For doses of all the above, see Directions for use of herbs for menopausal problems at end of chapter, page 101.

Self-help

Hot flushes may also be caused or heightened by episodes of low blood sugar, or HYPOGLY-CAEMIA. Try having frequent snacks, preferably consisting of whole grains and protein, to see if things improve; if so, see HYPOGLYCAEMIA. Flushes may be caused by deficiency of micro-nutrients in the diet: make sure your diet is opti-mally balanced and take a good multi-mineral with extra selenium and Vitamins A, C and E daily. ALLERGIES or food sensitivities may be a cause.

Taking a few commonsense measures will help: avoid tight clothing around the neck and wear lay-ers for easy removal. Take regular exercise. Try meditation, as well as other methods of relaxation. Try to avoid public situations where you are likely to get wound up for a while.

See also Nutrition in menopause (above).

Insomnia in menopause

This can be due to hormonal fluctuations and is particularly miserable if accompanied by night sweats. See treatment for Hot flushes (above).

Herbal treatment

Sedatives and hypnotics: Valerian, Passion Flower, Wild Lettuce, Oats, Californian Poppy or Hops, singly or combined as follows.

Formula for menopausal insomnia

Valerian	25 per cent
Passion Flower	25 per cent
Californian Poppy	25 per cent
Oatstraw	25 per cent

Total: 100ml a week. Dose: tincture, 15ml before bed and repeat with 10ml during the night if necessary. It may take several nights to a week before the full effect is felt. If there is no effect with-in a week then it will be necessary to take the tincture two to three times during the day as well to relax the mind for the night. Drink herbal relax-ing teas during the day. These herbs can also be used to treat anxiety and agitation.

(Proprietary brands such as Kalms or Quiet Life containing these or similar constituents are avail-able over the counter: check constituents. Take 2–4 tablets at night.)

- Use essential oils of Lavender, Chamomile and Rose in the bath at bedtime, 1 drop dispersed well, or 2 drops added to water in a vaporizer in the bedroom.

Self-help

To help yourself through a natural menopause it is really necessary to have some means of relaxation and rejuvenation. These could include biofeed-back, Alexander Technique, regular meditation, or prayer. Yoga and yoga deep breathing are tradi-tionally associated with peace of mind, suppleness and graceful ageing. Treat yourself to a regular massage. Do anything you find enjoyable and self-affirming but it is preferable to make a routine of it. You may be able to find a support group or if not start your own.

Remember that rest and exercise in the right pro-portions are necessary, especially for stress relief and good sleep.

Osteoporosis (brittle bones)

At menopause the chance of developing brittle bones increases, due to deterioration of bone structure as the result of loss of calcium, mag-nesium and other minerals from the bones; this may eventually cause fracture in later life. Cells called osteoblasts are responsible for forming new bone, utilizing magnesium and other minerals; cells called osteoclasts are responsible for causing resorption or breaking down old bone. As we age, osteoblasts slow down their activity, and osteo-clasts increase it. However, the good news is that as this is a dynamic process it can be changed.

With osteoporosis, collapse of the vertebrae of the back is common; the head of the femur in the thigh is the commonest long bone fracture. Hair-line fractures of vertebrae can be very painful. Around 2 million women in Great Britain may suf-fer from the condition to some degree. This figure comprises one-third to half of all post-menopausal women, but only a small number of these will have any treatment. Although men get osteoporosis as well, women after the menopause have ten times the risk as men of the same age.

Early warning signs of osteoporosis are those of calcium deficiency, such as nocturnal leg cramps, joint pain, transparent skin, restless behaviour and insomnia.

In severe cases, symptoms are very painful back-ache, especially in the upper back, loss of spinal movement and loss of height, up to six inches or more. Although the process of bone-thinning starts in the mid-thirties, there is a period of accelerated bone loss after age fifty of an average 1½ per cent a year for ten years. Prevention is much easier than cure, so it is best to take measures early.

To attempt to balance the picture, it has been

suggested that bad fractures in later life, especially of the hip, are not necessarily due to osteoporosis but may be due as much to awkward falls, through unsteadiness and poor sight.

Are you at risk of osteoporosis?

Risk factors to consider are age at menopause, a significant family history of post-menopausal fractures (osteoporosis may be genetic), a history of amenorrhoea (loss of periods), being underweight and small-boned, Caucasian and fair-skinned and having had no pregnancies. (There is evidence to show that women who breast-feed are less at risk from osteoporosis.)

Life-style factors such as physical inactivity, a poor diet low in calcium, heavy smoking and drinking all make osteoporosis more likely. By using scores based on the above factors predictions are made about likelihood of low bone mass, although no national screening is available in the same way as for cervical or breast cancer, for example. You may be offered a test using a bone scan or 'dual energy X-ray absorptiometry', although this is by no means widely available in the UK. Interpretation of the results depends largely on the operator and may vary between centres.

Women who are judged to be most at risk will probably be offered HRT. However, whether this creates more bone is a matter of controversy. (One recent article in the *Journal of the American Medical Association* states that HRT does not result in replacement of lost bone and if therapy is withdrawn, bone loss resumes.) Other treatments include high-level calcium supplementation or the hormone Calcitonin.

Strangely enough, there is new evidence to suggest that the contraceptive pill, early use of HRT and other hormonal treatments may be among the biggest causes of osteoporosis, causing zinc, magnesium and copper deficiencies in the long term, which disturb normal hormonal production. It is becoming clear that osteoporosis is due to nutritional deficiencies as much as, or more than, hormonal change.

The question of calcium

The amount of calcium absorbed in youth and middle age influences the outcome after menopause. Even so, it is suggested that an adequate and continuing amount of calcium in the diet, after menopause, *providing it is well absorbed*, will maintain the health of bones. The situation may be more complicated than just taking more calcium, how-

ever. Research in the naturopathic field suggests that metabolic dysfunction leads to inability to metabolize calcium. One study by Abraham (*Journal of Nutritional Medicine*, 1991, 2) showed magnesium supplements instead of calcium, taken by nineteen women over eight months, increased bone density by 11 per cent over those not taking it. Calcium supplements are often poorly absorbed, especially inorganic sources such as dolomite. Calcium should be combined with magnesium in the ratio 2:1. A supplement should ideally contain the other minerals and vitamins needed in the right proportions. Calcium taken alone depletes zinc and iron. Recent research suggests that mega-doses of calcium are not the answer to osteoporosis prevention. Interestingly, some women with osteoporosis have shown normal calcium levels in blood tests.

Try a supplement of 500mg magnesium, 10mg manganese, 30–50mg zinc, trace minerals including 3mg boron, and 1g Vitamin C daily. Essential fatty acids as found in Evening Primrose oil 2000–3000mg daily) and enough first-class protein (not necessarily animal) are also important for absorption.

Even better is to try to get your calcium and other minerals naturally, provided your digestion is good. Calcium from food sources is better, but only about 20–40 per cent of calcium in the diet is absorbed and this decreases with age.

Factors that influence absorption are:

1 Individual constitution: this influences efficiency of digestion in the stomach. Addition of natural enzymes such as from papaya and pineapple (papain and bromelain) would ensure efficiency.
2 Exercise: this needs to be regular and of the sort that puts the weight on long bones, such as brisk walking, dancing, gentle jogging, aerobics, use of a personal bouncer and yoga (thought to 'cement' calcium into bone).
3 Deficiency of essential micronutrients: magnesium, manganese copper, zinc, potassium, selenium and trace elements boron and chromium in the body.
4 Vitamins: Vitamin D is necessary for absorption and Vitamin C for formation of bone. Vitamin K accelerates bone formation.
5 Use of some orthodox drugs including steroids, contraceptive hormones, HRT, antacids and anti-epileptic drugs prevents uptake.
6 Chronic diseases, especially those of kidney, bowel and liver.

7 Certain foods, including coffee, tea, white sugar, chocolate, alcohol and those with high acidity, like rhubarb and spinach, if taken with calcium-rich foods tend to bind the calcium, making it unavailable. Smoking does the same as well as being as a risk factor for osteoporosis.

8 Lactose intolerance and other food sensitivities or allergies.

9 High phosphate content of food (usually in junk food).

10 Too much animal protein (as in cow's milk) decreases available calcium in foods. Vegetarians have been shown to be at less risk.

Milk and other dairy products are not necessarily the best natural sources of calcium. Milk is low in the magnesium needed to assimilate calcium, and there are other food sources that are higher. The following table suggests some other sources.

Calcium-rich foods

Kelp (Seaweed) per 100g	1093mg
Blackstrap molasses per 100g	579mg
Sardines per 100g	550mg
Dried figs per 100g	280mg
Almonds per 100g	250mg
Watercress per 100g	220mg
Sunflower seeds per 100g	100mg
Tofu (soya bean curd) per 100g	128mg

Comparison with dairy food

Cow's milk per 100ml	120mg
Cheddar cheese per 50g	400mg
Yoghurt per 100mg	180mg

Note: the calcium in sheep's and goat's milk and cheese has approximately the same food value, but it is easier to absorb because of the smaller protein molecules.

The RDA of calcium pre-menopause is 1000mg per day and post-menopause is 1500mg per day.

So it can be seen for example that by taking kelp in your diet, either dried (in food) or in tablet form, would give you about 50 per cent of the RDA to start with. It is also very rich in other minerals that are essential in menopause. Cooked speciality seaweeds (like Japanese nori) are also delicious added to food or crumbled over salads.

Herbal sources of calcium

These are generally more easily absorbed than inorganic minerals. The best sources are Nettles, Parsley, Raspberry Leaf, Alfalfa (add sprouts to salads), Comfrey Leaf, Cleavers, Red Clover, Oatstraw, Dandelion, as Dandelion coffee or fresh young leaves in salads, and Borage and Ribbed Plantain (eat the last two fresh or take as teas), Kelp (particularly rich) and Yellow Dock Root. Any of these can be powdered and taken in capsules (see page 10) or may be purchased ready made from specialist herbal mail order firms (see page 203).

Prolapse of womb

See under UTERUS PROBLEMS.

Sexual response in menopause

The fact that natural vaginal lubrication is less after menopause does not mean that desire is diminished, although this can vary. If your sexual relationship was a happy and satisfying one before, there is no reason why it should not continue so. Regular intercourse is the best way to maintain normal vaginal secretions. Libido depends to some extent on the hormone testosterone, present in women as well as men; some women have naturally less secretion of testosterone than others and find that their libido is diminished. Conversely, there are women whose secretion of testosterone goes up after menopause and who report they have never enjoyed sex so much!

As with men of the same age, intensity and duration of climax diminish and it takes longer to reach the plateau phase. The clitoris is more sensitive to touch because of general atrophy of tissue in the area, so gentleness is needed. Without regular intercourse the vagina will atrophy to half its former size.

Some women find a new freedom after menopause as there is no longer any need to be concerned with contraception. Others may decide that they are less interested in 'missionary sex' and look to other methods apart from penetration to satisfy themselves and their partners.

Herbal treatment

Herbal aphrodisiacs: it is worth mentioning these valuable herbs which increase libido, probably through their general tonic effect.

- Schizandra (Wu Wei Zi) not only enhances endurance but is said to increase sexual fluids and the lustre of the skin.
- Panax or Korean Ginseng contains plant sterols similar to testosterone. (*Caution:* this should not be taken if there is a history of high blood pressure and in any case should not be taken for longer than two to three months at a time by women.)

- Siberian Ginseng (*Eleutherococcus senticosus*) is generally considered to be more suitable for women, its plant sterols being nearer to the female hormones. Codonopsis (Dang Shen), known as Pseudo Ginseng, is less heating, which is important if you suffer from hot flushes. Ginseng is usually available as tablets, capsules, elixir or sachets of instant tea. It can also be found as tincture but is pricey if the best quality is to be obtained.
- Damiana is a nervine tonic which also strengthens the reproductive organs.
- Saw Palmetto, used mainly as a tonic for the male reproductive system, may be appropriate for women as well at this time of life.
- Cinnamon and Spearmint are reputed to increase libido and can be added during cooking or made into a tea.
- Black Willow should be mentioned for its ability to *decrease* sexual energy.

Skin and hair

As a rule, condition of skin and hair is an indicator of general health. In women, this is also connected to oestrogen levels. As hormones fluctuate at menopause, skin may become drier and hair brittle. Skin elasticity is lost gradually over the years from the mid-twenties on, as supporting collagen fibres break down and the fat layer beneath the skin thins. Many women fear these changes, but it should be remembered that lines and wrinkles that give a 'lived-in look' are a natural part of ageing. It is perfectly possible to look your age and still look good.

Understandably, if everything appears to be happening at once, the ageing process can be alarming. It is made worse by the process of oxidation in the skin by free radical molecules which cause damage in the tissues. These molecules are promoted by exposure to the elements, especially the sun, and also environmental pollution, smoking and alcohol.

However, there are measures you can take. Some women report that their skin and hair look much better as a result of HRT, although in the author's view this alone would seem to be insufficient cause to start it. Remember, HRT does not stop the ageing process. Unfortunately, some women report ageing alarmingly in appearance when they discontinue the treatment.

A type of skin discoloration, called Acne rosacea can be a result of hormonal imbalance. See under SKIN AND HAIR PROBLEMS.

If spots and whiteheads are a problem, see Acne vulgaris under SKIN AND HAIR PROBLEMS.

Self-help

Diet of course plays a major role in the appearance and quality of skin and hair. Nutrition should be first-class during menopause to provide all the nutrients needed, so include plenty of non-fatty protein, complex carbohydrates and essential fatty acids from nut and seed oils like safflower. Plenty of fruit, for Vitamin C and enzymes, is essential. Antioxidant vitamins can protect the face against the ageing process. Hydration is the key to radiant skin and there is no substitute for drinking lots and lots of water.

Herb and flower creams and oils are very good for skin repair and the wonderful aroma alone will make you feel better. Chinese women claim that the secret of youth and beauty is in the herbs they take. A few are mentioned here, and a Chinese herbal will give more information.

See also Oestrogenic foods and Plant hormones (pages 88 and 89).

Herbal treatment

- Chinese Angelica (Dan Gui), Schizandra (Wu Wei Zi), and White Peony (Bai Shao). You could try a ready-made Chinese preparation called Women's Precious which combines some of the above (see Directions for use of herbs for menopausal problems, page 101).

Local applications: Light water-based skin moisturizers to which you can add any of the following:

- Evening Primrose oil: 2–3ml to 50g cream.
- Marigold (Calendula) cream is excellent for cell repair.
- Essential oils, including Rosewood, Cedarwood, Lavender. Add a few drops of each to 50ml of a fine base oil such as grapeseed and smooth around danger areas. (Rose Absolute is precious and expensive but superb, as is Neroli, and only 1 drop is needed. You can add any of these to a basic skin cream. Note: Essential oils can be purchased in small quantities, 5ml or less.)
- Oils for the body: Wheatgerm, Avocado, Almond. Massage in after the bath and add a few drops to bathwater. Add a little to face cream for richness if skin is very dry.
- Cream containing natural progesterone from plants is considered excellent.

Supplements

Antioxidant Vitamins A, C, E combined formula with selenium.

Vitamin B$_6$. 5mg daily as part of B Complex.

Zinc: 25–50mg daily.

Vitamins A and E in face creams are antioxidant locally and repair skin. Flaxseed (Linseed) oil, high in EFAs: 2 teaspoons or 2 capsules daily.

Stress incontinence

See URINARY PROBLEMS.

Tiredness

Menopause can be a debilitating time. Although it is not certain whether this is purely hormonal or not, it is not surprising as readjustment of the body is obviously necessary. It may be to do with psychological loss and the subconscious grieving process going on – perceived loss of beauty, confidence and the person you once were can be shattering. You may be sleeping badly as well. If exhaustion does not improve, have a complete medical check-up to be sure you are not hypothyroid, which is associated with tiredness, increased susceptibility to disease, weight gain, constipation, dry skin and extreme sensitivity to cold. Anaemia (see page 43) and HYPOGLYCAEMIA are possible causes.

Self-help

Developing coping skills in various ways can ease tiredness. Learn to pace rather than push yourself, practise relaxation, learn self-affirming practices, exercise even if you do not feel like it, to help detoxify hormones. Deal with insomnia and night sweats if these are a problem: see Hot flushes above.

Make sure your nutrition is very good, take a multi-vitamin and mineral tablet daily. If you are hypoglycaemic, minimize this with diet (see Hypoglycaemic diet, page 143).

Supplements

Vitamin E, Vitamin C, Vitamin B complex, Evening Primrose oil, selenium and natural sources of iron.

Herbal treatment

Initially: Herbs to improve functioning of adrenal and thyroid hormones: include Ginseng, Capsicum in very small amounts, 1–2ml per 100ml as it is very hot, or ¼ teaspoon powder in water, Cola, Bladderwrack, most easily taken in tablet form as a dietary supplement, Sarsaparilla, False Unicorn Root and Chinese Liquorice.

Thymoleptics or nerve tonics: Lemon Balm, Vervain, Damiana, Rosemary, Wood Betony, White Poplar, Oatstraw, St John's Wort.

Chinese tonic herbs: Schizandra (Wu Wei Zi), Chinese Angelica (Dang Gui), Astralagus (Huang Qi), Codonopsis (Dang Shen), Atractylodes (Bai Zhu) and Peony (Bai Shao). These tonic herbs should only be used in moderate doses, but in China are taken for long periods. Often herbs are more effective after a cleansing and detoxification programme (see Colon Cleansing, page 146). In China expensive tonic herbs are often taken after a fast to increase the benefits. Ready-made Chinese tablets containing these herbs can be purchased from Chinese herbal suppliers. One of these is Women's Precious, another is the famous women's tonic, Soup of the Four Things.

The following formula has proved helpful:

Formula for menopausal tiredness

Dang Shen	25 per cent
Dang Gui	25 per cent
Sarsaparilla	25 per cent
Gan Cao (Chinese Liquorice)	25 per cent

Total: 100ml/g a week. Dose: tincture, 5ml three times daily, or infusion/decoction of dried herb in equal parts, 1 cup three times daily.

Urinary tract infections:

See URINARY PROBLEMS.

Vaginal problems

Atrophic vaginitis

As the tissues thin there is often a sensation of dryness and increased sensitivity, due to changes in the cells of the vaginal walls as they lose their protective acid mantle. Atrophy occurs as the vagina loses its elasticity and decreases in size. The older vagina is prone to changes in the natural bacterial population, which may present as thrush (see CANDIDIASIS) or as bacterial infection. There may be discharge and itching, particularly at the vaginal entrance or vulva. Intercourse may be painful because of the lack of lubrication, in which case try using KY jelly. The most effective treatment for the older vagina is regular and loving intercourse, specifically having orgasms, to keep the secretions flowing and the vaginal walls supple.

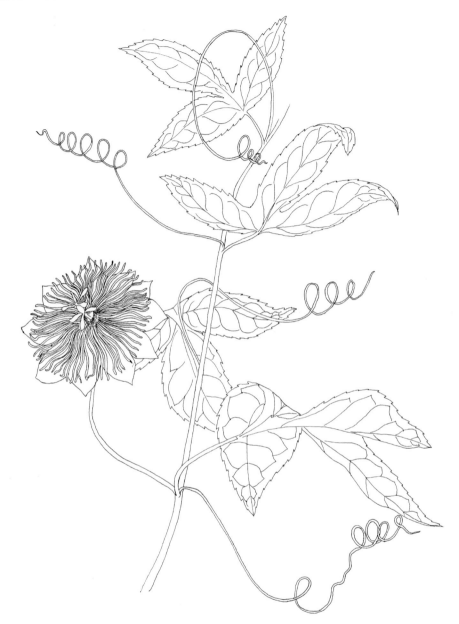

Passion Flower (*Passiflora incarnata*)

Herbal treatment

Herbal pessaries, or boluses, are made with powdered herbs added to a moisturizing base such as cocoa butter. They are formed in the shape of small cones when warm and when cool inserted into the vagina where they melt with body heat and release the herbs (see page 10 for directions on how to make them). It is easiest to put one in overnight; (protect your nightwear and bed linen). Douches can also be used to improve the vaginal condition, diluted well to avoid irritation: one part tincture to twenty parts of boiled cooled water or 30g herbs to

600ml boiling water. Leave to infuse for 2 hours, then add another 600ml boiled water.

Herbs for atonic vaginitis: Black Cohosh and Saw Palmetto have a reputation for improving tone.

Douche with tincture of Golden Seal, Red Clover, and Wild Pansy, equal parts. If there is infection, Myrrh or Marigold (equal parts) and add Thyme oil or Tea Tree oil (1 drop). Use diluted in proportions as above.

The same herbs, very finely powdered, if you can obtain them, can be added to pessaries made as above. Otherwise add tinctures, ½ml of each tincture to a pessary.

In an emergency try douching with diluted live yoghurt or put it on a tampon.

Hints on douching

Douching is most easily performed with a special douche kit brought from a chemist, consisting of a bag with its own tube and nozzle. If you lie on your back with legs raised and supported and suspend the bag above it is quite easy. The bathroom is the most suitable place to do this but it is important to be comfortable. A hand-held internal spray can be used on the toilet if preferred. In either case you should hold in the herbs for at least ten minutes.

If you don't feel like douching, make the herbs into a sitz bath (see page 12) and sit in it for 30 minutes at a time.

Success is determined by how regularly you use these methods. Although relief will be experienced right away, daily use is suggested for two weeks to ensure permanent results. See page 12 for further directions.

Local application: Aloe vera gel is healing and soothing. Herbs with a reputation for skin repair include Marigold, Red Clover, Comfrey and Marshmallow. (In tests Marigold cream has shown significant skin healing powers.) It is not easy to apply cream internally but you could use an applicator supplied with vaginal creams or spermicides. Try local applications of Evening Primrose oil or of Borage oil (Starflower oil) (both contain essential fatty acids (EFAs) for normal skin function) or a little Vitamin E oil. Use the fingertip to apply a little oil outside and inside the vagina daily.

Cream made from natural progesterone from plants is reputed to improve vaginal condition.

Vaginal discharge (Leukorrhoea)
See under VAGINAL PROBLEMS.

Varicose veins
See VARICOSE VEINS.

Vulvitis
See under VULVAL PROBLEMS.

Weight gain
See pages 70–72.

Hormone replacement therapy (HRT)

This is currently without doubt the most contentious women's health issue. Both sides of the argument are presented here.

HRT consists of synthetic oestrogens that mimic the female hormones, or so called natural (conjugated) oestrogen made from the urine of pregnant mares (the drug Premarin). Both are different in chemical structure from natural human hormones. Progesterone is now commonly included for the second half of the month to reduce the risk of endometrial cancer. Progesterone and oestrogen together are known as combined HRT. This causes the lining of the womb to break down and bleed once a month, but there is no ovulation. Women who have had a hysterectomy are sometimes recommended to take oestrogen only. These hormones do not mimic the finely tuned balance of premenopausal hormones, but may work by balancing out the tricky phase of oestrogen readjustment.

They can be administered as daily pills, injections, patches applied to the skin or as implants inserted underneath. There are pessaries or creams for vaginal use. If you decide to go on HRT for menopausal symptoms, it may be wise to try it just for the period of readjustment, usually about two years, which will allow monitoring. (*Caution:* you should be *weaned* off HRT, otherwise you may experience bad withdrawal symptoms.) It is as well to be aware that HRT was not designed to be taken on a permanent basis and does have side-effects, some of which are unknown, as there are as yet no studies of women who have taken combined HRT for half a lifetime. It is significant that in the UK, half of all women who are prescribed HRT stop it after six months due to side-effects. However, more women here try it than in the USA.

Advantages of HRT

1 *Prevention of osteoporosis.* If you are in the risk category it can reduce the likelihood of fractures by 50

per cent if taken for five years minimum. However, it will not work if started too late (over age sixty).

2 *Relief from hot flushes and night sweats.* These stop after administration of HRT although they will also stop on their own eventually.

3 *Depression and other emotional problems.* There is no proof that HRT has any effect on relieving distress, as low oestrogen is not directly connected with depression, although this is often given as a reason for going on it. In fact in the USA a warning is issued in every packet on behalf of the Federal Drugs Administration (FDA), that it should not be used as a treatment for emotional problems. The possible improvement in skin and hair appearance may contribute to feelings of greater well-being in some women.

4 *Vaginal dryness and discomfort during intercourse.* It is best to use the mildest preparation that works without causing any problems by absorption. This may be the best use for hormone replacement.

5 *Reduced risk of heart disease and strokes.* As cardiovascular disease is five times less common in premenopausal women than in men, but after menopause (by age seventy) the incidence becomes the same, it is suggested that HRT may guard against it. As heart disease is the major killer of post-menopausal women, it is worth considering carefully if there is a family history. (These benefits are lost if an implant is used.) Protection is by no means certain, however, as the studies showing it cannot be conclusive. There is evidence that women who have previously had heart attacks benefit from oestrogen-only therapy. However, progesterone can counteract the beneficial effect of oestrogen in protecting against heart disease and stroke.

Disadvantages of HRT
Side-effects
The use of combined HRT means the return of a monthly bleed similar to a period, although this may become very light after five years. Some women find the need for sanitary protection inconvenient. The effects of progesterone therapy for seven to thirteen days a month can include headache, depression, loss of energy and libido and other emotional symptoms similar to PMS (see page 16). Other reported effects are weight gain, fluid retention, breast tenderness, leg cramps and abdominal cramps. Although women are usually advised that these are likely to disappear when the body adjusts, this is not always the case. HYPOGLYCAEMIA is another side-effect of progesterone therapy.

Migraine may be the result of vascular over-reaction.

Long-term risks
As recently as 1969 many doctors were worried about the possible increased risk of heart attack, stroke, diabetes, breast cancer and endometrial cancer.

Studies of HRT suggest that after fifteen years the risk of breast cancer is increased by 30 per cent in oestrogen-only users but doubled by 50 per cent in those using the combination drug. There is no convincing evidence to implicate HRT in causing breast cancer in the short term, although this is relative.

Use of the combined drug decreases the risk of endometrial cancer from twenty times that of the untreated population if oestrogen treatment only was used, to one-third more than the untreated population in those taking it for ten years. In other words, an oestrogen-only drug trebles the risk, but even with progesterone there is still a long-term risk, and this continues for five years after the drug is stopped. Another larger study showed an increased relative risk of one and a half times after twenty years of oestrogen use. With implants progesterone must be continued for two years after oestrogen use is exhausted as cancer stimulation can continue during this period; however, not many women are willing to do this because of the side-effects.

The consensus of current medical opinion is that in the long term HRT increases the risk of developing breast cancer: a leading specialist has advised all women to have a mammogram before going on HRT. The current medical view is that progesterone protects against endometrial cancer.

The way it is prescribed affects the risks, as oral oestrogen passes through the liver, but implants under or on the skin bypass the liver. There is no doubt that artificial oestrogen is connected with the development of gall-bladder disease, doubling or trebling the risk. Women in their fifties and sixties find it aggravates existing gallstones, so those prone to them should take HRT in small doses, if at all, and then in patches or implants. Thrombosis and hypertension risks are also lessened with the later methods. However, this may lessen the positive effects of oestrogen on the cardiovascular system, including dilation of the arteries.

Contra-indications
Those who have breast cancer, endometrial cancer or a history of liver disease. Others who have to be

individually considered are heavy smokers, those with FIBROIDS, endometriosis (see page 24), otosclerosis, heart disease, or a history of thrombosis or hyperlipidaemia, especially if it runs in the family. High blood pressure is no longer considered a contra-indication.

Other causes for concern

This includes a growing worry over addictive-type behaviour reported towards HRT implants, including the need for ever-higher doses to maintain the same effect. (Up to 15 per cent of women may be affected in this way.) This seems to be because tolerance is produced by higher than normal levels in the blood. Women report the return of symptoms at increasingly frequent intervals. Oestrogens are known to be psychoactive, having powerful psychological effects. Few studies to date have been done in this area, so it is too soon to comment, but the possible implications are serious.

When coming off HRT, symptoms previously experienced often come back more severely. This is why it is necessary to wean off. Some women may seem to age alarmingly, in which case they should try a herbal oestrogenic mixture for several months.

Conclusions about HRT

The arguments need to be carefully considered in the light of your own particular case. Not all women have the same metabolism or genetic background and HRT may suit some much better than others. Some women cannot cope with a naturally managed menopause and the major commitment to life-style changes that this entails. There is a price to be paid for deciding for or against.

There can be no doubt that HRT has benefited the lives of many women, and produced spectacular results in well-being in some. Other women experience very unpleasant side-effects. The basic philosophy among some proponents of HRT, that the menopause is not an acceptable natural phenomenon, but rather a deficiency disease, is highly suspect. In common with others who advocate a natural approach to life, the author personally believes that the menopause is a natural event; apart from any other considerations it would be unnatural for women to go on bearing children well past the time allotted by nature because of other health problems which increase with age.

It is preferable to see HRT as essential in some women, for example those who have had an artificial menopause or who seem unable to produce oestrogen from any source apart from the ovaries, possibly for genetic reasons. These women could be compared to insulin-dependent diabetics.

These days the majority of women suffering with the menopause are having problems because of cultural, life-style, nutritional and other reasons, many of which can be avoided by taking action before the onset of the menopause. The cultural problems affecting women of menopausal age in our society may take much longer to be resolved; the individual woman can only come to terms with them in her own way.

Using HRT as a substitute for adopting a healthy life-style is a misguided viewpoint, and there may well be a change of attitude in the medical profession in another twenty or thirty years' time. It is sobering to reflect that the oral contraceptive has been around for at least two decades longer than HRT, and one leading specialist recently announced that it would be another twenty years before we know the full extent of the side-effects from oral contraception.

Lastly, there is the ethical question of whether it is right to offer women the promise of an 'elixir of eternal youth', either covertly or overtly. The campaign to eliminate menopause has become big business.

Directions for use of herbs for menopausal problems

Dried herbs by weight are taken either powdered and put into capsules (buy or powder your own); or as dried leaf, flowers, etc. in a standard infusion or decoction. Dosage below is per cup and 1 (small) cup = approx. 100ml water. As a rough guide when measuring quantities 5g dried flower or leaf = 1×5ml medicine spoon or a teaspoon; dried root and bark weighs more, so halve the quantity. It is easier to make 300ml at a time, which is sufficient for a day. A general rule is 30g dried herb to 600ml of water.

Tinctures of herbs are available ready-made. They contain alcohol, usually in proportion of 1:5, and are a concentrated form of herbal medicine. Doses below are given for tincture of this strength. Herbal tinctures are taken with water in the proportion of one part to at least eight parts dilution.

See pages 8–10 for further directions on preparation of all the above.

General Guide to Dosage: Total 100ml/g a week. Dose: tincture, 5ml three times daily, or decoction/infusion of dried herb equal parts, 1 cup three times daily. (Suggested dosages are *three times daily* unless otherwise stated. These are all within safe margins: *do not exceed*.)

After consideration of the actions of the herbs listed below it is recommended to combine four or five in equal parts to make a balanced prescription. The actions referred to are those with a particular affinity for the female reproductive system. If in any doubt follow suggested formulas or consult a medical herbalist. See List of Principal Herbs (page 198) for explanation of terms. Latin as well as common names are given for easy identification.

Key: **A =1–2ml/g; B = 3–4ml/g; C = 5ml/g; D = 6–10ml/g**

Agrimony (*Agrimonia Eupatoria*) Leaf
Dose: Tincture B, dried B or infusion
Actions: Mild astringent, haemostatic internally.
Indications: For excessive menstrual flow.

Angelica (*Angelica archangelica*) Root
Dose: Tincture B, dried herb B or decoction.
Actions: Anti-spasmodic. Bitter and aromatic. Emmenagogue. Tonic.
Indications: for delayed menstruation. Indigestion with flatulence.

Astralagus (Huang Qi) (*Astralagus membranaceus*) Root
Dose: Tincture C. Dried or decoction C–D.
Actions: Chi or energy tonic. Strengthens immune system.
Indications: Chronic problems. Tiredness. Weakness with diarrhoea. Sweating.

Atractylodes (Bai Zhu) (*Atractylodes macrocephala*) Root
Dose: Tincture C. Dried or decoction C.
Actions: Chi or energy tonic.
Indications: Tiredness. Sweating. Poor digestive functions.
Note: Used widely in China to help weight control.

Barberry (*Berberis vulgaris*) Bark
Dose: Tincture A–B. Dried or decoction A.
Actions: Liver tonic, hepatic. Cholagogue, increases digestive secretion. Beneficial reflex action on lower digestive tract, kidney, uterus and other abdominal organs.
Indications: Liver congestion, jaundice, gallstones.

Betony (*Stachys betonica*) Leaf and flower
Dose: Tincture A–C. Dried or infusion A–B.
Actions: Sedative. Bitter. Gentle tonic.
Indications: Conditions affecting the head: neuralgia, headache, migraine, lack of concentration, forgetfulness.

Birth Root or Beth Root (*Trillium pendulum*) Root
Dose: Tincture A. Dried or decoction A.
Actions: Anti-haemorrhagic. Uterine astringent.
Indications: Heavy bleeding during menopause.

Black Cohosh (*Cimicifuga racemosa*) Root
Dose: Tincture A. (Works best in alcohol.) Dried or decoction A.
Actions: Anti-spasmodic, anti-inflammatory and sedative. Nervous system tonic.
Indications: Cramps of toxic origin. Period pain.

Black Haw (*Viburnum prunifolium*) Bark
Dose: Tincture D. Dried or decoction B.
Actions: Uterine sedative. Anti-spasmodic. Astringent.
Indications: Period pain. Threatened miscarriage. After-birth pains.

Bladderwrack or Kelp (*Fucus vesiculosus*) Whole plant
Dose: Tincture C. Dried A as capsules or pills.
Actions: Anti-hypothyroid, anti-obesic.
Indications: Obesity, used as part of weight-loss programme. Tiredness due to sluggish thyroid.
Note: High content of minerals, especially calcium.

Blue Cohosh (*Caulophyllum thalictroides*) Root
Dose: Tincture A. Dried or decoction A.
Actions: Anti-spasmodic. Uterine tonic and stimulant but has a long-term relaxant effect. Emmenagogue. Oxytocic (increases contractions in childbirth).
Indications: Period pains. Painful cervical spasm.

Blue Flag (*Iris versicolor*) Root
Dose: Tincture B. Dried or decoction A.
Actions: Anti-inflammatory. Cholagogue. Stimulating and detoxifying action on gall-bladder and liver.
Indications: Hormonal problems of menopause related to poor liver function.

Borage (*Borago officinalis*) Leaf and flower and seed oil
Dose: Tincture C. Dried or infusion C–D. Oil in capsules. 500–2000mg daily.
Actions: Contains EFAs, particularly GLA, which are essential for biochemical actions in the body, forming prostaglandins. Anti-inflammatory action. Positive immune system action.
Indications: PMS. Period pain. Endometriosis. Menopausal symptoms.

Chamomile (German) (*Matricaria recutita*)
Flowers

Dose: Tincture B–D. Dried A–B.

Actions: Mild sedative. Anti-inflammatory. Anti-spasmodic.

Indications: Restlessness. Irritability. Insomnia. Digestive problems.

Chamomile (Roman) (*Chamaemelum nobile*)
Flower

Dose: Tincture A–C. Dried A–B.

Actions: Sedative, anti-spasmodic, anti-inflammatory, carminative.

Indications: Mental stress. Anxiety-related period pain. Endometriosis. Loss of appetite. Anorexia.

Chaste Berry (*Vitex agnus castus*) Berry

Dose: Tincture A. Dried or decoction A.

Actions: Works on the pituitary hormone LSH to increase progesterone levels in menstrual cycle. Probably has a balancing effect on other hormones. (One of the most important herbs for women.) Regulates menstrual cycle.

Indications: Irregular periods, painful periods, heavy bleeding, endometriosis, lack of periods. PMS, especially PMS(A). Enhances lactation. Menopausal symptoms.

Chinese Angelica (Dang Gui) (*Angelica sinensis*)
Root

Dose: Tincture C. Dried or decoction C.

Actions: Blood tonic, in Chinese terms, for 'deficient blood', tones and moves blood at the same time.

Indications: Menstrual irregularity and pain, where the woman is debilitated. Cessation of periods (with other herbs). Anaemia. PMS. Menopausal symptoms due to hormonal fluctuations.

Caution: Do not use in high blood pressure or in inflammatory conditions.

Cleavers (*Galium aparine*) Leaf and flower

Dose: Tincture D. Dried A–B. Fresh juice up to 15ml a day.

Actions: Astringent. Diuretic. Aids removal of toxic by-products in the body.

Indications: Enlarged lymph glands and sluggish lymphatic circulation.

Codonopsis (Dang Shen) (*Codonopsis pilosula*)
Root

See under Ginsengs.

Cola (*Cola vera*) Nut or seed

Dose: Tincture A–B. Dried as powder A–B.

Actions: Nervous system stimulant. Anti-depressive. Mood-enhancing.

Indications: Depression. Exhaustion. Muscle fatigue.

Cramp Bark (*Viburnum opulus*) Bark

Dose: Tincture C. Dried or decoction B.

Actions: Powerful anti-spasmodic, sedative, astringent.

Indications: All cramps, especially of uterus, in menstrual pain. Other uterine and ovarian pain. Threatened miscarriage. Heavy bleeding. Tones uterus so is used prior to childbirth.

Cranesbill (*Geranium maculatum*) Root

Dose: Tincture A–B. Dried or decoction A.

Actions: Astringent.

Indications: Heavy bleeding. Bleeding between periods. Menopausal bleeding.

Damiana (*Turnera diffusa*) Leaf

Dose: Tincture A. Dried or infusion B.

Actions: Nerve tonic. Thymoleptic (improves mood). Balancer for hormonal system. Reputed aphrodisiac.

Indications: Depression. Nervousness. Menopausal depression with Vervain.

Dandelion (*Taraxacum officinale*) Root and Leaf

Dose: Tincture C. Dried or decoction B–C. Leaf C.

Actions: Hepatic. Cholagogue. Bitter tonic to digestive system with reflex action on whole body. Gentle detoxifying agent. Leaf is diuretic for fluid retention.

Indications: Detoxification. Constipation. Debility. Hormonal fluid retention.

Echinacea or Cone Flower (*Echinacea angustifolia* or *E. purpurea*) Root

Dose: Tincture A. Dried A.

Actions: Anti-microbial and anti-viral. Positive immune system action.

Indications: Infection. Taken internally and used externally.

Evening Primrose (*Oenothera biennis*) Seed oil

Dose: Oil 1000–3000mg daily.

Actions: Contains EFAs which are essential for biochemical actions in the body, forming prostaglandins. Anti-inflammatory action. Positive immune system action.

Indications: Hormonal problems, including PMS(A) and menopausal symptoms. Oil as local application for skin problems.

False Unicorn or **Helonias (*Chamaelirium luteum*)**
Root

Dose: Tincture B. Dried or decoction A.

Actions: Important female herb. Oestrogenic. Hormonal balancer.

Indications: Uterine and general tonic. Indicated for hot flushes, menopausal depression, PMS, ovarian pain, heavy bleeding.

Fennel (*Foeniculum vulgare*) Seed

Dose: Tincture A–B. Dried or infusion A.

Actions: Diuretic. Anti-inflammatory. Carminative.

Indications: Hormonal fluid retention. Digestion.

Fenugreek (*Trigonella foenum-graecum*) Seed

Dose: Tincture B. Dried or infusion C. Can also be sprouted and eaten in salad.

Actions: Nutritive. Hormonal balancer in menopause. Rich in phytosterols. Reputed to raise oestrogen levels.

Indications: Menopausal symptoms related to oestrogen deficiency.

Ginger (*Zingiber officinalis*) Root

Dose: Tincture A. Dried or decoction A. For nausea A (dried) repeated hourly for up to six hours.

Actions: Gentle warming stimulant for all internal organs.

Indications: Flatulence, nausea and colic. Poor circulation and pelvic congestion.

GINSENGS

Panax Ginseng Root – Ren Shen (*Panax ginseng*) Root

Dose: Tincture or syrup B–C. Dried as tablets A.

Actions: Chi or energy tonic. Stimulant and rejuvenant. Reputed to promote longevity. Increases resistance to disease.

Indications: Chi deficiency diseases. Debility. Convalesence. Menopausal exhaustion.

American Ginseng (*Panax quinquefolium*) Root

Dose: Tincture or syrup D. Dried as tablets B–D.

Actions: Similar to above but milder and less stimulating for long-term use.

Siberian Ginseng (*Eleutherococcus senticosus*) Root (Not a true Ginseng)

Dose: Tincture D. Dried A–B.

Actions: Chi or energy tonic.

Indications: Low vitality and lack of endurance in women. Increases energy and stamina.

Codonopsis (Dang Shen) (*Codonopsis pilosula*) Root (Known as **Pseudo-Ginseng**)

Dose: Tincture D. Dried D.

Actions: Chi or energy tonic.

Indications: Use as milder substitute for Panax Ginseng for tiredness and debility.

Golden Seal (*Hydrastis canadensis*) Root

Dose: Tincture A–B. Dried or decoction A.

Actions: Stimulates uterine contractions. Antihaemorrhagic. Toning to uterus and other internal organs.

Indications: Period pain and heavy periods. Menopausal bleeding. Endometriosis.

Greater Periwinkle (*Vinca major*) Leaf and flower

Dose: Tincture C. Dried or infusion C.

Actions: Astringent. Anti-haemorrhagic.

Indications: Heavy periods. Bleeding between periods. Menopausal bleeding.

Hawthorn (*Crataegus oxyacanthoides*) Berry or leaf and flower

Dose: Tincture A. Dried or infusion A.

Actions: Circulatory tonic and restorative to heart. Leaf and flower indicated for circulatory insufficiency and high blood pressure.

Indications: Poor circulation. Pelvic congestion.

Herb Bennet or Avens (*Geum urbanum*) Leaf and flower

Dose: Tincture C. Dried or infusion C.

Actions: Anti-haemorrhagic.

Indications: Passive uterine haemorrhage. Heavy periods and menopausal bleeding.

Lady's Mantle (*Alchemilla vulgaris*) Leaf and flower

Dose: Tincture C. Dried or infusion C.

Actions: Anti-haemorrhagic. Hormonal balancer. Organ restorative for the uterus in many conditions.

Indications: Specifically for regulating menstrual cycle, relief of menopausal symptoms (with Motherwort), heavy periods. Locally as wash for vaginal/vulval itching.

Liquorice (*Glycyrrhiza glabra*) Root

Dose: Tincture B. Dried or decoction A–C.

Actions: Adrenal agent. Anti-spasmodic. Anti-inflammatory. Mild laxative.

Indications: In endocrine imbalance works synergistically with other hormones. Benefits any female condition where there is debility or exhaustion.

Caution: Liquorice should not be taken if there is high blood pressure.

Liquorice, Chinese (Gan Gao) (*Glycyrrhiza uralensis*) Root

Dose: As above.

Actions: As above, but as is roasted in honey, is more gentle and demulcent, and is less stimulating. In Chinese terms it enters all the energy channels of the body and is used in many formulas. Reputed to balance blood-sugar problems (hypoglycaemia.)

Caution: Liquorice should not be taken if there is high blood pressure.

Marigold (*Calendula officinalis*) Flower

Dose: Tincture 0.2–1.5ml. Dried or as infusion. A–B. Douche or cream.

Actions: Anti-inflammatory. Anti-fungal. Vulnerary.

Indications: Externally and internally for inflammation. Cuts. Burns. Ulcers, Candidiasis. Trichomonas infection. Atrophic vaginitis.

Motherwort (*Leonurus cardiaca*) Leaf and flower
Dose: Tincture C–D. Dried or infusion A–B.
Actions: Sedative. Anti-spasmodic. Hypotensive. Uterine tonic. Hormonal agent.
Indications: Menopausal symptoms (hot flushes, anxiety and depression). Nervous heart conditions.

Myrrh (*Commiphora molmol*) Tree resin
Dose: External application or douche: tincture diluted 1 part to 15 parts water.
Actions: Anti-microbial. Antiseptic. Astringent.
Indications: Vaginal discharge due to infection, candida.

Oat/Oatstraw (*Avena sativa*) Seed or leaf
Dose: Tincture A–C.
Actions: Anti-depressive. Nerve tonic.
Indications: General debility. Depression in menopause. Nervous exhaustion with insomnia.

Parsley Piert (*Alchemilla arvensis*) Leaf and flower
Dose: Tincture B–D. Dried or infusion B–C.
Actions: Diuretic.
Indications: Fluid retention. Kidney and bladder problems.

Passion Flower (*Passiflora incarnata*) Leaf and flower.
Dose: Tincture A–B. Dried or infusion A.
Actions: Sedative. Analgesic. Anti-spasmodic.
Indications: Insomnia. Neuralgic-type pain. Nervous tension.

Peony, White (Bai Shao) (*Paeonia lactiflora*) Root
Dose: Tincture B. Dried or decoction B.
Actions: Blood tonic. Emmenagogue. Anti-spasmodic. One of the most highly regarded women's herbs for regulating the female hormonal cycle. Relieves spasm and uterine cramps. Reputed in China to enhance beauty and longevity.
Indications: Menstrual dysfunction, uterine bleeding.

Raspberry (*Rubus idaeus*) Leaf
Dose: Tincture B–C. Dried or infusion C–D. Capsules or tablets B.
Actions: Hormonal precursor. High in vitamins and minerals.
Indications: Menstrual pain. Prevention of osteoporosis in conjunction with nutritional factors.

Red Clover (*Trifolium pratense*) Flower
Dose: Tincture A–B. Dried or infusion A–B.
Actions: Alterative, oestrogenic.

Indications: Chronic conditions of skin or internally. Vaginal itching as douche.
Note: High in essential minerals.

Rehmannia (Shu Di Huang) (*Rehmannia glutinosa*) Root
Dose: Tincture C. Dried or decoction D.
Actions: Chinese blood tonic for deficient circulation.
Indications: General debility. Anaemia. Palpitations. Scanty menstruation and exhaustion after childbirth. Combines well with Dang Gui (Chinese angelica).

Rosemary (*Rosmarinus officinalis*) Leaf
Dose: Tincture C. Dried or infusion A–B.
Actions: Gentle circulatory stimulant. Anti-depressant. General tonic. Anti-spasmodic. Anti-microbial.
Indications: Depression. Exhaustion. Headache.

Sage (*Salvia officinalis*) Leaf
Dose: Tincture A–B. Dried or infusion A–B.
Actions: Hormonal precursor. Reputed to be oestrogenic. Antiseptic.
Indications: Specifically for hot flushes of menopause. PMS late in life. Any condition where antiseptic internally or externally needed.

Sarsaparilla (*Smilax spp.*) Root
Dose: Tincture B–C. Dried or decoction A–B.
Actions: Reputed to be progestogenic. General tonic.
Indications: PMS. Menopausal depression and tiredness with other herbs.

Saw Palmetto (*Serenoa serrulata*) Fruit
Dose: Tincture A. Dried or decoction A.
Actions: Reproductive system stimulant. General tonic. Endocrine agent. Reputed to be progestogenic.
Indications: Menopausal symptoms.

Schizandra (Wu Wei Zi) (*Schizandra chinensis*) Fruit
Dose: Tincture C. Dried or decoction C–D.
Actions: Tonic for reproductive system. Increases vitality. Increases sexual secretions. Softens and beautifies mature skin taken internally.
Indications: Fatigue. Insomnia. Night sweats of menopause. Vaginal atrophy.

Shepherd's Purse (*Capsella bursa-pastoris*) Leaf and flower
Dose: Should be used *fresh*, or tincture made from fresh plant. Tincture A–B or A undiluted under tongue, in emergency. Fresh leaf infusion D.
Actions: Anti-haemorrhagic (vasoconstrictor and blood coagulant).

Indications: Uterine haemorrhage. Menopausal bleeding.

Skullcap (*Scutellaria laterifolia*) Leaf and flower
Dose: Tincture B–C. Dried or infusion A–B.
Actions: Sedative.
Indications: Nervous tension. Combines well with Valerian.

Squaw Vine (*Mitchella repens*) Leaf and flower
Dose: Tincture B. Dried or infusion B.
Actions: Uterine toner and relaxant.
Indications: Menstrual pain and irregular periods.

St John's Wort (*Hypericum perforatum*) Leaf and flower
Dose: Tincture B. Dried or infusion A–B.
Actions: Sedative. Analgesic and antiseptic locally.
Indications: Nervous tension. Overactive nervous system in menopause.
Caution: May cause photosensitive skin reaction in susceptible people, so do not apply before going out in strong sun.

Stone Root (*Collinsonia canadensis*) Root
Dose: Tincture C–D. Dried or decoction A–B.
Actions: Diuretic. Stimulates removal of uric acid and congestion. Tonic for all mucous tissues in the body.
Indications: Urinary stones. Liver congestion.

Valerian (*Valeriana officinalis*) Root
Dose: Tincture A–C. Dried or decoction A.
Actions: Tranquillizer. Anti-spasmodic. Hypotensive.
Indications: Stress, anxiety. Nervous exhaustion. Colicky pains. Period pain. Stress headaches. Palpitations. High blood pressure.

Vervain (*Verbena officinalis*) Leaf and flower
Dose: Tincture C–D. Dried or infusion A–B.
Actions: Gentle sedative. General nervous system tonic. Liver tonic.
Indications: Depression and exhaustion. Beneficial added to many herbal formulas for women to potentiate their action.

White Deadnettle (*Lamium album*) Leaf and flower
Dose: Tincture C–D. Infusion C–D.
Actions: Uterine anti-spasmodic. Anti-inflammatory. Catarrhal conditions of all mucous tissues.
Indications: Cystitis. Leukorrhoea and other vaginal discharges.

White Willow (*Salix alba*) Bark
Dose: Tincture B–D. Dried or decoction A.
Actions: Anti-inflammatory. Analgesic.
Indications: Symptomatic relief for painful conditions. (*Note*: aspirin was originally extracted from it.)

Wild Lettuce (*Lactuca virosa*) Leaf
Dose: Tincture A–B. Dried or infusion A–B.
Actions: Mild sedative. Hypnotic. Anodyne.
Indications: Insomnia. Anxiety with agitation.

Wild Pansy, Heartsease (*Viola tricolor*) Leaf and flower
Dose: Used externally or as douche. Tincture diluted 1 part to 15 parts water.
Actions: Local anti-inflammatory.
Indications: Menopausal vaginal atrophy. Vaginal candidiasis.

Wild Yam (*Dioscorea villosa*) Root
Dose: Tincture C. Dried or decoction A–B.
Actions: Progestogen. Anti-inflammatory. Anti-spasmodic.
Indications: Menopausal symptoms. Period pain. Uterine and ovarian pain, as a long-term treatment.

Yarrow (*Achillea millefolium*) Leaf and flower
Dose: Tincture A–B. Dried or infusion A–B. Fresh juice D.
Actions: Anti-haemorrhagic. Emmenagogue. Anti-spasmodic. Haemostyptic. General circulatory tonic.
Indications: Painful periods. Heavy bleeding. Atonic conditions of female reproductive system.

8   Tiredness and Chronic Fatigue Syndrome

Tiredness

Fatigue is one of the most frequent reasons for women's visits to the doctor.

It is a common condition which has a number of different causes. Many women feel constantly tired and run down and if there is no well-recognized organic cause they may be told by their doctor that there is nothing wrong.

Fatigue is defined as insufficient energy to carry out a task without needing to stop, rest or sleep. The commonest causes are lack of sleep or prolonged stress from either mental overwork or physical effort such as strenuous exercise.

If fatigue is continuous and not significantly relieved by rest or sleep, it may be chronic. (See Chronic Fatigue Syndrome below.)

Associated symptoms often include weakness, dizziness, headache, nausea, shaking, and feelings of irritability, ANXIETY or depression. In the majority of cases, diagnosis attributes the condition to primary psychiatric disorders such as depression. Among those causes that are more difficult to diagnose are hidden malignancies or infections, inflammatory disorders of unknown cause, thyroid disorders, multiple sclerosis and connective-tissue disorders.

Women are constitutionally more vulnerable to fatigue than men; the most common causes are menstruation, pregnancy and childbirth, and menopause (see previous chapters). Mothers with babies or young children at home are particularly at risk. It is known that working wives and working mothers may also be emotionally more vulnerable as they are subject to gender conflicts which can lead to a constant energy drain.

A number of studies show women to be overworked. Even those not working outside the home can spend up to seventy to a hundred hours a week on household tasks: cleaning, shopping, preparing food, doing laundry, gardening. Those with part-time or full-time jobs will also be doing a large proportion of these chores as well as looking after children when not working.

Fatigue is the result of an energy imbalance. Too much is being expended from the natural reserves and not enough conserved. If you think of energy as a pool, it is then obvious that draining it will leave it depleted and in need of filling up again. It is getting a balance that is important in overcoming fatigue. As women, we need to recognize that we are not automatons. We need to become sensitive to our biorhythms, not just the monthly cycle but our daily rhythms, so that we recognize a natural low and do not over-reach ourselves. At the same time, if we identify the causes of fatigue we can make choices about how to resolve it.

Drainers of energy are: poor sleep, hormonal imbalance, tensions at work, worries at home, poor dietary habits (fast foods), mental strain, EMOTIONAL PROBLEMS, occupational hazards, and lack of exercise.

Conservers of energy are: sleeping properly, lightening workload, more leisure time, resolving psychological conflicts, exercising, improving diet, giving up addictive habits, resolving work problems, asking for help, knowing when to say 'no'.

In the final analysis fatigue signals that something is wrong, and if the energy pool is allowed to get too low for too long, you could be vulnerable to a more serious condition, such as Chronic Fatigue Syndrome (see below).

Self-help

Try to conserve energy, particularly ensuring that you get more rest and sleep, for several weeks. If you still feel exhausted, visit your doctor or practitioner for a check-up to see that there is nothing physically wrong.

You could also try the following herbal tonics; start with a combination from Group A and progress to Group B if necessary.

A. Lemon Balm, Oats, Betony, St John's Wort, Vervain, Damiana.
B. Bladderwrack, Sarsaparilla, Liquorice, Panax Ginseng, Cola

(See Directions for use of herbs for chronic fatigue syndrome at end of chapter.)

Chronic Fatigue Syndrome (CFS)

This is a comparatively new and controversial phenomenon as far as modern medicine is concerned. However, it is not of recent origin; physicians have been trying to define it for several centuries.

Naming the disease

The first documented outbreaks were in the 1950s, occurring as small epidemics. In the UK it was called 'Royal Free Disease' following an epidemic viral infection among staff at the Royal Free Hospital in London. The main symptoms were extreme fatigue and muscle tiredness from which they did not get better in the normal recovery time. Later it was named Myalgic Encephalomyelitis (ME). Myalgic refers to inflammation affecting the muscles and encephalitic refers to the brain.

Naming the disease

Agreeing an appropriate label has proved controversial. The condition has been variously named Icelandic Disease; Post-viral Fatigue Syndrome (PVFS); Acute Onset Post-viral Fatigue Syndrome (AOPVFS); and a worldwide consensus has been reached recently with Chronic Fatigue Syndrome (CFS). PVFS is thought to be a separate problem as sufferers usually recover from it within a few weeks to a few months. According to recent criteria, CFS is not the same as ME. The core symptoms are the same, however, and some doctors and many patients in the UK still refer to the problem as ME. Although using CFS for clarity, the author takes the two labels to mean the same.

There have been other epidemic outbreaks all over the world in the last thirty years, leaving pockets of people suffering from CFS. The original epidemics were often related to poliomyelitis epidemics, occurring either before or after them. There have also been sporadic outbreaks and today CFS is becoming increasingly common in the general population. For example, in a recent survey of general practice in Scotland, in a sample of 200,000 people CFS was found in 1.3 per 1000 and affected all age groups and people in all walks of life. Significantly, about one-third of these patients were regarded by their practitioners as seriously ill.

Diagnosis

Initially there was doubt whether this was in fact a disease deserving a name of its own. Then the

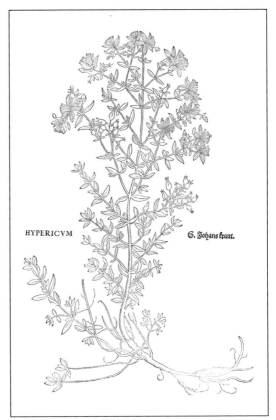

St John's Wort *(Hypericum perforatum)*

debate centred on the relative contribution of organic (physical) and psychological factors in the disease process. Recent studies have linked CFS with virological and immunological problems, which has given it credibility as an organic disease, and so it is not all in the mind. However, many of the patients suffer psychological disorders as part of the illness. The causation is still unproven and there is still no biochemical laboratory test for CFS.

Diagnosis is more often based on symptoms described by the patient. For this reason it has taken a long time to be recognized by the orthodox medical profession and is still considered controversial in some quarters. There is no doubt that patients are suffering, but the question is, from what?

The ME Association defines two paths of onset, an acute onset post-viral fatigue, and a slow, insidious onset, but it is only the acute onset that is medically recognized at present.

Symptoms

Those who develop CFS have often had a recent virus with flu-like symptoms, not necessarily severe. A number of other core symptoms develop later and are common to most sufferers. The following symptoms are based on a personal survey of patients who have come for herbal treatment following a diagnosis of ME or CFS. This accords with the general symptomatology.

Initial symptoms include sore throat, headache, nausea, abdominal pain, bowel problems, muscular pain with acutely tender spots in shoulders, arms and thighs, muscular weakness, dizziness and night sweats. Some of these may diminish after the initial stage, some may persist.

Primary (Major) Symptoms

1 Exhaustion, malaise, lethargy: overwhelming tiredness that has not been experienced before the onset.

2 Muscular symptoms: extreme muscle fatigue and pain (myalgia), made worse by exercise. The recovery time after exercise is much longer than normal. For example, whereas a healthy person will recover from normal exercise quite quickly, or at least after a night's sleep, a person with CFS will take days – or even weeks, if a relapse occurs. In the early stages sometimes the slightest effort, such as brushing the hair, can be exhausting.

3 Neurological symptoms: these may develop later and include sensations of pins and needles in limbs, other strange feelings like alternate heat and cold, twitching and spasm of muscles, problems with vision, even facial numbness and paralysis.

4 Mental and emotional symptoms: people report these as among the most distressing aspects of the condition. Symptoms commonly reported are, in order of frequency: loss of concentration, impaired memory, especially for recent events, anxiety, feeling dopey or 'spaced out', an atypical depression, weepiness and rapid mood swings, irritability, insomnia, other sleep disorders and panic attacks. (All these symptoms are worse premenstrually or post-stress.) Intelligence is not impaired, nor often is sense of humour and ability to enjoy life.

5 Less common symptoms include chest pain, breathing difficulties, palpitations, HYPOGLYCAEMIA, hyperventilation, URINARY PROBLEMS, joint pains, poor circulation, symptoms of CANDIDIASIS and ALLERGY, tinnitus (noises in the ears), unusual sensitivity to noise and light, and aphasia (dyslexia of the spoken word) where it is not possible to remember the right word or to get words in the right order.

Diagnostic procedure

It is important to get a diagnosis if you suspect CFS is your problem. If diagnosis is delayed, it will be more difficult to prove under current guidelines, and having the support of your doctor may be invaluable.

In order to make a diagnosis a doctor will first make a full examination for signs such as a sore throat, low-grade fever and enlarged lymph glands in the neck, armpits or groin. To confirm the diagnosis these signs should have been observed by a doctor on at least two separate occasions. Unfortunately for some of those who feel very ill there are often not many signs to see, specially if the acute early stage has been passed. In fact sufferers may look quite well. Careful questioning should follow. Your illness will need to meet certain criteria in order for the diagnosis to be confirmed. These are:

1 Previous activity levels should have been reduced by at least 50 per cent for six months: fatigue should be debilitating, affecting physical and mental functions, be worsened by activity and unrelieved by rest.

2 It must be possible to pinpoint the onset of the syndrome, such as from a viral infection *or* some other event: sudden onset of the illness occurs in 85 per cent of patients. However, for some it may not have seemed significant at the time and they will not be able to fulfil this requirement. The virus may commonly have affected either the respiratory system, with symptoms of flu, cold or labyrinthitis (viral ear infection), or the digestive system, with diarrhoea and vomiting (gastroenteritis).

3 There will be other minor symptoms present which must have persisted or recurred over six months, including fever, sore throat, enlarged lymph glands, muscle pain and weakness, and loss of mental abilities.

4 Other chronic clinical conditions which could cause fatigue must be excluded, including pre-existing psychiatric disease. This is done through medical history, examination and blood tests.

These criteria constitute the case definition recognized by the US Center for Diseases Control which is increasingly being applied in the UK. The current British system is similar but has a subtype for PVFS which requires laboratory evidence as well. This system of diagnosis has obvious limitations, in fact more than 30 per cent of patients may be excluded. Currently in the UK work is being done on a new clinical rating scale for evaluating symptoms. This will not only use wider criteria for diagnosis so that some of those previously excluded will be recognized, but it will be easier to differentiate CFS from other conditions more clearly.

Other causes of fatigue

Generally speaking, normal life exposes us to tiredness from three sources: inadequate sleep, unaccustomed physical exercise or prolonged mental effort. A number of well-defined illnesses also cause tiredness:

1 Muscular and neuromuscular disorders: polymyalgia rheumatica, fibromyitis, myasthenia gravis, multiple sclerosis.
2 Blood disorders: Anaemia (see page 43).
3 Hormonal imbalances: PMS (see page 16), Menopause (see page 85), Endometriosis (see page 24), under- or over-active thyroid.
4 Immune system disturbance: ALLERGY, auto-immune disease such as rheumatoid ARTHRITIS and AIDS.
5 Diabetes.
6 Liver function disturbance: caused by hepatitis.
7 Drugs, especially beta blockers. Also some over-the-counter drugs, drug addiction, smoking, alcohol and over-use of caffeine. Chronic caffeine withdrawal state.
8 HYPOGLYCAEMIA or low blood sugar.
9 Infectious illnesses caused by viruses or bacteria such as flu or colds, urinary tract infection (cystitis) or chest infections such as bronchitis. More rarely, brucellosis, tuberculosis, AIDS and parasitic infections.
10 Cancer: especially lymphoma and gastrointestinal tumours.
11 Dieting or nutritional deficiency.
12 Post-operative trauma and childbirth.
13 Psychiatric disease: depressive illnesses, generalized anxiety.
14 Neurological disease: Parkinsonism.
15 Kidney disease: uraemia.

The course of CFS

It takes time to recover from feeling tired and low after an infection like flu, but usually no longer than two to three weeks. In contrast, CFS is characterized by non-recovery after infection, and improvement is followed by relapse. Symptoms fluctuate, sometimes in a cyclical pattern, and are usually brought on by even trivial physical or mental overactivity. Improvement is usually slow. Statistics show that of the untreated population one-third recover in under two years, with most recovering between five and ten years, and the majority of those nearer to the five-mark. A small proportion of ME sufferers do not recover, or are left permanently with a low level of health.

From the author's personal observation, the average length of time suffered by those patients having herbal treatment is under a year, if they have been diagnosed early. Those who have suffered for four or more years can still make a substantial recovery, but more slowly. Rest is absolutely essential in the early stages and will influence outcome. Herbal treatment and nutritional guidance shorten the length of time as do some other alternative therapies. The usual pace is two steps forward and one back – but this is still progress!

Women and CFS

In a book for women it seems appropriate to devote a chapter to CFS as this disease strikes women down three times as often as men. They are usually in the twenty to forty age group, the most productive part of their lives in terms of work and family. Significantly the majority fall into the thirty to thirty-nine age group. This may be no coincidence, as unremitting stress is a factor in the development of this condition and failure to recover. Statistics show that women are more likely to carry on working and to keep looking after children even when they are ill. Even though 50 per cent of the work-force are women, they still do most of the housework and childcare as well. When they are older they are also likely to be carers of elderly parents. It is hardly surprising that they are under greater pressure than men with similar work commitments.

Women in the following occupations are most at risk either because of stress or repeated exposure to viruses:

1 Teachers.
2 Mothers with jobs.
3 Doctors, nurses and other health care professionals.
4 Farmers' wives and agricultural workers.
5 Shop assistants and those coming into daily contact with the public.

Suggested causes of CFS

There are many known neurological and psychiatric syndromes that can follow viral infections, so most scientists support the viral causation. Some researchers come down on the side of CFS being a persistent viral infection causing damage to the immune system. It is suggested that this causes inflammation in the central nervous system, although this is not proven. Metabolic disturbances affecting all the body's systems may occur because the control centre, or hypothalamus, in the brain is affected.

Another school of thought sees ME as being activated by various triggers, only one of which may be a virus. These are bacterial infection, allergy, candidiasis, environmental pollution, (particularly lead from traffic), carbon monoxide or heavy metal poisoning.

Dietary factors like vitamin and mineral depletion (especially of Vitamin C, Vitamin B, magnesium, selenium, chromium and zinc), poor diet, low stomach acid levels and intestinal parasites may contribute. Other factors are physical trauma, prolonged stress, psychological upset, hormonal change (menarche, childbearing and menopause) and overwork, particularly in those who push themselves very hard to succeed. A woman fatigued by one or more of these factors is more prone to contract ME.

From personal observation of many women, the author sees a combination of the two schools of thought as holding the key to ME.

More about viruses

Virology has proved that viruses can persist in the body and cause chronic disease. Certain viruses are able to interfere with cells' ability to produce specific substances such as hormones, neurotransmitters, cytokines and immunoglobulins. Increased levels of cytokines such as interferon have been noted. Part of the research is concerned with finding these 'markers'; however, they are not specific for a particular virus.

The enteroviruses, part of the RNA (ribonucleic acid) virus group, are suspected of being the culprits in CFS. Two of these are Coxsackie B and Echovirus. The enteroviruses principally affect the muscles and nerves. Organs affected include the heart and brain. Glands affected are thyroid, pancreas, pituitary and adrenals. The enteroviruses are spread through faecal contamination from sewage, polluted rivers, polluted beaches, drinking water and food. Poliomyelitis is one of this group of viruses.

Tests

The VP1 test which detects antibodies from enterovirus in blood is used in diagnosis, but it is non-specific for CFS. The involvement of another group, the DNA viruses, is also suspected. These include the herpes viruses, notably the Epstein Barr virus which causes glandular fever. (Nearly everyone has antibodies to this virus, so it is impossible to use this as a laboratory diagnostic test.) EBV may be involved as the trigger in a percentage of patients with CFS but it is now thought to be a separate problem. There is a possibility that EBV could be reactivated by stress and lead to CFS.

Other tests include muscle biopsy, using the PCR test for enterovirus, but this is controversial. The dispute revolves around what are normal findings in the muscle cells. Persistent viral infection in the nucleus of muscle cells has been proved but is still unspecific, as it may occur in other diseases. In one trial the incidence of enteroviral RNA was high: 53 per cent were positive. (It should be noted that it occurs in 15 per cent of the normal population as well.) Wherever it was found, damage was shown to the mitochondria or energy source inside the cell, which leads to abnormalities in cell energy production. It is suggested that damage of this sort in the central nervous system could lead to psychiatric abnormalities.

The technique of nuclear magnetic resonance imaging has shown excess lactic acid in muscles after exercise in a small study. This is a result of excessive glucose metabolism and a possible cause of muscle fatigue. More work is needed in this area, however. Brain MRI has demonstrated changes in brain tissue in patients with CFS, although this is not conclusive.

Electromyography has shown evidence of muscle dysfunction in CFS sufferers, notably a muscle membrane disorder and abnormal muscle fibres. These signs are not specific to those with CFS, however; other muscle dysfunction, such as myalgia, can cause such changes. Other research on muscle cells shows that there may be a possible imbalance of magnesium and calcium exchange across cell walls so that after exercise activity goes on in those muscles affected by chronic fatigue when they should be at rest. (This may show why intra-muscular injections of magnesium have proved helpful in one study.)

To differentiate CFS from other muscle diseases, more muscle studies need to be done, including neurological, biochemical and histopathological tests.

Summary

A persistent viral infection is caused by a virus living in the host's cells, which stimulates an immune response by the host's white blood cells, which, however, is not strong enough to kill off the virus. The immune system is then in a continual state of alarm. This could produce fatigue, muscle pains, nausea and other flu-like symptoms. (Multiple allergies are also commonly a result of this type of immune system response.)

Immune dysfunction is clearly implicated in CFS but it is not clear if this is a deficiency or hyperactivity. There is a case for CFS being a type of acquired immunodeficiency, like AIDS, though relatively benign. In this hypothesis the virally infected cells are not killed because there are not enough 'killer' T–cells. Other abnormalities of function found are altered levels of immunoglobulins, those guardroom soldiers of the immune system army; abnormal numbers, ratios and functions of lymphocytes, the scavengers, with raised numbers of those with immune activation; anti-nuclear and anti-thyroid antibodies, and raised levels of cytokines circulating in the blood (interferon). The current view on persistent virus is changing, and recent research proposes that instead, the virus has triggered a 'chronic immune system aberration'.

Coping with CFS

Most authorities agree that rest is the most important factor in the first phase. Once you have been diagnosed, you will need to monitor your activity carefully so that you know how much energy you have in a day and can expend it wisely, even if it is very little: at the beginning it may seem that just getting up in the morning takes all your energy. By being careful you will begin to build up some reserves. If you continually go to the limit of your strength, it will take much longer to recover, tempting as it is to do that extra activity. People differ in how badly they are affected. Some women are able to carry on with their jobs if their employers are flexible about hours, but need extra rest and sleep, for example naps in the middle of the day. Others will not be able to carry on working if their concentration and energy are too poor.

If you have children it is imperative that you have plenty of help. Don't be afraid to ask for it. In some cases a partner has to take over running the home. A willing mother or mother-in-law will be invaluable at this time, as will friends.

Because of the drastic changes in life-style, often due to loss of job and income, that CFS necessitates, and the frustration of being unable to lead a normal life, depression is often part of the condi-

tion. The evidence points to it being secondary to CFS rather than its cause, however. (In fact circulating cytokines in the blood can cause depression.) It is an atypical depression, quite unlike a clinical or endogenous depression, as there is a capacity for joy and pleasure at the same time.

Self-help

Gentle treatments aimed at supporting the body are the most effective in the early acute stage when treatment that overstimulates the immune system or overtaxes the muscles could be damaging. 'Graded activity' worked out by specialists may be inappropriate at this stage. If you are in bed for days or weeks at a time, do simple rotational movements of all the joints to prevent stiffening or get a helper to do *very* gentle massage. Work muscles very gently too. Complete physical inactivity is worse for the muscles than some movement. On the positive side take advantage of this period of enforced rest and take up an interest or hobby that will occupy you and keep your morale up. Relaxation methods, especially breathing techniques, are helpful, because while you are not active you may well be tense. Meditation, prayer and yoga are beneficial. Sufferers report feeling worse mentally and emotionally for being completely unstimulated, and a downward spiral can set in.

Recovery

After some time with sufficient rest there will be days of greater energy and well-being mixed in with bad ones. On a good day you will be tempted to do more, but if you do over-do it you will not take so long to recover, nor will the relapse be so bad. It is advisable to increase activities gradually, say 10–20 per cent at a time, and see how you react.

Some of the early symptoms have gone, but you will still be fatigued easily, perhaps have muscle pains and may be easily emotionally upset. Where you had only enough concentration to read for ten minutes before, you may feel all right if you read for half an hour. You are now in the second stage and with help have a good chance of getting better, as long as you do not over-reach yourself. It is necessary to be continually aware that you still have the condition and that you may need to go on pacing yourself for months. Graded exercises will be helpful now, but it is best to take advice on your own case.

On the psychological side, if you are a person who habitually overdoes things, now may be the time to face it. Sociologists suggest it is the modern cult of busyness, with over-commitment in too many directions, that prepares the ground for this condition. It is often people who find it difficult to say no, or push themselves too hard, who get ME. Apart from work, if there are other circumstances in your life that make you unhappy – an unsatisfying relationship for example – try to work it out now, as the emotional energy it requires may be preventing you from getting well. Counselling or psychotherapy may help.

Avoid the following as they may bring on a relapse: excessive mental stress, antibiotics, immunizations, anaesthetics and surgery (unless absolutely necessary), dental work, drinking alcohol, and any foods that you know worsen the condition.

Very gradually improve on what you can do. Just try one task at a time and when that is mastered, try another. Walk a little further each day. Do not suddenly do a major shopping expedition as you begin to feel better! Keep a diary so that you can see that there are good days and bad days and that the ratio of good does increase; in your blacker moments you can refer to it.

Join a self-help association or start your own self-help group: the ME Association (see page 202) has a wide network. Knowing there are others in the same situation helps. Make sure you have your GP's support. Practise any techniques that help you and that you enjoy. Don't lose heart, or patience. Optimism is important in recovery.

Orthodox medical treatment of CFS

There is no recognized orthodox 'cure' for CFS. Various drugs have been tried, but with no significant benefit over placebos. The lack of effective antiviral drugs makes orthodox treatment difficult, although the anti-herpes drug Acyclovir is sometimes used. Anti-depressant drugs such as Amitriptyline may be prescribed and in low doses have helped some but not all sufferers. This is not surprising as the type of depression linked with CFS differs significantly from clinical depression. It seems to help those whose symptoms are mainly neurological. In severe cases, psychotherapeutic treatments consist of cognitive behavioural therapy and counselling. Non-steroidal anti-inflammatory drugs have been used with varying degrees of success.

The most usual suggestion is rest, with graded exercise later and treatment of symptoms as needed. At the moment orthodox drugs are being used on a 'try it and see' basis, in much the same way as

'alternatives'; clinical research needs to be done on all methods that may benefit this distressing condition. Treatments with emphasis on nutritional measures, such as intravenous liver extract with folic acid and Vitamin B_{12}, and intramuscular magnesium sulphate, are used with varying degrees of success. Injections of immunoglobulins to stimulate the immune system have not been effective.

The use of essential fatty acids (EFAs) was tried in controlled randomized clinical trials in Glasgow. It was found that CFS patients had subnormal levels of EFAs, probably caused by viral infection; it was known that EFAs have anti-viral activity. These were given in the form of Gamma Linolenic Acid (GLA) from Evening Primrose oil (80 per cent) and EPA from fish oils (20 per cent) taken together as Efamol Marine. Up to 6000–8000mg daily were used. After three months 85 per cent of patients reported improved feelings of well-being, whereas only 17 per cent of the placebo group improved.

Even richer sources of GLA have been found in Borage oil (Starflower oil) and blackcurrant seed oil. 4000–5000mg GLA daily are recommended by herbalists for maximum effectiveness. (Efamol can be obtained on prescription.)

Alternative treatments for CFS

A large number of patients turn to alternative medicines for help. Apart from considerable anecdotal evidence, there is little documented evidence for efficacy due to lack of interest in research from the established scientific community, but what there is is significant.

Alternative medicine provides a range of treatments which support the body's ability to heal itself. In modern biochemical medicine an ancient tradition has been lost that all medicines have had in common since antiquity, that is, the concept of vitalism. Medical systems that see the body as sustained by a vital force include physiomedical herbal medicine, traditional Chinese Medicine (herbal medicine and acupuncture), Ayurvedic medicine and homoeopathy. This is important in its implications for management of and research into this condition. Could it be that mainstream medicine is missing the point?

Physical therapies that have proved helpful symptomatically are remedial massage and Alexander Technique. Bioenergetic methods such as applied kinesiology are particularly effective for CFS as they work in the field of energy rebalancing. In any case it would be wise to find a practitioner who has a good success rate for treating CFS and may use one or more techniques.

The following alternative treatments have all been used with some measure of success: food allergy desensitization; anti-candida treatment; nutritional therapy; vitamin and mineral supplementation (Vitamins A, B, C, D, E, potassium, magnesium, zinc); intestinal parasite (Giardia) treatment, probiotics (beneficial lactobacilli); EFAs as found in Evening Primrose oil, Linseed oil and Borage oil (Starflower oil), in doses up to 5g daily.

Herbal treatment of CFS

As this guide sets out to show, herbs can improve health. They are a living, vital source of healing substances and work by stimulating the body's own resources.

The immune system is encouraged to work properly again by specific herbs. The adrenals are boosted, the liver is supported in its functions, the nervous system is relaxed and the functioning of the brain and nerves improved. One of the most beneficent actions of herbs is their wonderful ability to improve well-being, and this is the first step on the road to recovery; although some of the symptoms are still there, there is a sensation of lifting spirits. This often happens within the first month of treatment, if all the other factors (dietary, rest, etc.) are being taken care of.

As it affects so many systems of the body, herbal treatment necessarily varies for different people and for the same person at different stages of illness.

Please take the following rules into account:

1 Only follow herbal treatment if you have been given a clear diagnosis of CFS or ME.
2 Do not self-diagnose. Ask your doctor or herbal practitioner about any symptoms you do not understand.
3 Stop treatment if you get worse or develop new symptoms.
4 It is advisable to consult a medical herbalist, at least initially, as there are so many factors to consider. Only general guidelines can be suggested here.

Actions of the herbs
For doses, see Directions for use of herbs for chronic fatigue syndrome, at the end of this chapter.

Digestive system
Liver herbs, taken because of their bitter action and major role in detoxifying and restoring all the body's organs: Milk Thistle, for its ability to repair the liver cells after viral damage; Gentian, which improves function and helps general debility: Dandelion Root for its detoxifying action and its reflex action on improving all the digestive processes. Barberry and Blue Flag have alterative properties; Wormwood improves appetite and helps nausea; Roman Chamomile is also excellent for nausea.

Immune system
Echinacea increases the white blood cell count, specifically that of the 'helper' T-cells. Others are Garlic, and Chinese herbs: Astralagus membranaceous, Atractylodes macrocephalia, Codonopsis, Ginseng, Siberian Ginseng, Pau D'arco.

Nervous system
Tonics: Vervain, St John's Wort, Oats, Lemon Balm, Cola, Rosemary, Gotu Cola.
Sedatives: Skullcap, Motherwort, Betony, Damiana.

Hormonal system
Evening Primrose, Borage (both rich in EFAs), Liquorice, Bladderwrack, Saw Palmetto, Sarsaparilla, Golden Seal, Chaste Berry.

Lymphatic System
Cleavers, Pokeroot, Wild Indigo, where there is sluggish lymphatic circulation leading to blocked drainage and persistent swollen glands and sore throat.

Muscular system
Devil's Claw, Guaiacum, and Celery Seed for inflammation (the latter can be drunk copiously as a tea). Add Prickly Ash to stimulate circulation to sluggish muscles. Herbal essential oils such as Rosemary, Wintergreen and Lavender in a base oil, for massage to ease sore muscles. Add Chamomile oil as an anti-spasmodic. Also use in baths. Other herbs that can be taken are Cramp Bark and Black Cohosh.

Colon cleansing
Red Clover, Barberry, Cascara, Golden Seal, Rhubarb, Yellow Dock, Burdock, Capsicum, Ginger.

Colon cleansing is effective if enteroviruses are

Never use immune system-stimulating herbs initially as this system is likely to be overactive already. Instead, build up your level of energy and repair some of the damage using liver herbs and those for the nervous system. When things have normalized somewhat, use the Immune system fortifying formula (see below).

If you are very depleted and the nervous system has taken a beating, gentle supportive remedies such as Oats give enough energy to relax and sleep, while St John's Wort repairs the nervous system (these are best as teas at this stage as tinctures contain a little alcohol, which will be poorly tolerated. Otherwise you can add boiling water to the tincture to evaporate the alcohol.)

Formula for exhaustion

Oats	25 per cent
St John's Wort	25 per cent
Vervain	25 per cent
Milk Thistle	25 per cent

Total: 100ml/g a week. Dose: tincture, 5ml three times daily, or infusion/decoction of dried herb in equal parts, 1 cup three times daily, or powdered in capsules, 2, three times daily (see pages 8–10).

In addition Garlic is an excellent anti-viral agent, either taken fresh (a clove a day finely chopped), or freeze-dried in capsules or as tablets. (Avoid Garlic Oil capsules as the Garlic content is often weak.) 3000–5000mg Evening Primrose oil or Borage oil (Starflower oil) daily is recommended. Dried Kelp tablets (6–10 daily) will provide essential minerals and build up the metabolism.

Aching muscles

Massage with herbal oils will provide relief and improve muscle tension. One or two of the following essential oils in a carrier oil are suggested: Basil, Bergamot, Chamomile, Eucalyptus, Geranium, Ginger, Lavender, Rosemary, Wintergreen: 2–3 drops of each oil are added to the base oil which should be warmed first.

St John's Wort oil relieves pain and irritation of the nerve endings as the result of pressure. Massage into the sacral area of the lower back. If severe, a compress of St John's Wort herb applied to the back will give relief (see page 11). Take St John's Wort tincture internally: 20 drops every few hours for pain relief.

For treatment of specific symptoms see HEAD PAINS, BOWEL PROBLEMS, ARTHRITIS, CANDIDIASIS, CYSTITIS, HYPOGLYCAEMIA and PMS (page 16).

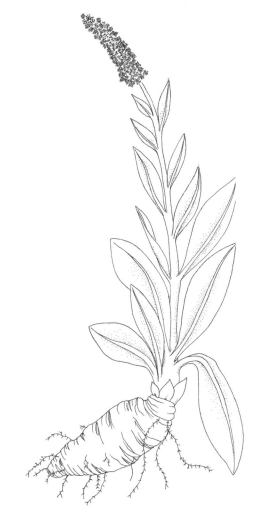

False Unicorn Root (*Chamaelirium luteum*)

involved, as an overloaded colon can maintain an unhealthy environment, encouraging the persistence of the virus. As well as taking the herbs, a daily rectal enema is sometimes useful, either a herbal or coffee enema to speed up the process of toxic release. You can monitor this by the amount of old faecal matter that is passed (see Colon cleansing, page 146).

First stage of treatment

Care needs to be taken not to overstimulate an exhausted body. This is especially important if you still have low-grade fever and flu-like symptoms.

Second stage of treatment

Immune system fortifying formula

Astralagus	20 per cent
Ginseng	20 per cent
Echinacea	20 per cent
Chinese Liquorice	20 per cent
Cola	20 per cent

Total: 100ml/g a week. Dose: tincture, 5ml three times daily, or infusion/decoction of dried herb in equal parts, 1 cup three times daily, or powdered in capsules, 2, three times daily (see pages 8–10).

This is recommended for 2–3 months followed by a break of a month. It can then be repeated if necessary. A similar proprietary Chinese herbal formula, called Immunoguard, is available from Chinese herbal suppliers. Do not take any formula for more than three months at a time without advice.

Over the longer term, a general formula taking a herb from each category (immune system, nervous system, etc.) depending on what is most affected, and changing it as necessary, is the most helpful for some sufferers. The following is a suggestion, or you could combine others from the list above (see Directions for use of herbs for chronic fatigue, at the end of this chapter).

For treatment of specific symptoms see A–Z Directory of Other Conditions (pages 151–92).

CFS formula

Echinacea	25 per cent
Barberry	25 per cent
Cleavers	25 per cent
Skullcap	25 per cent

Total: 100ml/g a week. Dose: tincture, 5ml three times daily, or infusion/decoction of dried herb in equal parts, 1 cup three times daily, or powdered in capsules, 2, three times daily (see pages 8–10).

Nutrition

Dietary changes may be necessary and bring about substantial improvement for some sufferers.

Food sensitivities
CFS has been equated in the past with total allergy syndrome or 'twentieth-century disease' as it is sometimes known. There is no doubt that classic allergy and atopic allergy are very prevalent in CFS. In one recent study 50 per cent of people with chronic fatigue were found to be reactive to a variety of inhalant or food allergens when tested by inoculation of these under the skin. In a normal population reactivity seldom exceeds 15–20 per cent in those tested.

CFS sufferers often tolerate wheat and dairy products poorly, perhaps due to the imbalance of immunoglobulins in the gut. If this seems to be your problem try an exclusion diet, leaving out one product at a time, each for a month (see Elimination diet, page 137), then challenging with the food. If there is a reaction leave that item out of your diet for at least six months, and then try again.

Problem foods
The foods most often observed to create problems are (in order):-

Wheat (includes bread, pasta and all the many foods containing wheat).
Other grains: corn, oats, rice.
Cow's milk, cheese and butter (but not natural yoghurt).
Yeast, yeast products and anything containing yeast.
Sugar, honey and other sweeteners.
Food additives and colourings.
Drinks containing caffeine: coffee, alcoholic drinks, colas, tea.
Chocolate.
Hen's eggs.
Some fruits: mainly citrus.
Tomatoes, peppers and potatoes.
Soya products.
Refined cooking oils.
Shellfish.

In practice the author has found that there are major and minor food sensitivities and the minor ones quite quickly diminish if the main culprits are avoided. In CFS food sensitivities are rarely full-blown allergies. If you think you have them but find it difficult to sort out what they are, a food allergy test may be the answer. This can be done in the orthodox way, by patch or skin-prick testing, cytotoxic tests, or less invasively, with applied kinesiology. There may be a candida hypersensitivity problem (it has been suggested by some authorities that up to 50 per cent of CFS sufferers have it, although others see it as much less). (See CANDIDIASIS for further information.) Although this is a benign commensal organism present in everyone, the immunotoxins released from an overgrowth of the yeast are harmful. If you suffer from thrush or have other symptoms of candida, it needs to be treated, but not with a very strict food exclusion diet; if you are already food-intolerant you are likely to react to the narrow range of foods imposed, until there is nothing left. (See Anti-candida diet, page 139). Sometimes desensitization to a particular food is necessary. This can be done by Enzyme Potentiated Desensitization (EPD), when very dilute amounts of the allergen are injected under the skin. It can also be taken orally in a homoeopathic dilution. (see ALLERGY.)

The cornerstone of the diet should be fresh and whole foods, organic if possible. This way you will avoid antibiotics in meat, pesticides and other chemicals added to food. (See Healthy wholefood diet, page 126.) The diet should be 50 per cent raw food, or work up to this gradually. When cooking, steam rather than boil to get maximum value. Nearly all vegetables are good except those mentioned above. Drink plenty of mineral water (or distilled if mineral is not tolerated). All sugars are to be avoided, as is anything refined or processed. If in any doubt, see Anti-candida diet (page 139). Avoid teas, except herbal, and stimulants: coffee, chocolate, cola, alcohol, tobacco. Avoid all non-essential prescribed drugs (these should be reviewed), over-the-counter drugs and recreational drugs.

Nutritional supplements

CFS sufferers often absorb nutrients poorly as a result of imbalanced metabolism, making vitamin and mineral supplements necessary. Weight loss and undigested food in stools indicate this. The RDA for healthy adults is no longer appropriate, so amounts recommended here are higher.

Recent scientifically validated research suggests that magnesium improves symptoms, and possibly shortages trigger the condition. A mineral analysis test before embarking on a course of mineral therapy would be advantageous. The test can be done from blood, saliva or hair. Private laboratories will do this, for example a reliable hair mineral analysis test is performed by ICAP (Inductively Coupled Argon Plasma Emission Spectroscopy). Larkhall Laboratories (see page 203 for address) provide these services to the public. Beware of dowsing or pendulum analysis as the results are very mixed.

All supplements should be hypoallergenic, free from gluten, sugar, yeast, soya products and grains.

Minerals

Calcium, magnesium, zinc, selenium, potassium, chromium and sometimes iron are taken as supplements. Beware of taking one without balancing it in the right proportion with the others as they should all be in correct ratio to each other in the body. Multi-mineral supplements bought over the counter from a reputable firm (see page 203) should be correctly balanced. If you are not sure what to take, check with a nutritionist or dietary specialist.

Vitamins

Vitamin C is taken for its anti-viral and positive immune system action. A positive relationship between Vitamin C intake and decrease in fatigue has been proved in several studies. It is also anti-oxidant and so minimizes damage to cells through free radicals, toxic by-products of cell metabolism. High doses up to 5g daily have been used by some nutritionists. Work up to this by 1g daily, but if you get diarrhoea, cut back to a comfortable level using the principle of bowel tolerance. Otherwise take up to 1000mg daily for a maximum of three months, then gradually reduce to 200mg daily for up to two years.

Vitamin B levels are often low, with B_6 and B_{12} being most frequently needed. B_6 is needed to metabolize the EFAs: deficiency affects mood, causing irritability and depression in particular. Vitamin B_{12} affects the nervous system, with fatigue, neurological and mental symptoms being caused by deficiency. Vitamin B_5 or Pantothenic acid plays a significant role in relieving stress-related illness and fatigue. A good multiple B vitamin should be taken containing 20–50mg of B_6 and B_5 and 3–5mcg of B_{12}, depending on severity, as this is often poorly absorbed from the intestine. In chronic ME it may be worth getting the blood levels checked for B_{12}; fatigue in some women responds well to injections of Vitamin B_{12} where it has been in short supply.

Fat-soluble Vitamins A, D, and E are often low. Vitamin A is required for repair of the immune system and resistance to infection. Beta-carotene from carrots is the best non-toxic source of Vitamin A – up to 20,000 IUs daily, as necessary. Vitamin D is needed to help in metabolism, and is present in vegetable and fish oils, or one hour's sunlight a day on the face alone will provide enough for the daily requirement. Vitamin E is another anti-oxidant; 200–400 IUs a day are recommended.

Probiotics, beneficial bacteria such as lactobacillus acidophilus and bifidus found naturally in live yoghurt or freeze-dried as a powder, are thought to be beneficial. Take 3–4 capsules daily. They help recolonize the gut and improve digestion as well as forming part of an Anti-candida diet (see page 139) and are used in the treatment of food allergies. Ask a healthfood shop to recommend a brand as some contain harmful *S. faecalis*.

Digestive enzymes: aids to digestion include natural vegetable enzymes as found in papaya (papain) and pineapple (bromelain). Hydrochloric acid tablets are sometimes recommended in ME because of lack of gastric acid, but it is powerful, so half the dose recommended should be taken, and only with food.

Caution: Avoid hydrochloric acid if you have a history of gastritis, stomach ulcers or ULCERATIVE COLITIS, or if in any doubt stick to the more gentle fruit enzymes.

Coenzyme Q10, which is naturally present in the body, is essential for production of energy on a cellular level. Some practitioners are enthusiastic about its benefits: 30–40mg daily is recommended by manufacturers.

Sufficient intake of amino acids is essential for health. Certain free-form amino acids, the building blocks of protein, have been found to be beneficial. Among these is Carnitine, an important source of energy for cells. Try 250mg daily with Vitamin C.

Directions for use of herbs for CFS

Dried herbs by weight are either powdered and put into capsules – buy or powder your own – or taken as dried leaf, flowers, etc, as infusion. The dose given is per cup and 1 (small) cup = approx. 100ml water. In measuring quantities, as a rough guide 5g dried flower or leaf = 1×5ml medicine spoon or teaspoon, dried root and bark weighs more, so half the quantity. It is easier to make 300ml at a time, which is sufficient for a day. A general rule is 30g dried herb to 600ml.

Tinctures of herbs are available ready-made. These contain alcohol and are a concentrated form of herbal medicine. Herbal tinctures are taken with water in the proportion of one part to eight parts dilution.

See pages 8–10 for further directions on preparation of all the above.

General guide to dosage:
Total: 100ml/g a week. Dose: Tincture 5ml three times daily, or infusion/decoction of dried herb, equal parts, 1 cup three times daily. (Suggested dosages are *three times daily* unless otherwise stated. These are all within safe margins – *Do not exceed*.)

After consideration of the actions of the herbs listed it is advisable to combine four or five in equal parts to make a balanced prescription. If in any doubt follow suggested formulas or consult a medical herbalist. See List of Principal Herbs (page 198) for explanation of terms.

Key **A = 1–2ml/g, B = 3–4ml/g; C = 5ml/g; D = 6–10ml/g**
Note: **The main therapeutic agents for this condition are <u>underlined</u>.**

<u>Astralagus (Huang Qi) (*Astralagus membranaceus*)</u> Root
> *Dose:* Tincture C. Dried C–D.
> *Actions:* Chi or energy tonic. Strengthens immune system.
> *Indications*: Chronic problems. Tiredness. Weakness with diarrhoea. Sweating.

<u>Atractylodes (Bai Zhu) (*Atractylodes macrocephala*)</u> Root
> *Dose:* Tincture C. Dried C.
> *Actions:* Chi or energy tonic. Immune system stimulant.
> *Indications:* Tiredness and debility. Sweating. Poor digestive functions.
> *Note:* Widely used in China to control weight.

Barberry (*Berberis vulgaris*) Bark
> *Dose:* Tincture A–B. Dried or as decoction A.
> *Actions:* Liver tonic, hepatic. Cholagogue, increases digestive secretions. Beneficial reflex action on lower digestive tract, kidney, uterus and other organs.
> *Indications:* Liver congestion, jaundice, gallstones.

Betony (*Stachys betonica*) Leaf and flower
> *Dose:* Tincture A–C. Dried A–B.
> *Actions:* Sedative. Bitter. Gentle tonic.
> *Indications:* Conditions affecting the head – neuralgias, headache, migraine. Lack of concentration. Forgetfulness.

Black Cohosh (*Cimicifuga racemosa*) Root
> *Dose:* Tincture A. (Works best in alcohol.) Dried or as decoction A.
> *Actions:* Anti-spasmodic, anti-inflammatory and sedative. Nervous system tonic.
> *Indications:* Rheumatic pain. Muscular rheumatism.

Bladderwrack or Kelp (*Fucus vesiculosus*) Whole plant

> *Dose:* Tincture B. Dried as capsules or pills A.
> *Actions:* Anti-hypothyroid, anti-obesic.
> *Indications:* Obesity, used as part of weight-loss programme. Tiredness due to sluggish thyroid. Myxoedema.
> *Note:* High content of minerals, especially calcium.

Blue Flag (*Iris versicolor*) Root

> *Dose:* Tincture B. Dried or as decoction A.
> *Actions:* Cholagogue – stimulating and detoxifying action on gall-bladder, liver and lymphatics. Alterative. Anti-inflammatory.
> *Indications:* Chronic congestion.

Borage (*Borago officinalis*) Leaf and flower

> *Dose:* Tincture C. Dried or infusion C–D.
> *Actions:* Contains EFAs which are essential for biochemical actions in the body. Anti-inflammatory action. Positive immune system action.
> *Indications:* Arthritis. Rheumatism. Myalgia.

Cayenne (*Capsicum minimum*) Fruit

> *Dose:* Tincture 0.2ml. Dried 30–120mg.
> *Actions:* Stimulant, anti-spasmodic. General stimulant by reflex action on the nervous system.
> *Indications:* Poor circulation. Functional sluggishness. Fatigue. Lethargy.

Chamomile (German) (*Matricaria recutita*) Flower

> *Dose:* Tincture A–B. Dried A–B.
> *Actions:* Mild sedative. Anti-inflammatory. Anti-spasmodic.
> *Indications:* Restlessness. Irritability. Insomnia. Digestive problems.

Chamomile (Roman) (*Chamaemelum nobile*) Flower

> *Dose:* Tincture A–B. Dried A–B.
> *Actions:* Sedative, anti-spasmodic, carminative.
> *Indications:* Mental stress. Nausea. Lack of appetite. Digestive problems.

Chinese Angelica (Dang Gui) (*Angelica sinensis*) Root

> *Dose:* Tincture C. Dried or as decoction C.
> *Actions:* Blood tonic. In Chinese terms, it both tones and moves blood at the same time. A powerful tonic and famous women's herb, used for many gynaecological complaints. Known as Women's Ginseng. Emmenagogue. Analgesic.
> *Indications:* Menstrual irregularity and pain, where the woman is debilitated. Anaemia. Loss of periods. Restores hormonal balance in PMS and menopause. Used as general tonic for fatigue. *Caution:* Do not use in high blood pressure or in inflammatory conditions.

Cleavers (*Galium aparine*) Leaf and flower

> *Dose:* Tincture D. Dried D. Fresh juice up to 15ml daily.
> *Actions:* Astringent. Diuretic. Aids removal of toxic by-products in body.
> *Indications:* Enlarged lymph glands. Sluggish lymphatic circulation.

Codonopsis

> (See **Ginseng**).

Cola (*Cola vera*) Nut or seed

> *Dose:* Tincture A–B. Dried as powder A–B.
> *Action:* Nervous system stimulant. Anti-depressive.
> *Indications:* Depression. Exhaustion. Muscle fatigue after illness. Neuromuscular dysfunction. *Small* doses for an accumulative effect.

Cramp Bark (*Viburnum opulus*) Bark

> *Dose:* Tincture C. Dried or as decoction B.
> *Actions:* Powerful anti-spasmodic, sedative.
> *Indications:* Spasmodic muscular cramps (with Prickly Ash). Apply locally to aching muscles.

Damiana (*Turnera diffusa*) Leaf

> *Dose:* Tincture B. Dried or as infusion A–B.
> *Actions:* Nerve tonic. Thymoleptic (improves mood).
> *Indications:* Depression. Nervousness.

Dandelion (*Taraxacum officinale*) Root

> *Dose:* Tincture C. Dried or as decoction C. Leaf C.
> *Actions:* Hepatic. Cholagogue. Tonic to digestive system with reflex action on whole body. Gentle detoxifying agent. Leaf is diuretic for fluid retention.
> *Indications:* Digestive problems and general debility.

Echinacea (*Echinacea angustifolia, E. purpurea*) Root

> *Dose:* Tincture A–B. Dried A.
> *Actions:* Anti-microbial. Anti-viral.
> *Indications:* Infection. Strengthens immune system. Externally as a douche, wash, etc.

Evening Primrose (*Oenothera biennis*) Seed oil

> *Doses:* Oil 2–3000mg daily.
> *Actions:* Contains EFAs which are essential for biochemical actions in the body. Anti-inflammatory action. Positive immune system action.
> *Indications:* Immune system dysfunction. Arthritis.

Garlic (*Allium sativum*) Bulb

> *Dose:* Tincture or fresh juice D. Dried as tablets B–C.
> Oil in capsules 2–4 daily. If used as fresh cloves, do not exceed C.

Actions: Stimulating tonic. Alterative and trophorestorative. Anti-microbial. Possible anti-viral action. Increases resistance to disease.

Indications: Weak digestion. Candidiasis. Infections.

Note: Locally irritant. Apply as oil of garlic, never apply fresh.

Gentian (*Gentiana lutea*) Root

Dose: Tincture A–B. Dried or as decoction A.

Actions: Bitter. Gastric stimulant. General stimulant by digestive reflex action.

Indications: General debility.

Ginger (*Zingiber officinale*) Root

Dose: Tincture A. Dried or as decoction A. For nausea (dried) A, repeated hourly.

Actions: Gentle warming stimulant for all internal organs. Carminative.

Indications: Deficient circulation and congestion. Relieves flatulence and colic.

GINSENGS

Panax Ginseng (Ren Shen) (*Panax ginseng*) Root

Dose: Tincture or syrup B–C. Dried as tablets A.

Actions: Chi or energy tonic. Stimulant and rejuvenant. Increases resistance to disease. Reputed in China to promote longevity.

Indications: Chi deficiency diseases. Chronic fatigue.

American Ginseng (*Panax Quinquefolium*) Root

Dose: Tincture or syrup D. Dried as tablets B–D.

Actions: Similar to above but milder and less stimulating for long-term use.

Siberian Ginseng (*Eleutherococcus senticosus*) Root

Dose: Tincture D. Dried A–B.

Actions: Chi or energy tonic. Increases energy and stamina.

Indications: Low vitality and lack of endurance.

Codonopsis (Dang Shen) (*Codonopsis pilosula*) Root

Dose: Tincture D. Dried D.

Actions: Chi or energy tonic.

Indications: Tiredness and debility. Use as milder substitute for Ginseng.

Golden Seal (*Hydrastis canadensis*) Root

Dose: Tincture A–B. Dried or as decoction A.

Actions: Anti-haemorrhagic. Mildly stimulating vaso-tonic with wide actions, chiefly on digestive organs and uterus.

Indications: Digestive disorders. Anorexia. Liver symptoms.

Gotu Cola (*Hydrocotyle asiatica*) Root

Dose: Tincture C. Dried D.

Actions: Important nerve tonic and alterative.

Indications: Stress. Insomnia. Emotional and other nervous system disturbances.

Liquorice (*Glycyrrhiza glabra*) Root

Dose: Tincture B. Dried or as decoction A–B.

Actions: Adrenal agent. Anti-spasmodic. Anti-inflammatory. Mild laxative. In hormonal imbalance works synergistically with other herbs.

Indications: Any female condition where there is debility or exhaustion.

Liquorice, Chinese (Gan Cao) (*Glycyrrhiza uralensis*) Root

Dose: As above.

Actions: As above, but as is roasted in honey, is much more gentle and demulcent, and is less stimulating. In Chinese terms it enters all the energy channels of the body and is used in very many formulas. Reputed to balance blood-sugar problems (hypoglycaemia).

Note: Liquorice should not be taken if there is high blood pressure.

Milk Thistle or Marian Thistle (*Carduus marianus*) Seed and fruit

Dose: Tincture B. Dried or as decoction A.

Actions: Hepatic. Organ restorative for liver. Bitter stimulant.

Indications: Debility with liver symptoms.

Motherwort (*Leonorus cardiaca*) Leaf and flower

Dose: Tincture C–D. Dried or as infusion A–B.

Actions: Sedative, anti-spasmodic. Hypotensive. Hormonal agent.

Indications: Tension. Stress-related problems.

Oats (*Avena sativa*) Seed

Dose: Tincture A–C.

Actions: Anti-depressive. Nerve tonic.

Indications: General debility and depression. Nervous exhaustion with insomnia.

Passion Flower (*Passiflora incarnata*) Leaf and flower

Dose: Tincture A–B. Dried or as infusion A.

Actions: Sedative. Analgesic. Anti-spasmodic.

Indications: Insomnia. Neuralgic-type pain. Nervous tension.

Pau D'arco (*Tabebuia impeteginosa*) Bark

Dose: Dried B–C, 2 tablets.

Actions: Anti-inflammatory. General tonic.

Indications: Immunodeficiency diseases. General weakness. Inflammatory conditions. Candidiasis.

Red Clover (*Trifolium pratense*) Flower

Dose: Tincture A–B. Dried or as infusion A–B.

Actions: Alterative.

Indications: Chronic conditions of skin or internally.

Note: High content of minerals.

Rosemary (*Rosmarinus officinalis*) Leaf
    Dose: Tincture C. Dried or as infusion A–B.
    Actions: Gentle circulatory stimulant. Anti-depressant. General tonic. Anti-spasmodic.
    Indications: Depression. Exhaustion. Headache.

Sarsaparilla (*Smilax spp.*) Root.
    Dose: Tincture B–C. Dried or as decoction A–B.
    Actions: General tonic. Hormonal agent.
    Indications: General debility.

Saw Palmetto (*Serenoa serrulata*) Fruit
    Dose: Tincture A. Dried or as decoction A.
    Actions: General tonic and alterative. Endocrine agent. Promotes tissue nutrition.
    Indications: Debility with sexual problems. Wasting diseases.

Schizandra (Wu Wei Zi) (*Schizandra chinensis*) Fruit
    Dose: Tincture C. Dried or as decoction C–D.
    Actions: Tonic for reproductive system. Increases vitality.
    Indications: Fatigue, with Codonopsis.

Skullcap (*Scutellaria laterifolia*) Leaf and flower
    Dose: Tincture C. Dried or infusion A–B.
    Actions: Sedative.
    Indications: Nervous tension. Stress-related problems. Combines well with Valerian.

St John's Wort (*Hypericum perforatum*) Leaf and flower
    Dose: Tincture B. Dried or as infusion A–B.
    Actions: Sedative. Alterative. Analgesic.
    Indications: Nervous debility and depression. Indicated specifically for nerve injuries and muscular twitching. Used locally for massage as St John's Wort oil.

Stone Root (*Collinsonia canadensis*) Root
    Dose: Tincture C–D. Dried or as decoction A–B.
    Actions: Diuretic. Stimulates removal of uric acid and congestion. Tones all mucous tissues in the body.
    Indications: Urinary stones. Liver congestion.

Vervain (*Verbena officinalis*) Leaf and flower
    Dose: Tincture C–D. Dried or as infusion A–B.
    Actions: Gentle sedative. General nervous system tonic. Liver tonic.
    Indications: Depression and exhaustion. Particularly beneficial for women.

Wild Indigo (*Baptisia tinctoria*) Root
    Dose: Tincture A. Dried A.
    Actions: Anti-microbial, antiseptic.
    Indications: Lymphadenitis. Chronic infections of the upper respiratory tract.

Wormwood (*Artemisia vulgaris*) Leaf and flower
    Dose: Tincture A. Dried or infusion A.
    Actions: Bitter. Tonic. Emmenagogue.
    Indications: General tonic by digestive reflex action. Poor digestion. Lack of appetite. Liver congestion. Anorexia.

Yellow Dock (*Rumex crispus*) Root
    Dose: Tincture A. Dried or as decoction A–B.
    Actions: General tonic and alterative.
    Indications: Tiredness. General debility. Anaemia.

9 Nutrition

'Let food be your medicine and medicine be your food.'
Hippocrates, 'The Father of Medicine', 460–377 BC

The field of nutrition is so wide that only a broad outline has been attempted here in order to provide some basic, general information and to show, hopefully, the benefits of healthy eating, especially as preventive medicine. The use of nutrition as a therapy is introduced and diets for a number of common medical problems and special needs outlined.

A brief history of nutrition

Humankind is ancient and our natural diet has evolved over millennia. We have become adapted over a very long time to certain staple foods that our primitive ancestors gathered, such as fruit, roots and nuts, and those they later farmed, such as other vegetables and grains. Animals were hunted, notably wild game and fish, but formed a smaller part of the diet. History shows that man ate raw foods long before he adapted to cooked.

There is debate over whether we have evolved as meat-eaters or vegetarians. Some argue that the length of our digestive tract makes us herbivores and others that our teeth distinguish us as carnivores; whatever our antecedents, since recent times we have eaten anything and everything. However, many people cannot tolerate modern agrochemical traces, drug residues, food synthesis and artificial additives in food. Modern food, particularly refined carbohydrates, presents other challenges. It is logical that if we start to follow a diet different from that evolved over millennia to suit us, we are going to encounter problems. Coupled with a more affluent, lazier life-style, this can be a recipe for ill-health and sometimes disaster.

For hundreds of years the staple diet of the British was bread, cheese, beef and beer. This gave an adequate intake of nutrients, especially if supplemented with home-grown vegetables. Fruit was rare and available only in season. Bread was made from coarse-ground flour, retaining its full quota of vitamins and minerals and 16 per cent of protein. It made up 70 per cent of the diet in some cases and provided reasonable nutrition. With industrialization white milled flour became widely available. The addition of white sugar and tea in place of beer worsened the situation. The process of refining food staples has continued until today; they are the basis of the Western diet. Factory farming and industrial food processing have developed to cater for the large, centralized populations of the post-industrial era.

The choice of diets currently available in the affluent West ranges from vegan (no animal-based foods at all), through vegetarian and 'wholefood' diets to the 'average balanced' heavily protein-orientated, omnivore diet with/without processed foods. The last diet, referred to as a Western diet, is far from the norm elsewhere as two-thirds of the world's population are vegetarian, and 70 per cent of mankind do not drink milk.

The science of nutrition

Nutrition as a subject did not really become established until the 1920s, with the discovery that vitamins were essential to life. Prior to that food was valued purely for its caloric value, that is, as a fuel to run the body. (See Vitamins and Minerals below.)

Food as energy
Nowadays a number of factors are taken into account in assessing nutritional needs, including the amount of fuel the body consumes in the form of carbohydrates, fats, proteins and alcohol. These

substances are converted in the body into energy for vital processes and physical activity.

Basal metabolic rate

A way of measuring the body's consumption of energy is by basal metabolic rate or BMR, the resting rate during which only energy for vital processes is used. Extra reserves of energy are required for physical activity. BMR is calculated by the amount of heat given off by the body per unit of body surface per hour (in kilocalories per kilo of body weight). When the intake of food and the energy needs are balanced, the body maintains its normal weight, but if the intake exceeds output then the extra has to be stored in the form of fat.

BMR varies with a number of factors and basal rates are now thought to be generally lower than they were previously: some women function perfectly well on a low rate. The BMR is lowered in obesity and starvation which is why most dieting to lose weight is unsuccessful in the long term. As food intake is reduced, so BMR is reduced in order to conserve energy and food then has a greater capacity to turn to fat. The best way to increase BMR is regular exercise and a nutritionally sound diet (see pages 72 and 75).

Food energy is calculated in kilocalories:

Examples of caloric values of foods (per 100g)

Potatoes	76kcal
Eggs	147
Beef	226
Herring	224
Sugar	394
Cheese	412
Cooking oil	899

Different food components provide different energy levels per gram of food eaten:

Carbohydrate	4kcal
Fat	9kcal
Protein	4 kcal
Alcohol	7 kcal

Composition of foods

Carbohydrates (sugars and starches)

Carbohydrate is a bulky, starchy, energy-sustaining food. A major component of the diet in the world today, it is provided by cereals and grains such as wheat, rice, oats, corn, etc. or by vegetables such as potatoes. When broken down, these complex carbohydrates yield glucose for energy. In primitive times they formed a large percentage of the diet, much of this in the form of roughage or fibre. This was healthy, as glucose and roughage combine together to release the glucose more slowly. The body, especially the brain, needs a constant supply to function properly. Today, much of the carbohydrate consumed is refined, the roughage having been removed, with inevitable loss of some vitamins and minerals in the process.

Simple carbohydrates or sugars come naturally from fruit or from milk lactose. A large proportion of sugar in the Western diet today is extrinsic sugar, or sucrose, made from refined cane sugar. This has increased enormously as a proportion of the British diet in the last seventy years, from twenty pounds per person a year to 120 pounds a year, which not only provides empty calories with low nutritive value but displaces complex carbohydrates from the diet by satiating the appetite. Sucrose is the basis of most junk food and is added to many convenience foods.

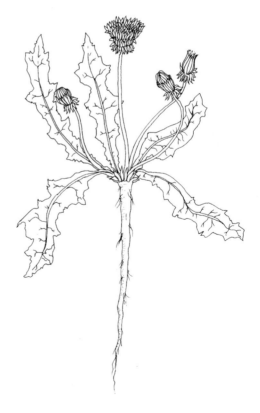

Dandelion *(Taraxacum officinale)*

Problems associated directly with high intakes of sucrose are dental decay and obesity. Hormonal problems such as hypoglycaemia and diabetes are also casually related. Very high intakes (in the region of 30 per cent) may be associated with raised blood cholesterol and atherosclerosis (leading to cardiovascular disease) and the gastrointestinal cancers. There are no known effects of high starch intakes.

It is preferable to take unrefined carbohydrates in the form of wholemeal bread, brown rice, etc. Natural sugars in fruit are best – honey makes a good substitute – or use brown, unrefined cane sugar in small amounts in cooking.

DRVs for carbohydrate

Extrinsic sugars 60g daily for an adult, or 10 per cent of total energy intake. Other carbohydrates: 37 per cent of total energy intake.

Fats

Fats provide a ready source of calories with high burn rate for fast energy. Fats should provide one-third of total calorie intake but in fact the total is much more than that in the average Western diet. (In the last fifty years intake has increased by 100 per cent.) They consist mainly of triglyceride and saturated and unsaturated fatty acids. Saturated fats come from animal sources: cooking lard, butter, cheese and meat. In the West over-consumption of saturated fats commonly occurs where milk, meat, butter and eggs provide most of the fat in the diet.

Unsaturated fats are from vegetable sources: vegetable oils such as olive, corn, sunflower, safflower, etc. Polyunsaturated fatty acids (PUFAs) are more beneficial than saturated, safflower being the best; however, when used in cooking, PUFAs should not be heated above 120°C as this alters the structure to a saturated fat. For the same reason, vegetable oils should ideally be 'virgin', cold-pressed rather than heat-extracted. Olive oil which is mono-unsaturated is thought to be the best oil in its class, and many nutritionists prefer it for salads and cooking. Hydrogenated fats (hardened vegetable oils as in margarine) are now thought to be harmful to arteries, and only non-hydrogenated margarines contain PUFAs.

The conclusions of a Government COMA (Committee on Medical Aspects of Health) panel on Nutrition in the UK in 1991 were: 1) The higher the blood cholesterol level in a population group the higher the risk of heart disease. 2) The intake of certain saturated fatty acids raises blood cholesterol levels. 3) EFAs lower blood cholesterol. 4) Trials to try to alter heart disease rates by reducing blood cholesterol levels have generally resulted in lower incidence. 5) The evidence available on the connection between cancer and saturated fats makes it wise to limit intakes.

Essential fatty acids (EFAs)

These are 'essential' because they are the only fatty acids that cannot be synthesized by the body and there must be a sufficient intake in the diet for normal cell metabolism, particularly for the brain and nerves. Total intake of these has not risen in line with other fats. They are found in the oils of seeds (sunflower, safflower) and in some fresh vegetables. Linseed oil and Evening Primrose oil are valuable additions to the diet to provide sufficient intake of EFAs, particularly important in acute and chronic disease states as the demand for tissue repair in the cells is increased.

Fish oils are high in EFAs of a different type which are thought to be beneficial in preventing cardiovascular disease. An increased intake of vegetables, seeds and oily fish in the average diet would satisfy the need for EFAs.

DRVs for polyunsaturated fatty acids = 6 per cent of energy intake (including EFAs 1 per cent linoleic and 0.2 per cent linolenic acid).
Mono-unsaturated fatty acids = 12 per cent of energy intake.
Saturated fatty acids = 10 per cent of energy intake.
Others = 2 per cent of energy intake.
Total fatty acids = 30 per cent of energy intake.

Protein

Protein is essential for body maintenance. There are two types, 'first-class' (complete protein) and 'second-class'. Protein consists of twenty amino acids, nine of which are essential and have to be present simultaneously to be used. First-class protein contains all of these and is found in eggs, milk, meat and fish. Second-class sources are in beans, lentils, grains and seeds. Vegetable sources do not contain all the amino acids, so they are usually combined in the vegetarian diet, for example as in lentils with rice, to give a complete protein. (The soya bean is the only source of complete protein, and soya products form a major part of the diet in China and Japan.) Vegetarianism is the most common diet globally and this way of eating is becoming increasingly common in the West for reasons of health as well as of compassion.

Protein deficiency is very rare in the West, but if you are vegetarian or vegan it is necessary to balance food more carefully. The vegan diet also lacks natural sources of Vitamin B_{12} and some minerals, so it may be wise to take supplements.

The protein content of the Western diet has increased in the last fifty years as a result of higher meat consumption, well over the DRV of 45g per adult female. Too much animal protein produces an end-product of uric acid from the kidneys that the body finds difficult to excrete. Many chronic, degenerative and inflammatory diseases such as hardening of the arteries, gastro-intestinal cancers and arthritis, the so-called 'diseases of civilization', may be attributed to overly high protein consumption among other things.

Dietary fibre (non-starch polysaccharides)

Dietary fibre or roughage consists of the outer husk of grains, for example of wheat, which is removed in the refining of flour. It is often replaced in the diet by addition of bran. Natural fibre is found in the skins of vegetables and fruits.

Fibre is important for regular bowel movement and in studies of people with high-fibre diets, is shown to be preventive of bowel disease. Among other things, it creates a wholesome micro-climate of bacteria in the bowel and reduces the food transit time, so less toxicity is produced.

Over the last fifty years the amount of fibre consumed in the average diet has decreased in proportion to the rise in fats and sugar. However, replacing it by the addition of bran is harsh on the digestion, and natural sources of fibre like wholemeal brown bread and vegetables are still best. The DRV is 30g.

What constitutes a healthy diet?

Studies of diet in primitive peoples in the world today show fewer degenerative diseases of all sorts. Significantly, these develop when these people move to civilization and take up a modern diet.

Aware of the growing connection of diet to disease, a National Advisory Committee on Nutritional Education (NACNE) report looked at all these factors. Its main recommendations were the following:

1 *Fat* intake should be reduced to one-third of total energy intake.

2 *Saturated fatty acids* should be only 10 per cent of total energy intake.

3 *Sugar as sucrose* should be reduced to half present levels, by eating fewer sweets and adding less sugar to food and beverages.

4 *Carbohydrate* intake should be increased by more than half, mainly by eating more unprocessed complex carbohydrates.

5 *Fibre* should be increased by nearly half to 30g daily, by eating more vegetables, pulses and wholegrains.

6 *Protein* intake should remain the same at 45g but should come less from animal and more from vegetable sources.

7 *Salt* should be reduced significantly to 5–9g daily.

8 *Alcohol* consumption should be reduced by one-third.

Note: Some dieticians say these recommendations are so far from our average normal diet that it is probably best to aim for these targets gradually over a period of a year.

Modern obstacles to a healthy diet

Although most people are assured that on an average diet they are getting an adequate intake of nutrients, malnutrition is not uncommon in the West. Where the diet consists of a lot of processed foods, relying on highly refined carbohydrate (white flour and sugar) and is poor in high-fibre carbohydrate like wholegrains, with few or no vegetables, there will be depletion of essential vitamins and minerals. Breakfast cereals, bread and margarine are fortified with vitamins by law for this reason. However, this is not enough to undo the deleterious effect of this type of diet in the long term.

Food grown on poor soil which has been depleted of natural minerals by chemically controlled farming techniques is arguably not the best source of nutrients. The use of herbicides, fungicides and pesticides has increased exponentially in the last three decades. Animals reared on synthetic foodstuffs and routinely doctored with growth hormones and other drugs are probably not in the best health either. We do not know what the long-term effects of agro-chemicals are, although the use of some pesticides is becoming increasingly suspect. Most of these are in the skins of fruit and vegetables and peeling removes 85 per cent. It is best to eat mainly organically produced vegetables and fruit, which are becoming increasingly available.

When food reaches the manufacturing and packaging stage, chemical additives are put in to preserve shelf life and enhance the appearance and taste of processed foods. Some of these so-called 'E' numbers are very suspect and are banned by law from children's foods. Processed foods also contain a high level of sugar and salt. In order to preserve them or keep them fresh in transit, foods are subject to canning, dehydrating, chilling, freezing and irradiation. Although most of these forms of preservation do no harm, they decrease the amount of vitamins available, and the process of irradiation to kill bacteria is too recent to know if it has harmful effects.

To contain its full natural complement of vitamins and minerals, food must be fresh, and eaten raw when possible.

Healthy wholefood diet

The following recommendations are recognized by the World Health Organization (WHO) as optimal for health.

1 Fruit and vegetables should make up about half of the daily diet in the form of five servings of fresh fruit and vegetables, as much of it as possible raw. For example, one piece of fruit, such as an apple or a small bowl of blackcurrants, raspberries etc. counts as a serving. Take fruit with breakfast cereals, in salads, fresh or lightly cooked for dessert. A small mixed salad or portion of cooked vegetable constitutes one serving. Almost all vegetables except potatoes can be eaten raw, so experiment: have a mixed salad with your main meal or as a starter, as well as lightly cooked vegetables, and include plenty of leafy green vegetables and oranges in your diet.

2 Protein and fat combined should make up less than one-quarter of the daily diet. Use polyunsaturated cooking oils such as sunflower, safflower and unhydrogenated vegetable margarine. Cut down on full-fat milk and hard cheese, cream, butter, fatty meat and eggs. Eat more fish and less red meat and make the meat organic where possible. Include vegetable sources of protein such as soya, pulses, nuts or seeds for at least three meals out of seven.

3 Slow-burning carbohydrate with natural fibre from porridge oats, rice and other grains and cereals, wholemeal bread, and organic potatoes should make up one-third of the daily diet.

Try to cut out cakes, pastries, biscuits, chocolate, etc. Where this is difficult follow the 'twice a week only' rule, so that the quantities eaten are not sufficient to cause a real problem.

4 Sufficient water is important – four to five glasses a day as well as other fluids. Avoid or cut down on fizzy canned drinks. Wean yourself off caffeinated drinks, or if you find this impossible, follow the 'twice a week only' rule.

5 Cut salt intake by half, to prevent heart disease, strokes and high blood pressure.

6 Keep alcohol to a minimum. Ideally have at least three days a week totally alcohol-free.

If you are one of those who feels that all the 'good' things are forbidden on this diet, allow yourself one day a week when you eat all the forbidden foods, and you will probably find after a while that they do not seem as appealing.

It may also make sense to take a small daily supplement of Vitamin C if you are not getting enough fruit, and Vitamin B complex if you are vegetarian. Mineral supplements, especially selenium and zinc which tend to be in short supply in some modern foods, are good health insurance. (See Nutritional supplements below for other vitamins and minerals.)

Preparing food

When cooking follow simple food conservation rules – grill rather than fry, use a vegetable steamer, or quickly stir-fry in a little vegetable oil, adding some water after a few minutes. Valuable minerals and vitamins are thrown away in cooking water and lost in frying. Use non-aluminium cooking utensils: stainless steel or glassware is best.

Changing diet

Bear in mind that it is necessary to take into account variations in dietary requirements according to metabolism and state of health. Some nutritionists believe in metabolic typing whereby according to a fast or slow digestion, people thrive variously on nearly all raw food to mostly cooked food. Experiment to see what feels right for you, otherwise see a nutritionist for professional advice.

Abrupt changes in diet should be avoided, and are best taken gradually. Remember that in sickness the body is less likely to cope with refined foods, additives, stimulants, etc. and also that a lot of raw food may be difficult to digest: try raw vegetable or fruit juices instead.

Dietary habits acquired in different cultures according to custom and climate may be difficult to change for all sorts of reasons, so go gently.

Nutritional supplements

Safety of vitamins

Vita means life. Vitamins are naturally occurring micro-constituents of food and are essential for life and well-being. They have a long benefit and safety record. If they are not present in food on a daily basis, deficiency states will occur after some time, with well-recognized symptoms.

There has been a growth market in self-medication with supplements in recent years, and with the accompanying increase in public and media interest, concerns have been voiced about what constitutes a 'safe dose'. As regards vitamins it follows that as they are found in a natural diet they must be beneficial rather than harmful if taken in equivalent doses as supplements. Vitamin supplements are widely used as preventive medicine, for example, Vitamin C for colds and flu. At normal levels adverse reactions are unknown, except in special cases: it is with much higher doses that the question arises. Unfortunately, there has not been enough research on some of the vitamins at high levels to prove their efficacy and safety, although dramatic therapeutic benefits have been shown in the last twenty years with some administration of higher doses, for example of Vitamin C in cancer.

Current legislation on vitamin supplements is being reviewed in the European Union with the aim of lowering the doses available of some vitamins over the counter, or even making them available on prescription only.

Recommended daily amounts

In the UK, the USA and Canada and some other countries a recommended standard of daily allowances (RDAs) for most vitamins and minerals has been in existence for some time. RDAs were set in order to minimize under-nutrition and are not necessarily the same across the board.

In 1991 new standards were suggested by the Committee on Food Energy and Nutrients in the UK, based on Dietary Reference Values (DRVs). They looked at both the high and the low limits and attempted to examine the relative risks and benefits of high levels of intake.

DRV is a general term used to cover up to four values for each vitamin and mineral. These are: 1) *Estimated average requirement (EAR)* – some people need more than this and some less. 2) *Reference Nutrient Intake (RNI)*, which in fact is higher than most people need but can be applied to all cases. 3) *Lower Reference Nutrient Intake (LRNI)*, only enough for those with lower needs. 4) *Safe Intake*, used for nutrients where there is not enough information to estimate requirements, adequate but not so large as to cause undesirable effects.

DRVs are intended to be applied to healthy people, so do not make any allowance for ill health. They are meant to be used as a point of reference rather than as fixed definitive values.

RDAs and DRVs provide a considerable margin of safety for most vitamins, and most people do not exceed the DRV for an extended period of time. Higher doses obtainable over the counter vary between ten and 100 times DRV. The water-soluble vitamins are particularly safe, except Vitamin B_6, because excesses are excreted. With the exception of adverse reactions, after long-term use of Vitamins A, D and E, there have been no reported side-effects at 100 times DRV. However, it is wise to keep doses within the 100-times limit pending more research. The risk of adverse reactions rises when excessively high doses are taken without professional advice.

Note: For the purpose of this guide, the DRVs given for vitamins and minerals are those of the RNI as this provides the needs of 90 per cent of the population.

Some vitamins are unstable and easily lost through storage, exposure to light, and cooking. Processed foods that have gone through all these stages may have lost most of their Vitamin B and C content. Tobacco and alcohol destroy vitamin absorption.

The myth of the well-balanced diet

The theory that the average mixed diet contains all the nutrients needed for health may hold true in some cases, but certainly not all, and not all the time. Absorption is affected by many factors, including efficiency of digestion and absorption, life-style, age, economics and general health.

Every human being is a unique physical and biochemical individual; in fact it has been shown that our stomachs are as individual as our fingerprints. Thus it is not surprising that at certain stages in their lives women may need supplements of vitamins and minerals, in particular women of childbearing age; women who are pregnant or nursing; adolescents; menopausal women; housebound, convalescent and elderly women; those who are athletic, under stress, or on prescribed drugs; women with poor absorption following pancreatic diseases, coeliac disease, gall-bladder and stomach removal; women who diet, snack, or eat overcooked or mostly processed food; women with poor digestion, poor appetite or dental problems.

Orthomolecular nutrition

This form of therapy treats disease with elements endogenous to the human body, using vitamins and minerals instead of drugs. Following this principle, higher than average doses for a short time may be suggested elsewhere in this guide for various problems where they have proved to be useful in practice. In general most doctors recognize that if a medical condition clears up with a supplement there was a need for it, but not many would consider using supplements as a therapy, although there is growing evidence that they work.

Use of vitamins

Vitamins are available in a number of forms – as capsules, tablets, oils, liquids and water-soluble powder. They are available on prescription, over the counter, or by mail order. Some are chemically synthesized, some are from naturally occurring sources, such as Vitamin D from fish oils, beta-carotene from carrots, Vitamin C from acerola cherries, etc. There are also food-state vitamins, which contain amino acids from protein and may consequently be more easily absorbed. Their content is nearer to the RDA and DRV recommended levels. (They may not be suitable for those with a reaction to yeast.)

Reputable combined multi-vitamin and mineral tablets should present the body with the right proportions of vitamins and minerals it requires on a daily basis, but the amounts can be confusing. When a vitamin or mineral is tableted with another substance, it is often not clear how much is represented by the active constituent, so check carefully. Note that some minerals are 'chelated' with an amino acid to help absorption, and the amount of mineral should be stated.

Vitamins

Vitamin A

This is essential for maintaining the health of skin and other tissue, such as the lungs, stomach, urinary tract and breast tissue. It is important as one of the antioxidant vitamins, beta-carotene, as a scavenger of free radicals, and also as part of the body's immune system. Being fat-soluble, it is stored in the body, so effects of complete deficiency in the diet do not show for many months. It is destroyed by smoking.

Best sources
This is found as retinol in the following foods of animal origin: cod liver oil, liver, margarine, butter, cheese, milk, eggs. It is also found naturally as beta-carotene, a precursor of Vitamin A, in orange and yellow fruits and vegetables, particularly carrots. (Note: it is inadvisable to eat liver when pregnant as the average portion contains four to twelve times the DRV of Vitamin A during pregnancy.)

Deficiency symptoms
Night blindness, burning and dry eyes, scaly, dry skin and scalp, poor nails and tooth enamel, brittle hair, respiratory infections, poor growth. Vitamin A deficiency is quite common, but rarely severe in the West. Stores in the body vary considerably between individuals.

Benefits
Consider taking it if you have a skin condition, gastric ulcer, malabsorption state such as irritable bowel disease, heavy or painful periods, PMS or fibrocystic breast disease. Beta-carotene may be protective against cancer and is helpful in cases of impaired resistance to infection.

Guidance on high intake
Beta-carotene is not toxic, but intakes of retinol in excess of need over a long time may lead to liver and bone damage. Symptoms are fatigue, loss of appetite, nausea, headache, insomnia, skin changes, loss of body hair. Regular intakes should not exceed 7500mcg daily for women. Avoid Vitamin A as retinol during pregnancy because it may cause birth defects; this does not apply to beta-carotene.

DRVs (mcg Retinol)
(6mcg beta-carotene = 1mcg retinol)
Women aged 15–50   600
Pregnant women   700
Nursing mothers   950

Vitamin B complex

This contains all the B vitamins in the right proportions. All the members of Vitamin B complex are water-soluble and eliminated naturally from the body if not needed.

Vitamin B₁ (Thiamine)

A daily supply is needed for the release of energy from carbohydrates. It is essential for the normal working of the nervous system. Alcohol impairs absorption.

Best sources

Found in wholewheat flour, wheatgerm, dried brewer's yeast and yeast extract, brown rice. Lacking in white bread and polished rice.

Deficiency symptoms

Results in beriberi, rare in the West. Extreme weakness, lethargy, anorexia, digestive upsets, weight loss, irritability, depression, poor memory, and neuromuscular symptoms.

Benefits

Consider taking if you are elderly, diabetic, being treated for depression and anxiety, are on HRT, taking diuretics, have cancer, liver or stomach disease. As prevention against deficiency, if you drink alcohol every day, are under physical or mental stress or eat processed and junk food.

Guidance on high intake

Any excess is excreted. Long-term intakes of 3g per day (about 1000 times the RNI) may be undesirable. No overdosage symptoms known, however.

DRVs

Women 0.80mg daily.
Pregnant women 0.90mg daily.
Nursing mothers 1.0mg daily.

Vitamin B₂ (Riboflavin)

It has an essential role in the release of energy from proteins, fats and carbohydrates. Intake is correlated to activity, more is needed by active women than sedentary. Absorption is impaired by alcohol, smoking and hormonal drugs. It is easily destroyed by light and food processing.

Best sources

Dried brewer's yeast and yeast extract, liver, wheatgerm and bran, eggs, cheese, yoghurt, soya products.

Deficiency symptoms

Tired, sensitive or bloodshot eyes with gritty sensation, cracks at corner of mouth, sore tongue, hair loss, dry face, dizziness and insomnia.

Benefits

Those with mouth or eye ulcers and gastric ulcers. Consider taking it if you are pregnant or breast-feeding, are elderly, on HRT. As prevention against deficiency if you drink alcohol every day or smoke.

Guidance on high intakes

Toxicity unknown. Absorption is limited by poor solubility, so it is unlikely that enough will be absorbed to be dangerous. Intakes of 120mg daily for ten months have shown no adverse effects. The urine becomes yellow when taking Vitamin B₂ but this is not harmful.

DRVs

Women 1.1mg daily.
Pre-conception and pregnant 1.4mg daily.
Nursing mothers 1.6mg daily.

Vitamin B₃ (Niacin, Nicotinic acid or Nicotinamide)

It plays a major role in the process of energy release in the cells of the body. It can be manufactured by the body in the presence of sufficient protein.

Best sources

Meat, milk, fish and wholegrains.

Deficiency symptoms

Mental changes, irritability, headache, memory loss. Skin changes on hands and face, sore tongue and gastrointestinal changes. Rarely seen except if there is poor protein intake and alcohol abuse.

Benefits

Breast-feeding women need extra Vitamin B₃ to maintain normal levels. May be helpful in schizophrenia, but only under the guidance of a medical practitioner. Has been used successfully to lower blood cholesterol. Consider taking if you are elderly, live alone or have a poor protein intake.

Guidance on high doses

3–6g of Nicotinic acid may cause changes in liver function tests, but these reverse when it is stopped. In excess of 25mg daily flushing and tingling of the skin may occur; this wears off after a day or two of taking it.

DRVs

Adults 6.6mg–12.8mg daily.

Vitamin B₅ (Pantothenic acid)

It is involved in adrenal function and the production of fatty acids and steroids. Found in very many foods, particularly eggs and wholegrains, so lack is unusual. Helps production of adrenal hormones and a healthy nervous system.

Deficiency signs

Tiredness and emotional symptoms. Known as the stress vitamin, it may help symptoms associated with prolonged stress.

Benefits

Alcoholics. Consider if you are stressed mentally/emotionally. Pregnancy and breast-feeding increase need.

Guidance on high intake:

None. Intakes of 10g daily produced only mild and reversible gastrointestinal disturbance.

DRVs

None: Requirements probably 3–7mg daily. Safe intake: adults 50mg daily or more.

Vitamin B₆ (Pyridoxine)

It is central to the body's protein metabolism, production of essential biochemicals and absorption of minerals magnesium and zinc. The amount needed relates to how much protein is eaten. It is fragile and easily destroyed by cooking and light exposure. Smoking and certain drugs impair uptake.

Best sources

Dried brewer's yeast, wheat bran and wheatgerm, yeast extract, wholegrain cereals, bananas, nuts, seeds and avocados.

Deficiency symptoms

Cracked lips, sore tongue, dry scaling skin on face, migraine, breast swelling and discomfort, fluid retention. Mild depression and irritability.

Benefits

Pre-menstrual syndrome. Morning sickness in pregnancy. Anaemia (with iron and copper). Consider taking if you are on contraceptive steroids, HRT, are pregnant or breast-feeding, diabetic or suffering from depression and anxiety.

Guidance on high intakes

Intakes in excess of 25mg daily may help counter some of the undesirable effects of contraceptive steroids in women. High intakes over 50mg–2g daily in long-term use have been associated with impaired function of sensory nerves, reversible on return to normal intake. 5–10mg daily may be needed in pregnancy and breast-feeding (do not exceed).

DRVs

Adults ages nineteen to forty-nine, 1.2–1.4mg daily.

Vitamin B₁₂ (Cobalamine)

It is needed for the functioning of all cells; helps produce the nerve sheath, maintain health of nervous system and produce red blood cells.

Best sources

Liver, meat, fish, eggs, cheese, milk. Vegans may need supplement.

Deficiency symptoms

Sore, smooth tongue, mental symptoms. Menstrual problems. Vitamin B₁₂ deficiency causes anaemia with neurological problems, usually due to malabsorption. Pernicious anaemia is rare, and due to an inherited inability to utilize B₁₂; injections are given regularly to correct it.

Benefits

Mental confusion, poor memory, tiredness, heavy painful periods. Consider taking if you are planning a baby, pregnant, elderly, a heavy smoker, or suffer from intestinal problems. Those on restricted diets, such as vegans.

Guidance on high intake

Vitamin B₁₂ is not dangerous; 3mg injected daily is not associated with any harmful effects. Hydroxycobalamine is the preferred form.

DRVs

Adults 1.5mcg daily.
Nursing mothers 2.0mcg daily.

Folic acid (part of the Vitamin B group)

Necessary for production of red blood cells. Requirements increase in pregnancy.

Best sources

Main source is leafy dark green vegetables, also yeast, liver, eggs and wholegrains.

Deficiency symptoms

Sore, smooth tongue, pallor, lethargy, weakness

and insomnia. Deficiencies are common in the general population, and associated with B_{12} lack, but only severe lack shows as anaemia.

Benefits

Folic acid has been proven to prevent birth defects like spina bifida. Supplements of 400mcg daily are recommended by the Department of Health for all women pre-conceptually and up to the fourth week of pregnancy at least; where there has been a previous birth defect, 5mg daily pre-conceptually and up to the fourth week of pregnancy, reducing to 400mcg after that. It is a useful supplement throughout pregnancy and breast-feeding. (See also Pre-conceptual care, page 32.)

The elderly may benefit and those people who do not bother to eat green vegetables. It should be taken with Vitamin B_{12}.

Guidance on high intake

Danger of high intakes slight (over 15g daily for adverse effects). Symptoms are loss of appetite, abdominal bloating, nausea, sleep problems. May cause reduced zinc absorption. Large amounts may hide symptoms of Vitamin B_{12} deficiency.

DRVs

Women 200mcg daily.
Pregnant women 400mcg daily
Nursing mothers 460mcg daily.

Biotin (lesser-known member of Vitamin B group)

Intakes of 10–70mcg daily normal. Up to 200mcg safe. Produced in the body by intestinal bacteria. Recommended to supplement live yoghurt or probiotics in anti-candida treatment.

Vitamin C

Humans, unlike most animals, whose tissues are saturated with it, do not synthesize Vitamin C and cannot store it, so have a daily requirement. It is anti-oxidant, provides resistance to infection, and is needed for normal brain function. Helps iron and folic acid absorption. Easily destroyed by storage and food processing.

Best sources

Mostly in fruits and vegetables: highest in blackcurrants, rosehips, broccoli, green peppers, green leafy vegetables and citrus fruits.

Deficiency symptoms

Scurvy. Weakness, anorexia, reduced growth and healing, susceptibility to infection, muscle and joint pains, swollen and inflamed gums with loose teeth, haemorrhaging of small vessels. Scurvy is uncommon but milder symptoms of deficiency are not.

Benefits

Important research on Vitamin C as a therapeutic agent in disease suggests high intakes are beneficial in some conditions. Research on Vitamin C for cancer shows benefit at very high levels. Important in preventing and treating infection; anti-viral, 1–2g needed to prevent colds (take at first symptoms).

Consider taking if you are on contraceptive steroids, corticosteroids, barbiturates, antibiotics, have a viral infection, have had recent surgery, have a gastrointestinal ulcer or iron-deficiency anaemia. Benefits those who are under stress, heavy smokers or drinkers, and the elderly. Lowers blood cholesterol in some cases. Pregnant and breast-feeding women need extra Vitamin C.

Guidance on high intake

Intakes of 3g or more may be associated with diarrhoea and abdominal cramps; if so, cut back to a level where these do not occur. Long-term intakes of over twenty times the DRV are associated with developing calcium oxalate kidney stones, in susceptible people only. Avoid if there is a history of kidney stones. Generally this is regarded as a very safe vitamin.

DRVs

Adults 40mg daily.
Pregnant women 50mg daily.
Nursing mothers 70mg daily.

Vitamin D (Calciferol)

As it is fat-soluble, reserves are stored in the body. Needed for calcium absorption and important for growth and maintenance of bone. Known as the sunshine vitamin, it is manufactured in the body from the action of sunlight on the skin. In the UK if the skin is exposed for an hour daily from April to October, enough UV light is absorbed from the sun for the summer and to last throughout the winter.

Best sources

Sun, fish oils. A little in eggs, milk and cheese.

Deficiency symptoms
Malformation in bone development leading to poor growth (rickets) and softening of bones (osteomalacia). Muscular weakness and spasm.

Benefits
Osteomalacia, osteoporosis (brittle bones) in older women. Pregnant and lactating women need extra. Those who may benefit are elderly women who do not go out much and Asian women who cover their skin in the sun. Babies and children may need supplements.

Guidance on high doses
As Vitamin D accumulates in the body, toxicity can occur at doses above 50mcg daily. Symptoms are anorexia, then nausea and vomiting with constant thirst and profuse urination.

DRVs
None for ages fourteen to forty-nine.
Adults over age sixty-five 10mcg daily.
Pregnant and nursing mothers 10mcg daily.

Vitamin E (d-alpha tocopherol)
A fat-soluble, anti-oxidant vitamin, found in all cell walls of body and responsible for healthy skin and blood vessels. The daily amount needed depends on how much polyunsaturated fat is taken in the diet.

Best sources
Nuts and seeds, pulses, cod liver oil, cold-pressed vegetable and nut oils.

Deficiency symptoms
Tiredness, irritability, muscle weakness, lack of libido.

Benefits
Many: prevents thrombosis, atherosclerosis, thrombophlebitis. Benefits those with varicose veins, menstrual problems, nerve, joint and muscular problems. May help post-gastric surgery, those with cirrhosis of liver, coeliac disease, cystic breast disease. Applied locally to heal scar tissue, stretch marks, burns and skin ulcers.

Guidance on high intake
No specific guidance available. Few adverse effects have been reported from doses up to 300mg daily. Suggested safe intakes are set at 100mg daily for women. Recommended intake at least 30mg daily. It can interfere with iron absorption so should be

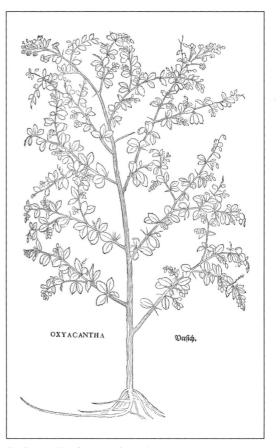

Barberry *(Berberis vulgaris)*

taken at separate meals. It should not be taken with anti-coagulant drugs without medical supervision. Diabetics should beware of hypoglycaemic attacks if taking high doses of Vitamin E.

Vitamin K
This is produced in the body from intestinal bacteria synthesis. It is involved in the process of blood-clotting of wounds. It is not taken as a supplement because of toxicity. To prevent haemorrhagic disease of the newborn it is routinely given by injection or orally at birth. Naturally occurring Vitamin K is free from harmful effects. Intake of 2mcg per kg is adequate.

Minerals

Use of minerals
Mineral means mined from the earth. These

elements are divided into metallic and non-metallic. Some minerals are also present in high quantities in the diet and in the tissues of the body: of these a constant replenishment in excess of 100mg each daily is needed. Others are found as trace minerals in the body and are needed in very small amounts in the diet.

Mineral content of foods reflects the soil in which they were grown. There are wide variables. Mineral absorption often requires certain vitamins to be available at the same time. It is also affected by competition among the minerals themselves; they often work in pairs. Any excess of one mineral over another will increase the chance of its absorption but limit its partner from being absorbed, which is how imbalances arise.

Minerals in food are lost during thawing from frozen, and during cooking they leach into water or fat and are lost to some extent in all refined and processed foods, losses of trace minerals being most significant.

Mineral supplements are often available chelated – combined with amino acids as carriers for better absorption and/or other complementary minerals and vitamins. Multi-minerals should be in the correct proportion if you buy from a reputable firm. They should ideally be taken with food.

DRVS are not given for the trace minerals cadmium, cobalt, fluorine, silica, strontium, germanium, molybedenum, boron and vanadium because of the tiny daily requirements. If you think you are likely to have a serious mineral imbalance, get a hair mineral analysis done and then see a nutritional specialist. Some mail-order supplement firms provide a nutritional questionnaire analysis.

Note: Where different DRVs of minerals for men and women are available, the women's figure is given here.

Calcium

Essential for blood-clotting and normal function of nerves and muscles. Abundantly found in bones and teeth. Co-factors Vitamins D, B_6, B_{12}, folic acid, magnesium and silica for efficient absorption. Absorption affected by oestrogen and parathyroid hormones. Dietary fibre inhibits uptake. Growing children, adolescents and older women have increased needs. Only 20–30 per cent of dietary calcium is absorbed.

Best sources

Hard cheeses, sardines and other small-boned fish, molasses, nuts, pulses, tofu, goat's and cow's milk, some herbs, and hard water. Nutritionists recognize that cow's milk is not the best source of calcium as it lacks the magnesium needed for its absorption and may lead to magnesium deficiency.

Deficiency symptoms

Rickets (children), osteomalacia, osteoporosis, poor sleep, muscle spasm, muscle weakness.

Benefits

It is better to have a diet rich in calcium rather than to take supplements. Ensure all the necessary co-factors are available as well. Should be taken in the ratio of two parts calcium to one of magnesium. There is no evidence to show that increasing dietary calcium decreases bone loss. (see Osteoporosis, page 93).

Guidance on high intake

Increased intakes lead to progressively reduced rates of absorption. High calcium and Vitamin D levels can lead to deposits in soft tissues such as the heart and arteries.

DRVs

Adolescents 800mg daily.
Women over age nineteen 700mg daily.
Nursing mothers 1250mg daily.
Best supplements: calcium citrate or amino acid-chelated calcium.

Magnesium

Necessary for the metabolism of protein and carbohydrate, for energy production. Co-factor for calcium, and Vitamins B_1 and B_6. Now thought to be just as important as calcium in maintaining healthy bones into old age.

Best sources

Soya beans, brewer's yeast, wholegrains, nuts, seeds, seafood, legumes, dried fruit, green leafy vegetables.

Deficiency symptoms

Mental problems, weakness, muscle cramps and tremor, irregular heart beat, menstrual problems.

Benefits

PMS, menstrual pain, low blood sugar. May help those with angina and atherosclerosis.
For mental problems take professional advice.

Guidance on high intake
Symptoms of excess are rare. Larger amounts pass through intestine unabsorbed.

DRVs
Adolescents 280–300mg daily.
Women 270mg daily.
Nursing mothers 320mg daily.
Best supplements: magnesium orotate or amino acid-chelated magnesium.

Phosphorus
Found mainly in bones, necessary for function of all cells, particularly nervous system. Deficiency rare, may result in muscle weakness and anaemia. Co-factor for calcium and magnesium.

Best sources
Foods with calcium and those rich in protein.

Guidance on high intake
Large doses may lead to increased need for calcium and magnesium. Excessive phosphorus in diet due to processed foods impairs uptake of calcium.

DRVs
Equivalent to calcium.

Potassium
Found in the fluid inside cells. With co-factor sodium it enables substances to move into and out of cells, and heart, muscles and nerves to function normally.

Best sources
Dried fruits, soya flour, molasses, wheat bran, raw vegetables, muesli breakfast cereal, fish and meat.

Deficiency symptoms
Muscle cramps, tiredness, headache, drowsiness, palpitations. Acute deficiency rare and may be caused by drugs like diuretics, steroids and overuse of laxatives, or following surgical operations on the intestine.

Benefits
An adequate intake is needed to balance sodium levels and remove excess salt from the body. In the Western diet there is too much sodium in relation to potassium. May help reduce high blood pressure. Supplements usually only needed in case of excess loss as above, in the form of potassium chloride. (It can be taken instead of salt, as Lo-salt or Ruthmol, when a low-salt diet is required.)

Guidance on high intake
Excesses are rare. Most of the daily intake is excreted in urine, but more than 18g daily is not recommended.

DRVs
Adults 3100–3500mg daily.

Sodium
Vital in the fluid balance of the body and in all nerve and muscle cell functioning. However, most people take a good deal more dietary salt than is needed for these functions.

Best sources
Salt, meat, bread, butter, cheese. Added to most processed foods.

Guidance on high intake
Excess may be detrimental to health although it is excreted very efficiently. Lowering intake may reduce prevalence of high blood pressure and heart disease in certain population groups. More than 2–3g daily may lead to high blood pressure in some individuals.

DRVs
Adults 1600mg daily.

Iron
An essential part of red blood cells, iron is recycled in the body. Infants, children, pubescent and child-bearing women all have increased needs. Absorption is about 15 per cent for the average mixed diet but less for those who do not eat foods of animal origin. Menstrual blood-loss adds to women's needs which are very variable. Co-factor molybdenum. Needs Vitamin C for absorption.

Deficiency symptoms
Iron-deficiency anaemia: tiredness, lack of energy, breathlessness, pallor, insomnia. Very common. Responds quickly to supplementation.

Best sources
Offal, particularly liver, sausage, fish, eggs, pulses, grains, wholemeal bread, molasses, nuts, seeds, green leafy vegetables and root herbs. Tannin in tea inhibits uptake: avoid drinking it with meals.

Benefits

Women of child-bearing age, especially those with heavy menstrual bleeding. 10 per cent of women have less than 12g/100cc blood and are sub-clinically anaemic. Vegetarians.

Guidance on high intake

Mostly rejected in faeces but constipation may develop. Too much iron inhibits zinc. A condition called siderosis, usually from too much cheap red wine, can occur – iron is found deposited in organs such as the lungs and heart. High intakes of iron are dangerous for a rare group with pathologically high rates of absorption. For a normal adult a single dose of 100g can be lethal.

DRVs

Adolescents 14.8mg daily.

Women aged nineteen to forty-nine 14.8mg daily. Pregnant and lactating women and those with heavy menstrual losses may need supplements if iron stores are low.

Best supplements: iron citrate or amino acid-chelated iron.

Zinc

Essential for the function of several enzymes. Important in many metabolic processes and for absorption of some vitamins and carbohydrate; builds healthy skin, hair and nails and a healthy reproductive system. Co-factor for calcium and phosphorus, accompanies them when they are lost. Absorption is approximately 30 per cent. A large intake of dietary fibre inhibits uptake.

Best sources

Oyster, fresh ginger, muscle meats, wholegrains, nuts and seeds, green vegetables, milk and eggs.

Deficiency symptoms

Skin disorders, alopecia (hair loss), loss of taste or smell, loss of appetite, anorexia, white spots on nails, infertility.

Benefits

All the above symptoms reversed. For vegetarians and others on restricted diets. May help eczema, some forms of dermatitis and allergies. Post-infection. Used in treatment of aluminium and cadmium toxicity. Consider taking with other appropriate minerals if having problems conceiving (see Pre-conceptual care, page 32).

Guidance on high intake

Nausea and vomiting produced by 2g of zinc. Antagonists are iron, copper and manganese: too much zinc interferes with the metabolism of these, but a high level of copper in blood inhibits zinc absorption. Long-term high intake in excess of 50mg daily may lead to copper-deficiency anaemia.

DRVs

Women over age fifteen 7mg daily.

Lactating women 6mg daily, up to four months, 2.5mg daily thereafter.

Additional amounts needed in pregnancy if stores low.

Best supplements: Zinc citrate, gluconate or amino acid-chelate.

Manganese

Important in normal growth and for enzymes controlling metabolism of fat and carbohydrate. Co-factor for Vitamins B, C and E and normal functioning of hormones and nerves. Antagonists are iron, copper, calcium and phosphorus, high levels of which inhibit its absorption.

Deficiency symptoms

Disc and cartilage problems, muscular problems, glucose intolerance. Associated with low fertility, birth defects. Low levels present in diabetes, heart disease, schizophrenia.

Best sources

Nuts and seeds, buckwheat, green leafy vegetables, black China tea, wholegrains. Deficiency quite common as poor levels in soil mean vegetables are low in manganese.

Benefits

Low blood sugar, with other factors; anaemia, infertility. (For schizophrenia, take professional advice.)

Guidance on high intake

Excesses rare but cause involuntary movement, rigidity of muscles.

DRVs

Adults 1.4mg daily.

Best supplements: manganese gluconate or amino-acid chelate.

Selenium

Important for normal functioning of heart, liver,

and immune system. Healthy bone, skin, nails and hair. Co-factor Vitamin E.

Best sources
Offal, sesame seeds, garlic, eggs, fish, vegetables.

Deficiency symptoms
Usually caused by low selenium soils. Arthritis and cancer may indicate deficiency.

Benefits
As anti-inflammatory for menstrual problems and arthritis. Works together with Vitamin E as anti-oxidant. Improves resistance to disease with zinc and Vitamin C. Role in cancer prevention. Relief of angina. Used in treatment of cadmium, arsenic and mercury toxicity. Consider taking if you are on contraceptive steroids or if you smoke.

Guidance on high intake
Hair loss, skin discoloration, brittle nails, fatigue, loss of appetite. Intake should not exceed 200mg daily.

DRVs
Adolescents 45mcg daily.
Women 60mcg daily.
Nursing mothers 75mcg daily.
Best supplement: as seleno L–methionine.

Copper
Essential for working of many enzymes and for normal blood cells and bone formation.

Best sources
Liver, shellfish, brewer's yeast, nuts, pulses, wholegrains. Most of that absorbed comes from copper water pipes or cooking containers rather than diet. Excess fibre inhibits uptake.

Deficiency symptoms
Copper-deficiency anaemia (rare), brittle bones, poor hair condition, irritability, low fertility.

Benefits
Those with malabsorption problems, on highly refined diets, or with chronic diarrhoea. May help rheumatoid arthritis. Copper bangles are a popular folk remedy for decreasing joint pain; this suggests it may be absorbed by the skin.

Guidance on high intake
Toxicity is rare. Poisoning with large doses gives rise to vomiting, pain, diarrhoea and coma.

DRVs
Adolescents 0.8–1.0mg daily.
Women 1.2 mg daily.
Nursing mothers 1.5mg daily.
Additional amounts needed in pregnancy if stores low.

Chromium
Essential for blood sugar and insulin regulation (forms glucose tolerance factor) – GTF. Increased levels of blood chromium are associated with decreased levels of diabetes and heart disease.

Best sources
Brewer's yeast, molasses, honey, wholemeal bread, nuts, shellfish, grapes. Poorly absorbed from diet, particularly refined foods.

Deficiency symptoms
Similar to those of low blood sugar (HYPOGLY-CAEMIA). Clouding of cornea of the eye. Low fertility.

Benefits
Some cases of hypoglycaemia (with other factors), some cases of juvenile and adult diabetes. Reducing blood cholesterol levels.

Guidance on high intake
No toxicity reported. GTF chromium is more effective and more easily absorbed than other forms, including food.

DRVs
Adults 25mcg +daily.
Best supplements: GTF chromium or chromium polynicotinate.

Iodine
Essential trace element for production of thyroid hormones which help control metabolism.

Best sources
Seaweed, particularly Bladderwrack (Kelp) as tablets, seafood, oily fish, iodized salt, meat, dairy products.

Deficiency symptoms
Iodine deficiency common in some areas of the world. Enlargement of thyroid gland in throat (thyroid deficiency goitre); slow metabolism. Probably too much iodine in the Western diet.

Benefits

Eliminates symptoms above. Bladderwrack seaweed used by herbalists to treat obesity.

Guidance on high intakes

Excessively high intake can cause hyperthyroidism. Intakes should be no more than 1000mcg daily.

DRVs

Adults 140mcg daily.

Therapeutic diets

A number of diseases are undoubtedly linked to nutritional patterns: obesity, dental decay, some cancers, particularly gastrointestinal, other digestive diseases, some respiratory diseases, circulatory problems due to atherosclerosis, allergies, alcoholism, diabetes, eczema and hyperactivity in children. There may be more. Among the common symptoms linked to foods are PMS (see page 16), HYPOGLYCAEMIA and migraine. The diets in this section are recommended because the author has seen how they have helped improve or eliminate symptoms in many cases.

Treatment of food allergy

True food allergies as they are currently understood are probably rare, that is, those that cause the body to produce an antibody response to the antigen (allergen), but food sensitivities or intolerances are much more common. Indeed there are so many that it is impossible to list them all here. Instead, a few of the main culprits are outlined, with suggested diets for avoiding them.

You may already suspect certain foods. Discovering those to which you are sensitive can be done by exclusion of and challenge with suspect foods, by a blood test or cytotoxic testing (see ALLERGY). When you avoid a food to which you are sensitive, you may feel worse for a week or so initially. This is due to removal of dependency and withdrawal symptoms sometimes occur. You may crave that particular food. If you challenge the body with the same food a month later and you are sensitive, you will probably experience the return of the same symptoms. Six months or more off a food may mean you reduce the reaction sufficiently to eat that food again, although some people have to avoid it permanently.

Desensitization to foods is possible by Enzyme Potentiated Desensitization (EPD) or by homoeopathic desensitization. This should only be a last resort however, and carried out under the guidance of an expert. Avoidance of foods is always a better way unless nutrition is compromised or the individual very severely affected. (See also ALLERGY for further information.)

Elimination

This is one way to identify food intolerances yourself. Try keeping an actual record of everything you eat, the time you eat and the time any symptoms appear, for two weeks. After this you can do a simple elimination diet for two to four weeks, avoiding foods you suspect from the diary, but only one at a time, until symptoms clear. You may need to do a more extensive elimination programme if symptoms do not clear on the diet. The classic elimination diet is based initially on water and only one or two foods known to be non-allergenic in most cases, adding one more at a time over a period of several weeks and carefully monitoring the effects; those foods that produce a reaction are eliminated from the diet. It is best to do this under the guidance of an experienced nutritionist or dietician. Remember, if you eliminate an item such as cow's milk, you need to avoid all the foods which may contain it as an ingredient, such as cakes, biscuits, etc. and probably all bovine products as well. If you react to one food, you may well react to others in the same family (see Food families below).

A drawback to elimination dieting is that the results are not always clear, although most major sensitivities should be spotted. In some cases it can take up to twenty-four hours for symptoms to show. Be aware of the phenomenon of 'masked food allergy' which means that because of adaptation, the body may feel better after a while on the very foods that make it ill; when you stop them you may have 'withdrawal' symptoms. If you get cravings for a certain item of food, then that item will usually be the problem.

Food challenge

If you reintroduce suspect foods, do so one at a time and only in a very small amount, for example ½–1 teaspoon initially, and watch reaction carefully. Intake can be gradually increased to the usual amount over a few days. If foods are known to cause severe reactions such as wheezing or asthma, do not reintroduce, and take medical advice.

Elimination and challenge diets are done in hospital under supervision if someone appears to react badly to a wide range of foods. Rest as much as possible when following these diets. If you have a strong reaction it is advisable to seek the advice of your medical practitioner. *Caution:* do not attempt these diets without the advice of a medical practitioner if you are suffering from a serious illness or are taking prescribed drugs.

Pulse test

The pulse test is sometimes used to see if reintroduction of a food increases your pulse rate. First, take your normal resting rate at the radial pulse on the inner wrist by counting the number of beats in a minute, which is usually around seventy beats. You need to be relaxed to do this. Try taking your pulse several times over an hour to check that it does not fluctuate much. If it is quite stable, take it ten, twenty, forty and sixty minutes after ingesting a new food. A significant increase in pulse rate, especially if maintained, is generally taken to be a general indicator of sensitivity.

Rotation diet

This is based on rotating different foods by taking just one food each from a selection of four to five different food each families every day throughout the week and not repeating it for at least five days. The diet is based on the principle that if you react to one food from a family, you may react to another from the same family to a greater or lesser extent: for example, milk and beef. Each food is only taken once in a week, to avoid the possibility of food sensitivities building up. It is healthy to rotate foods, whatever your diet; 'everything in moderation' is a good dietary rule.

To illustrate: on Monday choose from the fish family, either cod, whiting or plaice, and from the nightshade family, either tomato, red pepper, aubergine or potato. You then repeat with a different member of the same food family the following Monday. It makes it simpler to keep the same food families to the same days of the week. Rotation has the advantage of being less restrictive and can be carried on for longer than a classic elimination diet; six to eight weeks is ideal. Eliminate the suspect foods you discover for at least a month.

Below are examples of common food families. This is not a comprehensive list, but covers a lot of the foods we normally eat. You may want to add more to this list, or leave out any food if you never eat it. Once you are sure any food is safe carry on with it in your diet.

Food families

Carbohydrate: Grass family: Rice, millet, buckwheat, oats, wheat, wholemeal bread, pasta, brown sugar.

Vegetable: Lily family: onion, leek, garlic. *Parsley family*: carrot, celery, parsnip. *Mustard family:* turnip, broccoli, cauliflower, cabbage, Brussel sprouts. *Nightshade family:* potato, tomato, aubergine, green pepper. *Gourd family:* cucumber, courgette, squash. *Sunflower family:* lettuce, endive, chicory, sunflower seeds and oil.

Protein: Legume family: peanuts, peas, lentils, beans of all varieties including soya, soya protein and tofu. *Fish family:* cod, salmon and other true sea- or freshwater fish. *Crustacean family:* prawns, shrimps. *Bird family:* turkey, chicken, duck and eggs. *Bovine family:* Beef, cow's milk, cheese, butter, yoghurt. *Lamb family:* meat and liver. *Pig family:* pork, ham, bacon. *Goat family:* milk, yoghurt, cheese.

Fruit: Apple family: apple, pear. *Plum family:* plums, cherries, apricots, peaches. *Citrus family:* orange, grapefruit, lemon, tangerine. *Rose or berry family:* strawberry, raspberry, blackberry.

Drinks (see families above): apple juice, blackcurrant juice, orange juice, cow's or goat's milk, soya milk, black China tea, coffee, herb tea.

Miscellaneous: olive oil, wine vinegar, cider vinegar, mayonnaise, honey, margarine, pepper.

Suggested reading: R. Mackarness, *Not All in the Mind.*

Stone Age diet

Another way of dealing with food allergies, without going through the process of eliminating, is by returning to the diet of our forebears. You could try this for a month or two to see if it sorts out your symptoms before trying specific elimination diets. It avoids all modern pre-made, pre-packed foods and products of modern animal farming. It can be vegetarian or meat-eating. (For further information see Leon Chaitow, *Stone Age Diet.*)

Foods allowed

Meat, poultry and fish: from organically raised cows, pigs, sheep. Game birds from the wild. Free-range chicken not fed commercial poultry food. Sea fish (12–20 per cent of diet).

Dairy: a little sheep's or goat's yoghurt and cheese or raw, unpasteurized sour milk.

Eggs: Free-range only. No more than four a week. (Not if there is an allergy to eggs.)

Vegetables, fruit, beans and nuts: all sorts, but organic (50–60 per cent of diet).

Cereals: very small amount of rice, rye grain and oats.

Drinks: herbal teas, spring water, freshly squeezed fruit juice.

Foods to avoid

Dairy: cow's milk and butter, cheese, cream, yoghurt.

Cereals: wheat and all wheatflour products.

Drinks: No tea and coffee, including decaffeinated. Alcohol limited to 1–2 glasses white wine or beer. No spirits.

Sugar: none, neither white nor brown.

Salt: none, no processed foods or ready-made meals of any sort.

Biogenic diet

Biogenic means life-generating, and the diet is based on pure, organically grown foods. It is founded on principles laid down by Szekely, a nutritionist in the 1920s who claimed it originated with the Essenes in New Testament times and founded a colony that cured many chronic degenerative conditions. It has recently been revived and become popular with women as part of a weight loss programme. (See Chapter 6.)

Foods are classified as biocidic (life-destroying), biostatic (life-sustaining) and bioactive or biogenic (life-generating) in their effect on the body.

1 *Biogenic foods* (seeds, nuts, pulses, raw eggs), up to 40 per cent of diet.

2 *Bioactive foods* (raw fruits, vegetables and herbs, fruit), up to 50 per cent of diet.

3 *Biostatic foods* (wholegrain cereal, low fat dairy, free-range, game, etc.), up to 25 per cent of diet.

4 *Biocidic foods* (refined and processed) few or none.

Biogenic foods like sprouted seeds (alfalfa, etc.) may contain the necessary enzymes to help re-balance body biochemistry and bring about self-healing.

Further, the biogenic diet recommends avoiding food preparations such as drying and baking which remove water content. Seventy per cent of the water in the diet should come from uncooked foods, especially from fruit, and not from drinking fluids.

Anti-candida diet (Yeast-free diet)

The symbiotic yeast Candida albicans is normally present in the intestinal tract; it is only when it proliferates and becomes invasive that it can cause CANDIDIASIS and be responsible for a wide-ranging group of symptoms. A nutritional approach can return the mycelial or invasive fungus to the harmless form, and following a yeast-free diet can control it. A candida problem is usually associated with food intolerances. It is connected with Chronic fatigue syndrome (see page 108) in 50 per cent of cases. Herbal and vitamin therapy should be used in conjunction with the diet, for maximum benefit.

Advice on following the diet

Candida thrives on yeast-containing foods, sugar and glutinous grains, and is able to ferment and release alcohol from sugars. At the beginning all these foods need to be avoided, but as symptoms improve over time you can reintroduce some of them gradually. There should be at least a month between each stage of the diet. It is important to substitute permitted foods for forbidden foods. A common mistake is to stay on stage one of the diet for too long, as depletion of vitamins and minerals and weight loss can occur. A safeguard is to take a daily hypoallergenic multi-vitamin and mineral supplement.

Yeast and yeast spores are widespread in the environment. Limiting them in the diet minimizes them but does not eliminate the problem. Try to minimize by refrigerating food as much as possible.

Foods to avoid

1 Yeast and yeast-containing foods: avoid brewer's yeast, commercial leavened bread, and bakery products. Yeast extracts: marmite, vegetable stock, Bisto, Bovril. Soya milk. Vitamin supplemented foods. Packet and tinned soups, snack foods (potato crisps, dry roasted nuts).

All alcoholic drinks: avoid beer, wine, cider, home brews, spirits.

Fungi: avoid all types of mushroom and foods containing mushrooms, such as vegetable stock cubes and foods containing dried mixed vegetables.

Fermented foods (which contain moulds): avoid all cheeses, including cottage cheese, and sour cream.

Yeast is widely used in food preparation and flavouring, so read labels carefully. It is also the basis for many vitamin and mineral preparations, including the B vitamins and selenium. (Hypoallergenic Vitamin B preparations are yeast-free.)

2 Sugar: avoid white, brown, cane, molasses,

maple syrup, honey, glucose syrup, saccharine sweeteners. All sweets and chocolate. Sugar is added to many commercial foods such as soups and baked beans.

3 Mould-containing foods (pickled, dried, smoked, or cured): avoid vinegar, pickled onions, relishes, sauerkraut, salad dressings, soya sauce. Bacon of all sorts, cured ham, pastrami, salami, sausages, kippers, smoked and rollmop herrings. Smoked chicken and turkey. Hot dogs. Nuts, including peanuts. Dried fruits: prunes, raisins, figs, dates, apricots, etc.

4 Gluten-containing foods: avoid wheat, rye, oats, barley. Some people have to avoid potatoes, rice and corn as well, in the initial stage. Starch is added to many foods as thickening. Avoid breaded and battered foods.

5 Milk (pasteurized) and milk products need to be limited or avoided. Moulds and bacteria breed in it readily. Live natural yoghurt is an exception as it contains beneficial bacteria.

6 Vegetables: avoid cabbage family and tomatoes. Peel skins of fleshy vegetables and fruits as moulds accumulate on skin. Avoid all dried beans, kidney, aduki, blackeye, butter, mung, lentils, etc.

7 Avoid berry fruits, citrus fruits, bananas and grapes. Some sources cut out all fruit, however if you limit it to four to five pieces a week, this is effective in most cases. Avoid canned and frozen fruits and juices.

8 Herbs and herbal teas: if old these breed moulds, use date-stamped or fresh only.

9 Miscellaneous: avoid safflower and sunflower oils, nut oils, margarines. Also avoid citric acid, which is added to foods as preservative.

10 Antibiotics: avoid commercially farmed beef and pork which contain antibiotic residues. Also avoid penicillin and other antiobiotic drugs.

Suggested diet stage 1
(None of the above.)
Poultry, plainly cooked. Eggs. Seafood, fish. Lamb, rabbit. Natural live yoghurt, small amount. Butter, small amount. Brown rice, wild rice, millet, buckwheat. Yeast-free rye crispbread, rice cakes. Corn pasta or buckwheat pasta. Most vegetables, plenty of garlic. Small amounts of apples, pears, peaches, apricots. Olive oil. Herbal teas, spring water, coffee substitutes.
Supplements: Vitamin C, Vitamin B complex, zinc, biotin, garlic capsules, lactobacillus acidophilus as powder or capsules.

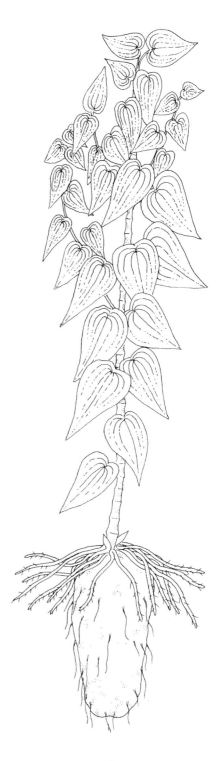

Wild Yam (*Dioscorea villosa*)

Suggested diet stage 2

Reintroduce these foods but not in excess or candida regrowth could occur: Beans, soya, blackeye,
aduki, chick peas, lentils. Citrus fruits. Oats, oat
bran, oatcakes. Goat's milk and cheese. Gouda and
Edam cheese. Nuts. Sunflower, pumpkin, sesame
seeds. Soya products including tofu.

Suggested diet stage 3

Reintroduce these foods in moderation: Wheat,
wheatgerm and bran. Unleavened Greek bread,
soda bread. Cornmeal (maize), corn oil. Berry
fruits, dried fruits. Cow's milk and Cheddar
cheese. Occasional organically farmed red meat.
Soya sauce. Safflower and sunflower oils, margarine. Decaffeinated coffee and weak black tea.
Freshly squeezed fruit juice.

Note: You have now built up a diet that is varied
without yeast or sugar-containing foods; if a food
is not on this diet, don't eat it.

As you reintroduce foods in the second and third
stages of the diet, you may find some to which you
have an intolerance. Avoid them for four to five
days and then challenge with the suspect food: if
the reaction returns you are hypersensitive to that
food, so avoid it. Try to rotate foods so that you
don't build up a sensitivity to them and eat everything in moderation.

   When the symptoms have cleared up, you will
still have to be careful of what you eat, but over
time you will be able to introduce more variety
into your diet. If you do stray back on to sugary
and yeasty foods you may find yourself as badly
off as before, but you will know how to deal with
it next time.

Recommended reading: Dr R. Trowbridge, *The Yeast
Syndrome*.

Milk-free diet

Conditions that may benefit from the diet are
eczema and other SKIN PROBLEMS, respiratory
conditions, such as ASTHMA and bronchitis and
catarrhal problems, chronic tonsillitis, sinusitis, ear
infections, and digestive problems characterized
by excessive production of gas causing discomfort.

   Although dairy products are considered staple
food in the Western world, two-thirds of the
world's population do not eat them, and in fact do
not have the lactase enzyme needed to digest
them. Children after weaning are prone to lose this
enzyme with resultant milk sensitivity. If you

remember that cow's milk is designed for calves
in the same way that mother's milk is designed
for human babies, and the two differ considerably,
it is not difficult to see why problems arise.
Some 'atopic' children who develop eczema in
infancy and asthma later on are allergic to the milk
protein but may be able to tolerate goat's or
sheep's milk which has a different type of milk
protein.

   The two dangers of a milk-free diet are protein
deficiency (only in vegetarians who use dairy
products as their main source) and calcium
deficiency. Vegetarians need to make sure they are
getting enough protein from eggs, nuts, seeds,
beans and soya products. Many other foods are
high in calcium, and it is in many cases better
absorbed, so not so much is needed. Remember
that the more calcium one takes in the form of milk
the less is absorbed, and that it is not a prime
source because the relatively high protein in it
binds the calcium, making it less available.

   If you discover that you are sensitive to milk
products, try eliminating them from your diet for
at least a month. After this, you could try goat's
milk and if you still react, substitute soya milk.
Remember that you may be sensitive to other
foods in the same family, for example beef.

Foods to avoid

Cow's milk, fresh or dried, including skimmed or
low-fat milk, butter, cheese, cream, yoghurt. All
foods containing casein and caseinates, whey, lactose, lactic acid and milk sugar. Read food labels!

   Bakery products, margarines, beverages containing milk, milk chocolate, sweets, some medicines and all kinds of processed foods.

Suggested calcium-rich menu

Breakfast: Fresh or stewed dried fruits. Muesli with
either fruit juice or soya milk. Wholemeal bread
with vegetable margarine. Egg or baked beans.
Porridge with soya milk and molasses. Herbal
tea, China tea or Luaka Ceylon tea.

Lunch: Mixed salads including watercress and
parsley. Tuna fish, sardines, tinned salmon,
beans, nuts, peanut butter, prawns, egg.
Sandwich with above and vegetable margarine.
Baked potato with above. Piece of fruit. Fruit
juice or herbal tea, Luaka Ceylon tea.

Evening meal: Vegetarian savoury from soya protein or tofu, kidney beans, lentils or nuts. Fish,
prawns, liver. Mixed salad with sunflower and
sesame seeds. Brown rice, buckwheat, whole-

wheat pasta. Desserts made from dried apricots, figs and dates. Dandelion coffee or herbal tea. China tea.

In cooking use: Herbal salt, Tamari soya sauce, nutritional yeast, Vecon or other yeast-based vegetable stock.

Supplements: Kelp tablets, brewer's yeast tablets.

Gluten-free diet (wheat-free)

Gluten is a sticky protein found in grains, mainly wheat, also rye. Many people have an intolerance to gluten. Oats, maize and rice contain little gluten and may be tolerated better. Those who are most affected are sufferers from sprue or gluten enteropathy, who must avoid it altogether. Other conditions that may benefit from avoidance are digestive problems, ARTHRITIS, PMS (see page 16), fatigue (see page 107) and CFS (see page 108). There are a host of symptoms associated with wheat intolerance. If you find you are sensitive, try excluding foods containing wheat for a month. Read all labels carefully as wheat is a hidden ingredient in many foods. Take Vitamin B complex to make up for any nutrient loss.

Recommended reading: Rita Greer, *Wheat, Milk and Egg Free Cooking* and Robin and Sheila Gibson, *The Complete Wheat Free Cookbook*.

Arthritis diet (alkaline diet)

Conditions that may benefit from the diet are osteoarthritis, rheumatoid arthritis, fibrositis, rheumatism and lumbago, polymyalgia rheumatica, gout and some other problems affecting the joints and muscles.

In degenerative and inflammatory conditions a well-balanced diet which maximizes vitamin and mineral content is essential. Avoiding certain foods that are acid-forming in the body and junk foods with high phosphate content can alleviate pain and stiffness. Improving elimination of waste products is also essential, and an alkaline diet can help.

(Allergies may be implicated in rheumatoid arthritis as it is an auto-immune condition. You can find out which foods affect you by eliminating them one by one, or you can have a food-sensitivity test.)

Some foods are not what you would think of as acid in nature but produce acid ash in the body when they are digested. Alkaline foods which consist mainly of vegetables and certain fruits and grains produce an alkaline ash in the body.

Foods to avoid

Fruits: Citrus (oranges and grapefruit), strawberries, raspberries, blackcurrants, blackberries, gooseberries, plums, pineapple, rhubarb.

Vegetables: Tomatoes, spinach, pickled beetroot, pickled onions.

Meat: Pork, bacon, ham, gammon and pork sausages. Preserved cold meats. Beef, including beef burgers and hot dogs.

Refined flour: White bread and bakery products made from white flour (these also contain a variety of 'E' numbers). Wheatflour or starch used as thickeners and fillers in other foods and drugs. White pasta.

White sugar: and all products containing it. Jams, and other preserves with sugar. Sweets and chocolate.

Beverages: Coffee and tea and cola drinks with caffeine.

Processed foods: Fast foods. All chemical preservatives, artificial colours, and flavourings.

Condiments: Salt, pepper, vinegar, ketchup, salad cream and other sauces.

Other: Lard, suet, cooking fat, gravy mixes, meat stock.

Foods to limit

(Some can take these in moderation, i.e. once or twice a week. Others need to cut them out altogether.)

Dairy foods: Cow's milk and milk products including butter, cheese, cream, yoghurt. Eggs.

Alcoholic drinks: all (except a little white wine).

Grains: Rye, oats, white rice, 100 per cent wholemeal bread.

Foods allowed

Fruits: Grapes, melon, pears, apples, bananas, peaches.

Vegetables: All except those in 'Foods to avoid', above.

Meat: Lamb once or twice weekly, chicken or turkey two to three times weekly.

Fish: White fish such as haddock, cod. Oily fish such as mackerel, herring. No shellfish.

Lentils, pulses, beans, nuts.

Dairy: Goat's milk, cheese and yoghurt. Eggs two to three times weekly.

Grains: 100 per cent wholemeal bread, preferably organic. Wholemeal pasta. Organic brown rice. Sugar-free muesli.

Sweeteners: Honey in moderation, molasses, sugar-free jam. Raisins, sultanas, figs, dates.

Beverages: Herbal tea, Luaka tea, dandelion coffee, Bambu or Barleycup coffee substitutes, soya milk, grape juice or celery juice.

Condiments: Ruthmol salt. Tofu salad dressing.

Other: Olive oil, sunflower or safflower oil, vegetable stock.

See ARTHRITIS for vitamins and minerals.

Hypoglycaemic diet

This is aimed at stabilizing blood-sugar levels. The many physical and mental symptoms of low blood sugar or reactive hypogylcaemia are caused by inappropriate hormonal reactions and are relieved by eating. (See also HYPOGLYCAEMIA.) Treatment is through dietary correction. This diet is also suitable for diabetics. *Note*: Hypoglycaemia in a diabetic may be a medical emergency.

Reactive hypoglycaemia is usually brought about by over-consumption of refined carbohydrates (refined flour products and sugar), which because they are quickly digested cause a rapid rise in blood sugar after which levels fall quickly again to a low level. It is this see-saw reaction that is the problem. The symptoms are usually felt one to three hours after a meal. A glucose tolerance test is diagnostic of the condition.

If people with a hypoglycaemic tendency do not correct their dietary habits they run the risk of eventual pancreatic exhaustion and possibly diabetes. It can be controlled and even cured by dietary means.

The treatment involves eating a well-balanced diet consisting mainly of protein (preferably of vegetable source) and fat with some unrefined carbohydrate, at frequent intervals, with as many as five small meals daily. This type of diet is broken down slowly by the body to yield glucose without dramatically raising the blood sugar. If three main meals are taken then a snack every two hours is necessary to avoid sudden drops of energy.

Foods to avoid completely

Refined and processed foods: Including white bread, pasta and rice.

Sugar: Honey, syrup, molasses, etc. Sweets, chocolate and all types of confectionery.

Bakery goods and desserts: Cakes, biscuits, pastries, puddings, pies, cereals with sugar, ice-cream, jam and marmalade.

Snacks: Crisps and other snack foods.

Miscellaneous: Tomato ketchup, relishes, pickles, mustard, sauces. Salt.

Medication with caffeine: Cough syrups, laxatives.

Drinks: All stimulants: Tea, coffee, alcohol, chocolate drinks and cocoa. Diluting juices, canned soft drinks.

Herbs: Ginseng, Pau D'arco, Guarana.

Foods allowed

Unrefined carbohydrate: Oats, brown rice, other wholegrains. All types of lentils, beans, peas and nuts. Wholegrain rice cakes, oatcakes and crispbreads without salt or sugar. Unsweetened muesli, porridge.

Protein: Nuts, nut butters, tofu and soya protein, baked beans without sugar, eggs, milk, yoghurt, cottage cheese, fresh and tinned fish (in moderation).

For sweetening: Unsweetened jams and pure fruit juice concentrate (in moderation).

Vegetables and fruit: All except those mentioned below as limited.

Drinks: Herbal teas, coffee substitutes, vegetable juices, cow's milk, soya milk, spring water.

Miscellaneous: Potassium salt (Ruthmol, Lo-Salt). Home-made vinaigrette with olive oil. Margarine.

Snacks: Nuts, fruit, yoghurt, milk or soya milk. Crispbreads with protein (see above).

Limited intake (two to three times weekly)

Unrefined carbohydrate: Wholemeal bread (one slice a day).

Protein: Fresh meat, fish and poultry. Full-fat cheese such as Cheddar. Butter.

Vegetables and fruit: Potatoes and sweet potato. Bananas, grapes, plums and dried fruit (dates and raisins, prunes).

Drinks: Unsweetened fruit juices.

Suggested menu

Breakfast: Porridge or sugarless muesli with fresh fruit and milk or soya milk, or boiled or scrambled egg, or baked beans with 1 slice wholemeal bread or rye crispbreads. Herbal tea or coffee substitute.

Lunch: Lentil soup or minestrone soup with beans or tuna fish, salmon or cottage cheese salad, or avocado or prawns. Rice cakes, rye crispbread or 1 slice bread if not had already. Piece of fruit or unsweetened yoghurt. Fruit juice and water. Coffee substitute.

Evening meal: Vegetable savoury with nuts or beans, or piece of chicken or poached fish, with brown rice and salad or vegetables. Dessert of stewed fruit and yoghurt. Herbal tea.

General advice

Avoid stress and exhaustion as this contributes to the problem. Don't rush meals, and chew well. Practise relaxation techniques. Get plenty of sleep. Exercise is important, particularly if you tend to be overweight, but not to the point of exhaustion. Meals should not be too large or taken too late at night.

Supplements

Multi-vitamin: 1 daily.
Vitamin C: 1000mg daily.
Multi-mineral: 2 daily plus chromium: 100mcg daily.
Vitamin B complex plus extra Vitamins B$_5$ (Pantothenic acid): 500mg daily.

Food-combining diet

This is based on the principles laid out fifty years ago by naturopath Dr Hay who recommended combining in the same meal foods that are digested together easily. Those that are not digested easily in combination are taken at separate meals. The diet was based on the principle that the enzymes needed to digest different foods, for example starch and protein, require different digestive mediums to work efficiently. By following this simple food plan many digestive problems have been helped. The same sensible principles are embodied in the eating habits of some cultures, such as the Jewish Kosher diet.

Medical conditions that may benefit are: gastric and duodenal ulcers, colitis, IRRITABLE BOWEL SYNDROME and CONSTIPATION, food ALLERGIES, chronic catarrhal problems, weight problems (see page 00), ARTHRITIS and other inflammatory conditions. It is suggested that the diet may not only prevent inflammation in the digestive area but may help decrease inflammatory reactions in other areas of the body.

Guidelines

1 Do not mix starchy foods or sugary foods with protein.
2 Do not mix milk with protein or starch.
3 Acid fruits are eaten with protein meals and sweet fruits with starchy meals, otherwise eat fruit separately from the main meal.
4 Vegetables and salads are considered neutral or alkaline.
5 Have one starch-based, one protein-based and one alkaline meal a day.
6 Avoid processed or refined foods.
7 Allow at least four hours between starch- and protein-based meals.

Table of compatible foods (Combine 2 with 1 or 3 but not 1 with 3)

1 *Protein foods*
Meat of all kinds, poultry and game birds.
Fish of all kinds.
Eggs.
Cheese. (Milk and yoghurt combine best with fruit and should not be served with a protein-based meal.)
Fruit: Apple family, Rose/berry and gooseberry family, citrus family, gourd family (melon), plum family.
Miscellaneous: salad dressing, vinaigrette with oil and lemon juice.

2 *Neutral foods*
Nuts: Legume or pea family, walnut and cashew family.
Fats: Butter, egg yolk, vegetable oil – olive, sunflower, sesame.
Vegetables: Nightshade (tomato) family, *except* potato. Mustard family (cabbage), lily family (onion), parsley family (carrot), beet family, fungi family (mushroom).
Salads: Aster family (lettuce), Laurel family (avocado) and above.
Miscellaneous: Salad dressing – mayonnaise or salad cream.

3 *Starch foods*
Grass family: wheat, barley, corn, rice, oats, rye, millet. Bread, flour products, oatmeal.
Fruits (sweet fruits): Currant family, grape family (raisins/other dried fruit), palm family (bananas).
Vegetables: Potatoes, Jerusalem artichokes, sweet potato.

For further information see Kathryn Marsden, *Food Combining in 30 Days.*

Fasting

Fasting means going without food and taking only liquids for a day or more. This may consist of only water, or more usually fruit juices and water. However, fruit-only fasts are easier to follow than just liquids to start with. The principle behind fasting is that as the digestion is given a total rest the body's energy can be diverted elsewhere into beneficial healing. It also allows detoxification, that is, getting rid of waste matter that has been stored in the body, in the liver, fat cells and large intestine, waiting for an opportunity to be released.

It is particularly recommended for certain digestive diseases such as IRRITABLE BOWEL SYNDROME, CONSTIPATION, DIVERTICULITIS, cancers of the gastrointestinal tract and ULCER-ATIVE COLITIS. Other chronic conditions that may be helped are skin diseases like eczema and psoriasis, catarrhal problems, rheumatoid ARTHRITIS. Many long-standing problems may be alleviated by judicious fasting when all else has failed. Weight loss is not usual if you keep up your fluid intake because the weight loss that occurs in the first week of a diet is mostly fluid.

Naturopaths recommend fasting one day a week, providing you are in good health, to allow the body to detoxify and undo the effects of an overly rich diet, pollution by pesticides and environmental chemicals. For maximum benefit one week two to three times a year is ideal, but you may find it easier to fast for one to two days to begin with.

Some basic rules to follow when fasting are:

1 Don't fast without medical advice if you are seriously ill, underweight, or on orthodox drugs. Do not attempt if you are hypoglycaemic.
2 Drink plenty of water.
3 Keep your blood sugar up. If feeling faint or shaky have a drink of water with a spoonful of honey or glucose.
4 Keep your bowels open: drink prune juice or if necessary take a herbal aperient.
5 Rest or relax during a fast, which is best done at home. Cultivate feeling good about fasting; this is not a punishment but a treat that you are giving your overtaxed body – pamper yourself with baths, music, pleasant walks, and anything that makes you feel good.

Detox symptoms are usual during the first day or two. These may be mild – headache, coated tongue, aching joints, fatigue – or more pronounced, depending on your state of health. If you feel very uncomfortable, slow down the rate of toxic release by eating some fruit – apples and pears or grapes are best. On days three to five you should start to feel really good, full of energy. When you stop feeling good is the time to stop, for you are then no longer fasting but starving: this may be on day seven on a first fast.

When you break the fast it is important to do so by eating only raw fruit and vegetables for a couple of days, then go on to cooked vegetables and soups, and finally add some protein like yoghurt or cottage cheese and grains like porridge or bread. Allow a week to return to your normal diet.

If you are serious about fasting it will pay to invest in a juice extractor.

Types of fast
Water: Don't fast on water alone if you have not fasted before. The body will be flooded with toxins from ingested pollutants as heavy metals, pesticides, etc. are released, and the detoxification symptoms will be severe.
Fruit: Any sort of fruit may be eaten but it is best to stick to one type at a time as mixing them decreases the activity of their enzymes. Be sure to scrub fruit well, or peel it if it is not organic. However, eating peel and pips gives maximum benefit. Be sure to chew very thoroughly. Remember to drink plenty as well, either spring water or juice. For a grape fast, you may eat 1.5–2kg of grapes daily and at least 2.5 litres of water, on a fast lasting one to seven days. You may eat 2kg of other fruit daily, taking a piece frequently.
Citrus juice fast: Freshly squeezed oranges, lemons, grapefruit. Enough to make 2.5 litres a day, to which you should add 1.2 litres of water. Aim to drink a glass of juice an hour through the day on a fast lasting two to five days. Break the fast with carrot juice and raw carrots. This fast is superb for colon cleansing as it has a scouring action on the gastrointestinal tract. Do not follow it if you suffer from irritable bowel, acidity, ulcers or colitis; follow the grape fast (see above) instead.
Vegetable juice fast: Freshly extracted carrot, parsley, celery, beetroot juice are especially beneficial, but any vegetable except potato can be used. This is an alkaline fast. Aim to drink a glass every two hours, 2.5–3.5 litres a day. Contains more food value than fruit, so is suitable for those who are in poor general health. For a fast lasting from one to five days. (Fasting on vegetables such as carrots is not recommended except for the dedicated, as it is not easy to eat through 4lbs of raw carrots.)

Anti-cancer diet
A combined organic vegetable and fruit juice fast with added supplements is used in some natural cancer treatment clinics. (See Dr Max Gerson, *A Cancer Therapy – Results of Fifty Cases*, and other

books by the Gerson Institute for further information and guidance on fasting for cancer.) Prevention of cancer is largely dietary as up to 60 per cent of cancers are thought to be connected to foods or additives ingested as well as environmental carcinogens.

Additives to avoid

Cyclamates and saccharine sweeteners, nitrites and nitrates used in food preservation, and sulphates. All 'E' numbers forbidden in children's food, including all artificial colourings.

Note: If you are receiving treatment for cancer seek professional advice before changing your diet drastically.

Foods to avoid

Coffee and tea, chocolate and cola.
Alcohol.
Milk, butter and cheese.
All meats except poultry reared on organically grown feed.
Smoked fish and any smoked or cured foods.
Toasted, fried and roasted foods.
All fast foods, junk foods and ready meals.
Refined foods (biscuits, cakes, sweets, or white flour bakery products).
Salt and sugar (brown and white).
Vegetables and fruits: Citrus. Nightshade family: potato, aubergine, tomato and green pepper. Radishes, horseradish.
Peanuts, cooking oils and hydrogenated fats (especially reheated cooking oils).
Spices such as cayenne or chilli, curry powder.
Tobacco.

Foods to include

Most herbal teas. Fruit juices apart from citrus, all fruits, especially grapes. Most vegetables, especially raw in salads. Vegetable juices, especially carrot and beetroot. Pulses, beans (not too many). Sprouted seeds and pulses, alfalfa, lentil, etc. Organic grains including brown rice. Millet.

Foods allowed in moderation (twice a week)

Organic wholewheat bread. Sunflower and olive oil. Free-range eggs. Soya milk and soya products. Fresh deep-sea fish, cod, whiting, haddock, etc.

Environmental pollution

Research points more and more to polluted air and water as causes of disease in the late twentieth cen-

tury, so minimize the effects of these as much as possible, especially if you live in a city. The planet is suffering, and if trees and animals can die from pollution, so can we. Radiation from nuclear power is known to be carcinogenic, and there is no general consensus on safe levels at present. Proximity to overhead power lines is thought to be harmful and possibly carcinogenic. Avoid or minimize sources of heavy metals. Get out into unpolluted country air as much as possible to exercise. (See Bibliography, page 204) for further sources of information on these topics.

Colon cleansing

According to naturopathic theory, what goes on in the bowel can cause symptoms elsewhere in the body, so colon cleansing may be indicated when there is sluggish liver function as well as bowel toxicity. Symptoms may be general fatigue, headache, poor concentration, irritability, constipation, mildly aching joints and PMS. Iridology or iris diagnosis is a good diagnostic tool to show the scale of bowel toxicity. The iris of the eye is examined under high magnification as it is believed to reflect the state of the internal body organs.

The bowel contains billions of bacteria needed to break down the remains of our food. In a healthy bowel these are mostly beneficial bacteria such as lactobacillus acidophilus, holding the pathogenic bacteria in check. However, in an unhealthy bowel the harmful bacteria can gain the upper hand and produce harmful toxins. Hostile viruses can also take up residence in the gut, from where they may invade the body.

When performing a colon cleanse, it helps to use a rectal enema once a day to remove old faecal matter. Usually old black or sticky mucous matter is released and this speeds up the process. A coffee enema (not instant) or herbal enema such as Dandelion root are used to stimulate the colon. These are absorbed internally by the bowel and transported via the portal blood system to help stimulate toxin release from the liver as well.

Scrupulous cleanliness must be maintained, with all items sterilized by boiling before and after use.

Dandelion root enema: 50g dried root to 1.5 litres water. Make a decoction (see page 9). Leave to cool to blood heat. Fill the enema bag, lie down with the bag suspended above you, and insert the nozzle. Allow it to empty slowly (it should have a valve so the flow can be adjusted), using only half the contents until you get used to the sensation.

Hold for ten minutes. The operation is best performed in the bath.

Caution: Do not attempt without medical advice if you suffer from colitis. Do not perform for more than a week at a time.

A colon cleanse is ideally done in conjunction with a citrus juice fast and a herbal bowel corrective formula.

Dr Christopher gives this helpful formula:

Herbal bowel corrective
1 part Barberry Bark
2 parts Cascara Bark
1 part Cayenne
1 part Ginger
1 part Golden Seal
1 part Raspberry Leaf

All the herbs are powdered and put into small capsules. (This formula or similar can be purchased ready-made from some supplement firms.) Take 2 three times a day with food initially, you can take up to 6 three times a day if necessary to produce a good bowel movement three times a day. Do not take enough to produce diarrhoea, cut back to a comfortable level if this happens. Copious movements should be produced initially and will decrease as time goes on. It may take six to nine months to eliminate all the old matter and get the bowel working normally again. The author has used this formula with many patients over the years with good effect.

Supplements
Psyllium seeds or husks: a mucilaginous bulking agent that helps remove waste products along with it. Take 1 teaspoon to start with, working up to 3 teaspoons over a week, in a glass of water ten minutes before meals and follow with another glass of water.
Fresh garlic or dried garlic capsules: 2–3 daily.
Probiotics or lactobacillus acidophilus, mixtures of beneficial bacteria normally found in the colon: 1–2 three times daily. Take advice on a recommended probiotics brand from a health store.
Cayenne pepper: ¼ teaspoon to start with, working up to 1 teaspoon, in water twice daily with meals. This stimulates the whole digestive tract to work better. *Do not take* if you suffer from ulcers or colitis. (Can be purchased as tablets: 1–2 twice daily.)
Olive oil in orange juice: 2 teaspoons daily in a glass of fresh juice, work up to 1 dessertspoon daily. Best administered lying down on your right side on an empty stomach last thing at night. Take if you have liverish symptoms.

You can take these supplements for up to six months with the herbal bowel aid. You may want to follow the Colon diet or Liver diet (see below) for part of this time. (Recommended reading: B. Jensen, *Tissue Cleansing Through Bowel Management*.)

Colon diet
Conditions helped are atonic or sluggish bowel, CONSTIPATION and DIVERTICULITIS. Most of these conditions are only known in affluent Western societies as the result of diets over-rich in protein and lacking fibre. It is natural to have a bowel movement after each meal, as an infant does, but most people have only one a day, some even less. This leads to a build-up of waste matter, toxicity and poor functioning of the digestive tract. Bowel movements should be soft and well-formed. If they are hard and difficult to pass, this may be due to inadequate amounts of natural fibre in the diet or too many mucus-forming foods, such as dairy and meat. Five to six servings daily of natural fibre from fruit and vegetables and wholegrains are now recommended, which brings us nearer to the diet of people elsewhere in the world who do not suffer from bowel disease. Drinking insufficient water is another contributory factor: hot beverages do not provide fluid in a form the body can immediately use. Only water does not need to be digested. Bad bowel habits learned as a child, such as not going to the lavatory as soon as the urge is felt, are part of the problem, and tension is also a factor. A herbal bowel corrective may help, see BOWEL PROBLEMS.

In treatment of IRRITABLE BOWEL SYNDROME a high-fibre diet is usually recommended. This should not consist of wheat bran, which irritates the bowel, but should be rich in wholefoods and fibre from the skins of vegetables and fruits. In inflammatory bowel disease (ULCERATIVE COLITIS) a low residue or soft diet is recommended, although including some bulk can help to 're-educate' the bowel. Introduce oatmeal, oat bran and some vegetables, particularly raw grated carrot. Try some variety in raw vegetables and see which you can tolerate. Intolerance of dairy products, gluten in wheat, and citrus fruits are among the causes of irritable bowel and colitis. A relationship between food intolerance and bowel flora has been identified recently, particularly in relation to irritable bowel syndrome. Shifts in the population of bowel flora in response to certain

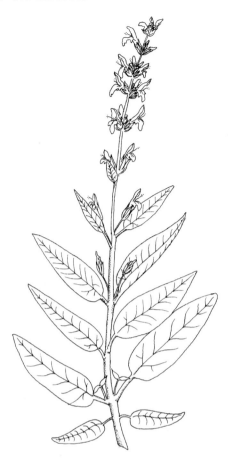

Sage *(Salvia officinalis)*

foods may bring on symptoms. You may benefit by excluding dairy and wheat products for a while and then trying them again to see the effect. Avoid tea as tannins are constipating, and coffee is a stimulant that can cause diarrhoea.

Liver diet

The liver has an enormous daily task to fulfil, being responsible not only for many of the processes of chemical breakdown in the body but for maintenance of many metabolic functions. As all our food is dealt with and converted to energy, alcohol, drugs and chemical pollutants have to be detoxified. It is no wonder that the liver can sometimes work below par. This may not be reflected in liver function tests but you will feel less than well in yourself. Conditions that may be helped are sluggish digestion with 'liverishness' (a general feeling of being below par with digestive symptoms, possibly yellowish skin), and poor liver function leading to hormonal imbalance, including PMS (see page 16) and menopausal hot flushes (see page 87), and gallstones, HYPOGLYCAEMIA and obesity (see page 68). Fortunately the liver has an amazing capacity to regenerate its own cells, and a dietary and herbal tune-up will enhance this capacity.

Avoid fatty foods and alcoholic drinks. Your diet should be light on protein, (recommended daily amount 45g). Grill lean meats. Eliminate cooking oils, butter, cheese, milk and cream altogether. Cut out caffeinated drinks. Dandelion coffee made from roasted Dandelion root is an excellent substitute for real coffee and is one of the best things for the liver. Follow the principles suggested in the Healthy wholefood diet (page 126). Take plenty of fibre-rich foods including wholegrain cereals and raw vegetables. The enzymes in raw food help digestion. Drink plenty of spring water.

Try the diet for a month and monitor improvements. If you are suffering from liver disease take professional advice from your doctor or a medical herbalist.

As an aid to liver function take olive oil and fresh garlic in lemon juice once daily in the morning. Put 4 teaspoons olive oil in a blender with 2 cloves of garlic and the juice of 2 lemons and add sufficient water to fill a wine glass. Drink back quickly. Ideally lie down on your right side for half an hour after drinking to allow it to work. Chew parsley, coriander seed or aniseed, or suck an aromatic clove afterwards if you don't want to be antisocial. This is a great liver cleanser and stimulant and particularly good if you suffer from gallstones. Spring is the ideal time to do a liver cleanse, which is best performed for two weeks. For added benefit fast one day a week on juices (see Fasting above).

There are many excellent herbal liver tonics, among them Milk Thistle, Dandelion Root, Barberry, Wormwood, Gentian. A decoction made from equal parts, with a small piece of Liquorice and Ginger added, drunk before a meal, stimulates and regenerates liver function.

See under BOWEL PROBLEMS for herbal treatment of digestive problems.

Part Two

A–Z Directory of Other Conditions

This self-help directory provides herbal, nutritional and life-style advice for gynaecological and common ailments. It is cross-referenced to the rest of the book. References in SMALL CAPITALS are to entries in the Directory. For preparation of herbs see pages 8–13.

ABDOMINAL PAIN

Gynaecological abdominal pain

(Pain occurring between the navel and the groin)

Acute

Pain that starts suddenly and becomes acute quickly, in the lower abdomen if not pregnant, may be caused by FIBROIDS, SALPINGITIS (inflammation of the Fallopian tubes), PELVIC INFLAMMATORY DISEASE, rupture of OVARIAN CYST, endometriosis (see page 24) or appendicitis. Any of these may present as an emergency.

During early pregnancy pain may be caused by miscarriage or ectopic pregnancy (foetus in the Fallopian tubes), degeneration of a FIBROID (see pregnancy – abdominal pain in, page 42), kidney inflammation or appendicitis. Treat any pain in the first trimester of pregnancy that does not clear up in two hours as an emergency.

During late pregnancy the pain may be caused by onset of labour, placental separation, ruptured uterus, haemorrhage of ruptured stomach rectus muscle, kidney inflammation, or appendicitis. Braxton Hicks contractions (see page 43) should not be painful. Treat all pain in late pregnancy as an emergency.

Chronic

Recurrent lower abdominal pain in women maybe caused by PELVIC INFLAMMATORY DISEASE, endometriosis (see page 24), uterine tumours and uterine prolapse (see under UTERUS PROBLEMS), OVARIAN CYST, or pelvic adhesions following surgery.

Other causes of abdominal pain

The abdominal area extends from the diaphragm (ribs) to the groin. Pain from the digestive organs is likely to be felt in the upper abdomen, between ribs and navel, and is commonly referred to as tummy ache. It is not easy to put pain into words – it may be felt as sharp, mild or severe; a cramp, dull ache or colic – but an attempt has been made here to indicate the different types and their causes. It is beyond the scope of this guide to cover all possibilities, however, and it is essential to take medical advice.

Acute

Severe and sudden pain may be due to rupture of an organ (spleen, aorta, or as a result of ectopic pregnancy) or perforation of the bowel (by peptic ulcer or ulcerated colon) producing tearing, agonizing pain followed by shock, and requiring immediate hospitalization and surgery. It may be due to peritonitis (inflammation of the lining of the abdominal cavity, with fever, vomiting, and possibly shock and collapse), caused by the above, or by appendicitis (right-sided lower abdominal pain), or gall-bladder pain, (right-sided upper abdominal pain, felt also in the back) or inflamed Fallopian tubes with severe, sharp pain, much worse for movement. Other causes are obstruction of intestine or bowel (with abdominal distension, inability to pass wind, vomiting and constipation) or pancreatitis (left-sided upper abdominal pain radiating to the back).

Colicky-type pain (intermittent painful spasms) may be from the colon, bowel, gall-bladder (biliary colic), uterus or kidney ureter (renal colic) resulting in legs drawn up and collapse if severe.

Other causes of acute pain in the abdomen are gastroenteritis (food poisoning with DIARRHOEA and vomiting), CYSTITIS, heart attack or pneumonia. If the cause is not obvious, a laparoscopy to see into the abdominal cavity is often performed in hospital before deciding on the course of treatment.

It is often difficult for a doctor, however practised in diagnosis, to differentiate the cause of pain, so if you have experienced great distress for more than one hour, do not delay, or wait for a doctor or try to treat yourself – call an ambulance.

Chronic

Long-standing, recurrent abdominal pain may be caused by indigestion, gastritis, gastric and duodenal ulcer (pain after eating with the former and relieved by food and antacids in the latter), DIVERTICULTITIS, IRRITABLE BOWEL SYNDROME (with spasms), ULCERATIVE COLITIS (with DIARRHOEA and/or CONSTIPATION, pain relieved by passing stool – and blood or mucus in stool with ulceration).

As a general rule, any pain that does not clear up warrants a medical opinion.

ALLERGY

It is suggested that as much as half the world's population suffers from allergies. In the Western world the incidence is growing rapidly and in its most extreme form it may be referred to as 'Twentieth-century Disease'. Two types of allergy have been observed in practice. Orthodox medicine defines true allergy by an antigen–antibody reaction in the blood: that is, the immune system has produced an antibody to a particular allergen or antigen, be it a food, an inhalant or another environmental trigger. A substance called histamine is produced in large quantities, causing fluid to leak out of tissues and resulting in the well-known allergy symptoms of swelling and redness. Anaphylaxis, an extreme response of this sort occurring throughout the body, can be life-threatening due to shock.

The other type of allergy reaction that is widespread today is an intolerance or sensitivity below the level of the immune system which perceives it as an invader and mounts a response, resulting in some very uncomfortable symptoms.

Many of the things that cause these reactions, such as tobacco smoke or car exhaust fumes, are not particularly good for anyone, but they are tolerated and do not bother most people. For some, however, an overload may produce uncomfortable symptoms such as a stuffy nose, sneezing fits or headache, or a worse reaction such as breathlessness and wheezing. Skin reactions are common, for example to tomatoes, strawberries or various other plants, nickel, wool, soap powders and other household chemicals; those affected break out in a rash when touching them. Other common inhaled allergens are pollens and grasses, and gas vapours from central heating appliances. Almost anything can produce a sensitivity reaction if the body disagrees with it. Some unfortunate people suffer multiple sensitivities to many foods and environmental allergens, and spend their lives avoiding those that are known; this can be time-consuming, uncomfortable and expensive.

Some people are allergic types and so are more likely to develop sensitivity; there is usually a genetic connection and other close family members are often known to suffer as well. Atopic eczema, ASTHMA, allergic rhinitis, urticaria and hayfever are common in this group. Common allergens for these sufferers are animal hair and feathers, house-dust mite, pollens and grasses. Reactions usually manifest in childhood. Food reactions in this group are often due to a leaky bowel as a result of early weaning or introduction of the infant to certain foods too early; dairy and wheat products are common culprits.

In the other types of sufferer – usually adult – it is suggested that chronic ill health, stress and/or poor diet or CANDIDA infestation, coupled with over-exposure to certain environmental triggers, may lower immunity sufficiently to start off an allergic reaction. Adaptation to allergens we react to is continually taking place in the body, for example cells in the lungs will change in response to cigarette smoke. It is when the invasion exceeds the body's ability to cope that allergic problems begin. There may be multiple intolerances, especially to foods, which may be cyclic – coming and going depending on how often the person is exposed to them. The symptoms that present are many, and although they most commonly affect the skin, nose and lungs, they may affect all the systems and parts of the body. As this reaction is far wider than may be explained by the classic antigen–antibody response, it is thought that there is some other mechanism at work.

Some of the main symptoms most commonly associated with allergy are listed here. If you suffer from more than five, especially the first five, then you are probably allergic, and you should see an allergy specialist or clinical ecologist.

1 Swelling of tissues due to fluid, particularly facial with puffy eyes, and swollen hands, abdominal bloating.

2 Streaming eyes, or alternatively stuffy head, both without a cold. Frequent sneezing.

3 Skin reactions, rashes including eczema, dermatitis, itching, hives, extreme dryness.

4 Persistent fatigue that does not improve with rest.

5 Perspiring without exertion or increased room temperature, in absence of other illness.

6 Abdominal symptoms, diarrhoea, flatulence and constipation, particularly if alternating.

7 Mental and emotional symptoms, irritability, mood swings, feeling dopey or spaced out a lot of the time, poor concentration for mental tasks.

If extreme there may be short-term memory loss.

8 Tinnitus (ringing in the ears).

9 Muscle aches and cramps, muscles abnormally tired after moderate exertion.

10 Palpitations, especially after eating, racing pulse and breathlessness.

Allergy tests

Tests can be performed to ascertain your major sensitivities. The main ones are:

Skin prick and patch testing

These are available on the NHS. In the prick test the suspected food or other substance is placed on the skin and pricked in, and the result observed after ten to fifteen minutes. In the patch test the suspected allergen is left on under a plaster for twenty-four to forty-eight hours and the results observed. A local skin reaction such as a red weal is considered an allergic response. This is 40 per cent accurate for substances known to produce an allergic skin reaction, but not for foods which generally produce a reaction when eaten.

RAST (radio absorption testing)

Also available on the NHS, this is a blood test to find antibodies in the blood for confirmation of 'classic allergy'. It includes usually only four to five foods.

Cytotoxic testing

An alternative test that is not widely available. It is done by taking a sample of blood and seeing how the white blood cells react to substances introduced to them under the microscope. This is probably the most accurate test available, and laboratories report approximately 80 per cent improvement in symptoms if patients follow the findings of the test; it does however depend on the accuracy of the individual technician.

Sub-lingual testing

The allergen, diluted in drops, is placed under the tongue and the pulse rate tested. It is not highly accurate because other factors may raise the pulse rate.

Applied kinesiology (muscle testing)

Suspect foods are placed in the mouth and muscle responses tested. A weak response is considered indicative of allergy. It is non-invasive and may provide a good result. Accurate testing is only as good as the sensitivity of the practitioner, so look for someone qualified and experienced.

Vega testing

This measures the electrical response of the skin in response to known allergens. Ampoules containing the allergen are used so they do not come into direct contact with the skin. It relies again on the skill of the operator but can be accurate in the right hands.

Treatment of allergy
Self-help

Detection may be done by elimination diet followed by challenge (see Treatment of food allergy, page 137). This is best carried out on the advice of a dietician or nutritionist, although you could try a modified elimination diet yourself (see Elimination diet, page 137), using the pulse check as a method of measuring your allergic response. Treatment is mainly by exclusion of a food or avoidance of the known allergen. Start by restricting or avoiding the suspected food or environmental allergen. Get rid of feather pillows, take measures to decrease house-dust, house dust mite, etc. Minimize environmental pollution. (See books on allergy for other preventive measures.)

Vitamin supplements (see page 127) raise general health. Make sure they are hypoallergenic. Include time-release Vitamin C (up to bowel tolerance levels then cut back to a comfortable level). Vitamin A as beta-carotene, at least 5mg daily, and Vitamin E, 200–400 IUs.

Desensitization

This is a method used by clinical ecologists (specialists in treating allergy). It is done by injecting a very dilute solution of the allergen, or by taking it in drops under the tongue, to try to neutralize sensitivity. In the author's view this should only be done as a last resort, and avoidance of foods is always the preferred method, unless nutrition is severely compromised. An exception would be if it is impossible to avoid a particular environmental allergen, such as lead from car exhaust pollution. Side-effects to desensitization injections are possible, individuals often feel awful afterwards, and the allergy may return after a while. Further, removal of one allergic response could allow another to take its place. However, some individuals do report up to 75 per cent improvement in symptoms. An alternative is desensitization by homoeopathic dilution of the allergen taken orally. This is not true homoeopathy but has far less possibility of side-effects. If desensitizing, treatment to strengthen constitution is always advisable, and you should consult a medical herbalist.

Herbal treatment

It is essential to bring about an improvement in overall health or constitution at the same time as following the self-help measures outlined above. Allergies fall into one of two categories, either due to a deficient immune system, or a faulty life-style and eating habits over a number of years, or maybe a combination of both. It may be necessary to work mainly on the immune system or else to concentrate on a clearing-out and eliminating process using alteratives. These are herbs which beneficially change organ responses, working primarily on the eliminative channels: Red Clover, Raspberry Leaf, Burdock, Oregon Grape, Plantain, Echinacea (Cone Flower), Garlic.

The following formula, based on the above, may be helpful:-

Formula 1 for allergy

Red Clover	30 per cent
Echinacea	30 per cent
Burdock	20 per cent
Garlic	20 per cent

Total: 100ml/g a week. Dose: tincture, 5ml three times daily (unless allergic to alcohol), or infusion/decoction of dried herb, 1 cup three times daily, or powdered in capsules, 2, three times daily. (This may need to be continued for several months, although improvement in symptoms should be felt sooner.) In addition, Garlic can be taken as capsules or tablets.

Herbs for immune system

Atractylodes, Astralagus, Pau D'arco, Panax Ginseng, Codonopsis, Siberian Ginseng, Schizandra, Liquorice, Golden Seal, Bear's Lichen (Usnea).

The following formula, based on the above, may be helpful:

Formula 2 for allergy

Codonopsis	30 per cent
Schizandra	20 per cent
Astralagus	20 per cent
Atractylodes	15 per cent
Liquorice	10 per cent
Ginger	5 per cent

Total: 100ml/g a week. Dose: tincture, 5ml three times daily (unless allergic to alcohol), or infusion/decoction of dried herb, 1 cup three times daily, or powdered in capsules, 2, three times daily. *Note:* This is a warming formula in Chinese terms and should not be used if there are acute, inflammatory allergic symptoms such as tissue swelling. Wait until these have died down, or use Formula 1 for allergy above.

Then, depending which systems are most affected, the following can be used.

Herbs for digestive system

Golden Seal, Astralagus, Marshmallow, Chamomile, and astringents, Agrimony or Cranesbill.

Herbs for eyes, nose and lungs

Eyebright, Plantain, Elderflower, Chamomile.

Herbs for skin

To purify blood and improve skin: Sarsaparilla, Nettles, Chamomile, Yellow Dock.

Applications for local relief

- Chamomile (anti-allergic and anti-inflammatory): dried flowers as infusion for steam inhalant for upper respiratory tract; or skin washes; or added to creams as tincture, 2ml to 25g, or oil 1–2 drops to 25g.
- Marigold cream (anti-inflammatory).
- Chickweed cream (anti-itch).
- Peppermint (cooling and anti-itch) added to creams, as tincture or oil as above, or infusion of leaf as a wash. Can be used with Chamomile Flowers in the bath for soothing sore skin.

Note: There is a possibility that you may react to some of the herbs if you have multiple allergies, although this is more unlikely than a reaction to foods, because we usually react to those allergens we are exposed to most often. As a precaution, however, combine fewer herbs and monitor your reactions carefully; ideally see a medical herbalist.

APPLIED KINESIOLOGY or VEGA TESTING (see above) could be used to see which are safe.

ANGINA PECTORIS (CHEST PAIN)

Cardiovascular disease is the major cause of death in post-menopausal women in the UK. Serious heart disease should be dealt with by a qualified physician or practitioner; always inform your doctor if you are taking herbal remedies.

Angina is chest pain caused by ischaemic heart disease which occurs when not enough blood reaches the heart. This is usually the result of plaque build-up (atherosclerosis) narrowing the arteries to the heart.

Other causes of chest pain are ANXIETY, indigestion, acid reflux from food pipe, muscle strain, rib fracture, referred pain from upper back, gastritis, peptic and duodenal ulcers, gall-bladder colic, lung infection, severe anaemia, or myocardial infarction (heart attack).

The pain of angina is described as a dull, crushing, squeezing or pressing sensation. It is felt centrally in the chest behind the breast-bone and moves up to the throat area and down the left arm. It is often caused by exercise and emotional factors. It ceases when you stop exercise, rest or calm down, unlike the pain of a heart attack. Other symptoms may be difficulty in breathing or dizziness. If the pain does not stop, treat it as an emergency.

Angina varies in severity, being known as unstable if it happens when taking minimal exercise or at rest. A test known as an angiogram may be used to ascertain the extent of the damage to the arteries.

Severe angina may predispose the patient to a coronary heart attack. Considering this, and the extent to which the person's life is disrupted, angioplasty (widening the arteries) or a coronary bypass operation may be suggested. Orthodox treatment consists of nitroglycerine and sometimes beta-blocker drugs to slow the heart down, and hospital bed-rest for serious cases.

Self-help
A normal life-style should be followed as far as possible, with gentle exercise, such as walking every day; swimming and yoga are also beneficial. Try to reduce stress. It is essential to give up smoking and if you are overweight you should try to reduce. Hormonal contraception or replacement therapy is not advised. Dietary measures such as a low-cholesterol diet have been shown to improve angina.

Add oat bran, and soya lecithin to your daily diet. To reduce cholesterol levels eat foods high in natural fibre – mainly skins of vegetables and fruits. Cook with garlic and add it to salads. Add fresh lemon juice and eat plenty of all kinds of fruit. Eat fatty fish like herring.

Avoid saturated fats – butter, cheese, cream, fatty meat. Grill, do not fry or roast. Avoid salt and salted and sugary foods. Cut out coffee and white bread altogether.

Supplements
GLA from Evening Primrose oil and EPA from fish oils: 1000–2000mg daily of each. Vitamin C: 250–500mg daily in divided doses.
Garlic capsules: Full strength, such as Cardiomax, 1 daily.

Herbal treatment
Any herbal treatment will need to be carefully monitored by a herbal practitioner, as orthodox heart drugs may well be prescribed. Any herbs should be given as part of a wider treatment; a medical herbalist may use a number of different herbs. *Note:* Self-medication with herbs is not a substitute for any drugs you have been prescribed by your doctor for angina.

To improve the condition in the long term the following may be taken: Hawthorn Berry tincture, 1–2ml three times daily, or as a decoction, 1–2g per cup, three times a day. A pleasant wine may be made of the berries by steeping them in a good red wine for two to three weeks, then 1 tablespoon two to three times daily is taken. Follow directions for making tinctures on pages 8–9.

ANXIETY

See under EMOTIONAL PROBLEMS.

ARTHRITIS

Arthritis is a degenerative and inflammatory condition of the joints. There are two main types, Osteoarthritis and Rheumatoid arthritis. Other conditions affecting the joints include spondylitis, osteoporosis, gout and types of arthritis associated with colitis, psoriasis and connective tissue disease. Rheumatic diseases are systemic, that is, they can affect many other parts of the body as well as the joints. The main symptoms of arthritis are pain and stiffness, loss of movement and signs of inflammation around the joint, such as heat and redness.

Osteoarthritis (OA) is caused by a degeneration of the joint surfaces where they articulate, due to wear and tear, usually connected with ageing or injury. Most people over sixty have some arthritis. It may affect one or more joints, generally the weight-bearing ones, but the vertebrae bones of the back and the finger joints can be involved. Stiffness and pain, worsened by cold and damp, are the common symptoms. The pain tends to worsen as the day goes on. Diagnosis is by case history and later by X-ray of the joints. Analgesics are the orthodox treatment, with orthopaedic surgery in severe cases.

Rheumatoid arthritis (RA) is an inflammatory condition caused by an abnormal immunological reaction, where the body attacks itself unwittingly, eventually destroying the internal structure of the joints and tissues around them. At one time or another most joints are affected, usually a pair of joints at a time, such as the knees, shoulders or ankles. Deformity in the knuckles of the fingers is common. Joints are swollen, red, and sore to touch when inflamed. Pain is usually worse on rising and improves a little with movement. Other symptoms which may or may not be present are anaemia, dry eyes, swollen glands, skin ulcers, lumps or nodules. Fever and tiredness are often present in the early stages. More serious, but fortunately rare, complications can occur.

Diagnosis is by blood tests for antibodies (rheumatoid factor) and for levels of inflammation (ESR test). The cause is not known, although infection, prolonged stress and dietary factors such as food sensitivity may be triggers. Women are affected three times more than men, commonly from around age forty.

There is no orthodox cure, only drugs to alleviate inflammation and pain. A small proportion of women recover spontaneously when they are post-menopause. Alternative medicines generally improve the condition and in some cases halt the disease. Acupuncture, osteopathy and physiotherapy give relief to many, as well as herbal medicine.

Self-help
Gentle exercise to keep joints mobile is important in RA, and a regime of 'arthrobics' for OA is beneficial.

The diet should be as alkaline as possible, avoiding acid foods and those that create excessive acid waste products. If you suspect you are sensitive to any foods, try eliminating those items. If you suffer from RA, get an ALLERGY test (see above). Maximize your vitamin and mineral intake from fresh foods. Check if you have any deficiencies by hair or blood mineral analysis.

See Diet for arthritis (alkaline) or Milk-free diet (pages 142 and 141).

Supplements
Correct deficiencies of minerals, following a test. You will need to take them for up to six months, then repeat the test. As a precaution in the meantime take selenium and zinc which are often deficient.

Also, depending on severity:
Vitamin C: 500mg twice daily for a month, then cut down to 250mg daily. Vitamin E: 400 IUs twice daily. Vitamin B complex: 25–50mg daily plus extra Vitamin B$_5$ (pantothenic acid): 50–100mg daily. Cod liver oil (Vitamin A+D): 2–6 capsules daily depending on strength. Vegetable oils, safflower and sunflower, 1 dessertspoon daily (add to salads). GLA from Evening Primrose oil: 1000mg twice daily or Borage (Starflower) oil: 500mg twice daily.

Herbal treatment
Combine from the following (all doses are for tincture or standard infusion three times daily):
Anti-inflammatories:
Either Devil's Claw (RA) or Bogbean (OA) 3ml/g and Celery Seed, 5g, as tea.
With
Analgesic (as needed): White Willow Bark, 3ml/g.
Add
Diuretics: (for tissue decongestion): Birch or Meadowsweet, 3ml/5g.
Add
Circulatory stimulants (as needed): Prickly Ash or Ginger, ½ml/1g.

Note: Maximum dose of tincture should not exceed 20ml daily (140ml a week).

Liniments (for pain relief externally): Rosemary, Wintergreen and Lavender essential oils in carrier base oil, 1 drop of each in 1 per cent dilution, or add to Comfrey ointment. Massage in twice daily. Bladderwrack poultices made from powdered seaweed, used nightly. Cayenne or Fresh Horseradish as hot compresses (see page 11 for directions on making)

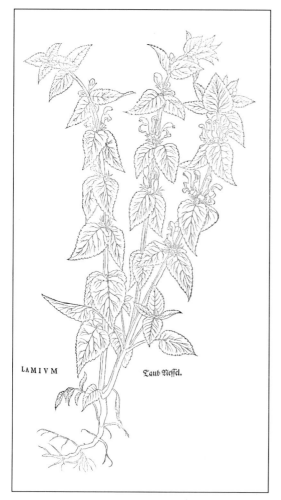

White Deadnettle *(Lamium album)*

Some quite good proprietary brands of herbal tablets and liniments for arthritis are available over the counter – check constituents (see page 203 for suppliers).

ASTHMA

Symptoms are wheezing, coughing and shortness of breath. There are two types of asthma. One begins in early childhood and is often connected with allergy; there may be allergy in the family and the child may also suffer from eczema at some point: this type often comes in bouts and usually improves with age. The second type, late-onset asthma, occurs without any family history, often coincides with chest infections and after repeated episodes can become chronic. Hayfever is often a problem as well.

An asthmatic attack can be worrying or even frightening. It can last for variable lengths of time and as it is made worse by fear and tension, a vicious circle is set up. Causes are certain allergens, such as house dust, or house dust mite, grasses or pollens, or sensitivity to certain foods. Other factors are exertion, excitement and cold air. EMOTIONAL PROBLEMS are connected with onset of asthma in some cases. A severe attack (status asthmaticus) is a medical emergency; an ambulance should be called right away. It is more difficult to breathe out than in during an attack, because of closing of the air passages. Treatment is usually hospitalization.

Orthodox drugs used to treat asthma such as Salbutamol are administered by inhaler and if this does not work, steroid inhalers and stronger bronchodilators and during acute episodes, oral steroid drugs are used.

Self-help

Try a dairy-free diet initially for a month, as sensitivity to dairy products are known to worsen asthma in many cases. (See Milk-free diet, page 141.) Sensitivity to chicken or wheat may also be a factor. Aim for as healthy a diet as possible, low in sugar and animal fat. Avoid all harmful food additives that may cause asthma, especially monosodium glutamate in processed and packaged foods and in Chinese food.

Take regular exercise such as walking briskly or swimming to reduce symptoms. You can build up to aerobic exercise which improves functioning of the lungs. Practise relaxation methods daily, particularly breathing exercises, and put these to use during an attack. Sitting up and trying to stay calm will ease an attack.

Find an allergist to help sort out environmental and ingested allergens to which you may be reacting, or you may be able to do this yourself: see Elimination diet (page 137). Control your environment and desensitize to those things you cannot avoid (see ALLERGY above).

Supplements

Zinc: 10–20mg daily. GLA as Evening Primrose oil: 2000–4000mg daily. Vitamin C: 500mg daily. Vitamin E: 600 IUs daily. Magnesium: 100mg daily, balance with calcium, 200mg daily. Garlic tablets: 1–2 daily.

Herbal treatment

Herbal treatment aims not to replace drugs but to improve condition of the lungs, by relaxing spasm and getting rid of build-up of catarrh. In time it may be possible to cut drugs down. Inform your doctor if taking herbal medicine and do not discontinue any drugs suddenly or without advice. Consult a medical herbalist if you suffer severely. Combine from the following (all doses are for tincture or standard infusion, three times daily, and herbs underlined are first choice):

Bronchial anti-spasmodics (to relax broncial tubes):
Either <u>Cramp Bark</u>, White Horehound, Thyme or Angelica Root, 2–5ml/g
With
Expectorants (to clear lungs):
Either <u>Euphorbia</u>, Coltsfoot or Liquorice and Garlic, 2–5ml/g
Add
Demulcents (to soothe): Marshmallow Root or Irish Moss, 5–10g as cold decoction sweetened with honey (see page 9 for directions).
Essential oils as inhalants, 1 drop of each in a bowl of hot water: Peppermint, Eucalyptus, Aniseed and Thyme to prevent attack. Inhale deeply for 10 minutes.

Note: Maximum dose of tincture should not exceed 20ml daily (140ml a week).

BACKACHE

Gynaecological causes of backache in women are period pain (see page 22) uterine or vaginal prolapse (see under UTERINE PROBLEMS), PELVIC INFLAMMATORY DISEASE, pelvic tumours, pregnancy (see page 44), and post-natal injury (see page 63). See under individual entries for treatment. If the backache is due to injury, treatment is best administered by an osteopath or chiropractor. In addition, herbal anti-inflammatory Devil's Claw may be taken, 5ml three times daily or as tablets or capsules over the counter, 1–2 three times daily or follow packet directions. When menopausal symptoms or menstruation are the cause this is often due to low oestrogen levels. Herbs to stimulate oestrogen production include Black Cohosh, Liquorice and False Unicorn Root. (See Directions for use of herbs in menopause, page 89.) Try Wintergreen, Penny Royal, Lavender and Chamomile, 1 per cent essential oils in carrier herbal oil, preferably St John's Wort oil, for massage.

BOWEL PROBLEMS

Conditions affecting the small intestine and colon, as well as the rectum or bowel, are IRRITABLE BOWEL SYNDROME (spastic colon); inflammatory bowel disease (ULCERATIVE COLITIS AND CROHN'S DISEASE); coeliac disease, DIVERTICULITIS. The main symptoms are DIARRHOEA, CONSTIPATION, discomfort or pain. Note that pain originating in one area can often be felt in another or be generalized in the abdomen because of the common nerve supply to many abdominal organs, so make sure of the diagnosis before treating yourself. See also other causes of ABDOMINAL PAIN.

Herbal treatment for digestive problems

Herbs used for digestive ailments work superbly well in bowel problems, and the following principles have been proven in practice by the author over a number of years.

Look for underlying factors in selecting herbs: for example, if irritable bowel is mainly due to tension and stress, use a combination of sedative herbs, although an anti-spasmodic for pain may also be needed. Specific treatment is under individual ailments listed: thus see under Irritable bowel syndrome (below), then refer back here to combine from the following (all doses are for tincture, three times daily, or dried herb as infusion/decoction, 1 cup three times daily; herbs underlined are first choice).

Anti-spasmodics:
Either <u>Peppermint</u>, Angelica Leaf or Liquorice, 2–4ml/g
With
Anti-inflammatories:
Either <u>Chamomile</u>, Meadowsweet or Golden Seal, 2–4ml/g.
Add
Carminatives (for relief of flatulence and dyspepsia): <u>Fennel</u>, Lemon Balm, Aniseed, Dill or Ginger, pleasant as an infusion, combine two or three, 3–5g per cup.
Add
Sedatives (as needed): <u>Chamomile</u>, Catnip or Valerian, 3–5ml, or Hops 1–2ml/g.
As needed:
Demulcents (to soothe): <u>Marshmallow Leaf</u> or Slippery Elm, powder of either, 5–10g as infusion or Slippery Elm dissolved in warm milk/soya milk, two to five times daily, depending on severity.

Bulking agents: <u>Beetroot fibre</u>, 1 tablespoon daily or Psyllium husk, 5g working up to 15g, three times daily with a glass of water, followed by another glass of water right away.

Immune system-enhancers:
Either <u>Echinacea</u>, Garlic or Barberry, 2–3ml/g daily. Garlic can taken as capsules or tables, 1–2 three times daily; or 1–2 small chopped fresh cloves, daily with food or drink.

Hepatics (for liver):
Either <u>Dandelion</u>, Burdock, Wormwood or Gentian, 1–2ml/g, to stimulate the bowel to work better by reflex action.

Note: Maximum dose of tincture should not exceed 20ml daily (140ml a week). Many herbal proprietary brands are available over the counter for digestive problems: check the constituents with the above.

Irritable bowel syndrome (IBS)

IBS is three times as common in women as in men. Another term used to describe it is spastic colon. Bowel movements alternate between bouts of CONSTIPATION and DIARRHOEA with discomfort before passing a motion. There is usually uncomfortable flatulence and distension. Other symptoms may be tiredness, depression and anxiety, although it is hard to tell which comes first. It is multi-factorial, sometimes following gastroenteritis or other infections. IBS is common with post-viral fatigue syndrome. Other causes include stress, lack of digestive enzymes, spastic bowel tone and food intolerance particularly of milk and cream, gluten in wheat and other grains, oranges and coffee. See Colon diet (page 147).

Self-help
Include plenty of fibre in the diet and drink plenty of water. Soft mucilaginous bulk such as Psyllium seed/husk will iron out bouts of constipation and aid smooth bowel movements – be sure to take plenty of water with it. Avoid any food or drink, such as coffee, that stimulates excessive contraction of bowel. Try the Elimination diet (see page 137) to identify problem foods. Abdominal and pelvic exercises and yoga (see pages 195 and 38) will help strengthen and tone the area and promote normal intestinal contractions.

Herbal treatment
Combine from each of the following herbs: Antispasmodics, carminatives, sedatives for nervous overstimulation. Include mucilages and bulking agents as tinctures and/or infusions to stop spasm, calm wind, gently relieve tension and soothe sensitive membranes (see Herbal treatment for digestive problems, above).

Supplements
Lactobacillus acidophilus, to repopulate the bowel with ecofriendly bacteria. Vitamin B complex with extra biotin and Vitamin B$_5$ (pantothenic acid) for proper intestinal function.

Ulcerative colitis and Crohn's disease

Inflammatory bowel disease (IBD) is the term used to describe chronic inflammation of the bowel, which falls into two categories, ulcerative or mucous colitis or the potentially more serious Crohn's disease.

Ulcerative colitis gives rise to inflammation of the large intestine with spasmodic pain, DIARRHOEA and sometimes blood or mucus in the stools. Other symptoms are tiredness and debility; under-nourishment and anaemia are complications. Crohn's is characterized by severe pain, diarrhoea and bleeding affecting the small and large intestine, accompanied by bouts of fever, weight loss and exhaustion. IBD is most common between the ages of fifteen and thirty-five. Many theories abound as to causation of IBS, including heredity, nutritional deficiency, iatrogenic disease (side-effects of drugs), immune system malfunction, stress, allergies and infection. Orthodox treatment is by anti-inflammatory drugs followed by a course of steroids if that is not successful. There are often problems in coming off high doses of steroids, and weaning off very gradually is necessary. Herbal medicine can be very useful in this case, but take professional advice.

Self-help
A well-balanced diet plus supplements and possibly an Elimination diet (see page 137) to pinpoint food intolerances. Gluten in wheat and other grains is a major culprit, as are dairy products. Take advice and follow the diet under supervision if the colitis is severe. Dietary arachidonic acid, as found mainly in red meats and poor-quality vegetable margarines, should be avoided as it is known to cause intestinal cramping. A natural

fibre diet in moderation is often helpful. Avoid wheat bran. Treatment needs to be long-term: consult a medical herbalist, but in the meantime the following will help symptoms.

Herbal treatment
Anti-inflammatories are the first-choice herbs, with plenty of mucilaginous and soothing herbs, plus Anti-spasmodics and immune system-enhancers especially Garlic. (See Herbal treatment for digestive problems, page 158.)

Supplements
High-potency vitamin and mineral supplements daily, especially Vitamins C, D and E. Minerals may be poorly absorbed in IBD and zinc, potassium and iron supplements needed. 'Food state' vitamins are ideal as absorbed more easily. Fish oils containing EPA and DHA, as in Omega 3 oils, reduce inflammation.

Diverticulitis

This is exclusively a disease of the Western world. It is associated with degeneration of the colon with age and a diet low in fibre and high in refined foods. There is a tendency to CONSTIPATION with small hard stools due to excessive absorption of water. Due to the effect of straining, the colon balloons out into pockets (a diverticulus) which become inflamed and sometimes infected, giving rise to pain, usually on the left side, and on passing motions. Other symptoms may be abdominal distension, nausea, and vomiting and fever if infection is present.

Self-help
Drink plenty of water – at least 2 litres daily – to accompany a diet high in natural fibre from vegetables and fruit.

Exercises help, particularly for the abdominal muscles which stimulate the bowel to work properly. See also Fasting (page 144) which is very beneficial for this problem, allowing the bowel to rest and heal. Try fasting for two to three days initially with fruit juice and fruit, then one day a week for six months. With persistence, the right herbs and careful diet, this problem can be cured. Lactobacillus treatment is useful because a diverticulus often harbours harmful bacteria. Remember, if you have suffered from diverticulitis for years, it will take an equivalent number of months to clear.

Herbal treatment
Anti-inflammatories, anti-spasmodics, and mucilage, particularly Psyllium husk or seed with plenty of water. Sugar beet fibre is preferable to wheat bran fibre, 1 tablespoon daily. To heal, Garlic is excellent: best as 1–2 chopped fresh cloves daily (add chopped parsley if you want to be sociable), or 2 strong capsules daily. *Liver herbs* are particularly beneficial (see Herbal treatment for digestive problems, above).

Supplements
Take Vitamin C to bowel tolerance level for healing (or 1–2g daily for a maximum of two months), particularly if infection is present.

Constipation

This is a widespread problem in Western society. It is generally defined as having less than one bowel movement daily. In fact some people go for two to three days without a movement, which is building up problems for a later date. Constipation can be uncomfortable and gas may build up, causing a lot of wind to pass. Causes are primarily dietary, although stress, nervous tension and lack of exercise contribute. Lack of bowel muscle tone in older women is helped by small regular doses of bitters.

Self-help
Exercise daily – running, jogging, aerobics, dancing, or any other exercise that involves vigorous movement. Correct by increasing the amount of natural dietary fibre from the skins of fruits and vegetables and from wholegrains, such as brown rice and muesli breakfast cereal. Try 2–3 glasses of prune juice initially for relief of stubborn constipation; if this does not work, use the herbs listed below. Try to regulate the bowel naturally through diet. Aperients are gentle laxatives and may be taken in the early stages when re-educating the bowel; always start with the mildest. The strongest laxatives should be taken only in dire need and not on a continual basis.

Herbal treatment
(All doses are for tincture, three times daily, or infusion/decoction of dried herb, 1 cup three times daily.)
For tense bowel:
Either Cramp Bark or Valerian, 2–4ml/g
With

Bitters (to restore bowel tone):
Either Wormwood or Yellow Dock, 1–2ml (fifteen minutes before meals).
If these are not helpful, then:
Aperients:
Either roasted Dandelion Root coffee 1 cup three times daily, or Rhubarb or Liquorice, 2–3ml/g daily.
Or
Laxatives:
Linseed, 1–2 teaspoons soaked in water or added to cereal or 2 teaspoons made into infusion.
Or
Cathartic:
Senna, 2–4 pods soaked in 150ml hot water overnight, take a cup on rising. This should be used only as an emergency treatment. *Note:* Add a small pinch of Ginger powder to this to prevent griping.

Diarrhoea

Caused by hyperactive intestinal activity (peristalsis). It is commonly a symptom of food poisoning, gastroenteritis or gastric flu, in which case there is vomiting as well. Other causes are IRRITABLE BOWEL SYNDROME and ULCERATIVE COLITIS, or gynaecological problems such as Endometriosis (see page 24), inflammation of the Fallopian tubes, or PELVIC INFLAMMATORY DISEASE. In most cases it is necessary to look for the underlying cause.

Herbal treatment
In simple cases the following herbs are effective. Try pure Slippery Elm powder dissolved in warm milk several times a day, to soothe and slow down the bowel. Simple infusions of astringents like Agrimony or Raspberry Leaf tea, 5g per cup three to four times daily, or Red Raspberry Tablets, work quickly. Back this up with Garlic as a natural antibiotic when there is infection. Anti-spasmodics are also helpful (see Herbal treatment for digestive problems, above).

BREAST PROBLEMS

The main problems that affect women's breasts and that are dealt with in this section are Fibrocystic breast disease and Breast cancer.

The breast consists of glandular tissue designed for lactation, with many small ampulae leading to ducts which open on the nipple. The ampulae enlarge with milk production under the influence of the hormone prolactin. Breasts vary greatly in size – bigger breasts usually have more fatty tissue around the glands. Often one is slightly bigger than the other, and this is quite normal.

Women of all ages should be alert to any changes in their breasts. Monthly Breast self-examination (see below) is important so that any changes (or dysplasia) are spotted as soon as possible. Breast cancer is the commonest malignancy in women, especially those in their fifties and sixties.

Nodular or lumpy-feeling tissue before a period is normal, due to hormonal stimulation, and should disappear afterwards, although if it happens every month it may leave some fibrous tissue, or be due to Fibrocystic breast disease.

Fatty lumps or fibroadenoma are most common, and harmless. A benign fluid-filled cyst usually swells pre-menstrually and may be tender. Breast cysts are very common and are associated with the contraceptive pill or HRT. Lumps will often prove benign but it is sensible to have them examined if you find anything unusual. The orthodox procedure is a mammogram X-ray of the breast or thermography to assess temperature changes. A more effective alternative is a needle biopsy of the cyst to remove some cells for examination. A fluid-filled cyst is aspirated to remove the contents.

All women in the UK between the ages of fifty and sixty-four are at present being offered breast-screening by mammogram every three years. Women over sixty-five will not be routinely invited for screening although they can request it.

Breast self-examination

The ideal time to examine your breasts is after a period. You should be looking for any change in the size of your breasts and the way they hang, also any unusual puckering or dimpling of the skin. To do this, stand in front of a mirror and compare your breasts which should move freely as you raise your hands above your head. Next, lie down in bed or in the bath and examine each breast individually. Using a firm, circular motion with the flat of your fingers, stroke around the breast clockwise. Look for any lumps that are solid and do not move with the breast, as these may be tethered to the tissue below. Normal breast tissue moves freely and you should be able to roll any cysts between finger and thumb; they are round and smooth, not rough and craggy. Feel for the glands under your arms, which drain away any unwanted debris from breast tissue; normally you should not be able to feel them, and if you can, you may have an infection. Examine the skin to see if there are any changes, for example in colour or texture, particularly a stippled or 'orange-peel' look. When examining the nipples look for any changes in the way they normally sit or in their colour. Any discharge from the nipple, especially if bloody, should be reported to your doctor immediately.

Fibrocystic breast disease

Part of a breast may become hard and tender following development of cysts, especially before a period. According to naturopathic theory, women who develop cysts are not metabolizing and eliminating their food properly, usually because they are eating more than they need and the metabolites produced then become stored in the body tissues. The quality of food is important too, with an excess of animal proteins (meat and dairy foods) being contra-indicated. Women with cysts also have a tendency to sluggish liver and constipation. The lymph circulation which clears cellular debris is usually sluggish as well. Poor general circulation may be a problem in women with cystic breasts; indications are VARICOSE VEINS, haemorrhoids and cold extremities.

As it is thought that cystic breasts increases the risk of breast cancer by two or three times it is well worth clearing up.

Self-help
If you suffer from cysts every month, avoid fatty foods, especially pre-menstrually, as breast tissue is sensitive to fat. Methylxanthines in coffee, colas and chocolate stimulate their development so should be eliminated. Avoid sugar. Come off the contraceptive pill or HRT as the disruption caused by artificial hormones, particularly oestrogen, stimulates cysts.

Dietary change aimed at cleansing the tissue at a cellular level is essential. Take the measures described above, and aim to eat as many potassium-rich fruits and vegetables, such as celery, as possible, preferably raw. Drink plenty of water.

Try a raw-food diet for two to three weeks, repeated several times over a six-month period. (For further information see Leslie Kenton's *Raw Food Diet* and Liver diet (page 148)).

Stress is also implicated, as with so many female dysfunctions when the delicate hormonal balance is upset. Increase your exercise levels to improve circulation, and if you lead a sedentary life start to exercise now. Lymph circulation is helped enormously by using a bouncer or mini-trampoline for a few minutes every day.

Supplements
Try the following for one month:
Vitamin E as alpha-tocopherol: 400–1000 IUs daily. (This brought an 85 per cent improvement in one study.)
Vitamin A as beta-carotene: 12mg or 25,000 IUs daily.
Vitamin B complex: 100mg daily.
Selenium: 200mcg daily.
Evening Primrose oil: 500mg twice daily.
Iodine as iodized salt or as kelp tablets. (If it helps, carry on for another month, but do not take for longer than two months at this level without professional advice.)

Herbal treatment
This treatment will not remove breast cysts quickly, but over time will soften and shrink them. Importantly, it will prevent recurrence.
Combine from the following (all doses are for tincture or infusion three times daily):
Hepatics (for the liver):
Either Burdock, Dandelion Leaf, 2–5ml/g or Barberry, 2ml/g
With
Lymphatic cleansers:
Either Cleavers, Birch or Meadowsweet, 5ml/g
Add
Circulatory herbs (as needed):
Either Hawthorn Berries, 1–2ml/g or Ginger, 0.25ml/g
Add
Astringents (as needed):
Either Agrimony or Herb Bennet, 5ml/g
Add
Hormonal balancers:
Either Lady's Mantle, Wild Yam or Raspberry Leaf, 5ml/g.
Note: Chaste Berry is contra-indicated for this condition. (For further information see Directions for use of herbs in menopause, page 101.)

Suggested formula

Dandelion Root	20 per cent
Cleavers	20 per cent
Raspberry Leaf	20 per cent
Lady's Mantle	10 per cent
Agrimony	10 per cent
Rhubarb	10 per cent
Ginger	10 per cent

Total: 100ml/g a week. Dose: tincture 5ml three times daily, or infusion/decoction, 1 cup three times daily.

Breast cancer

This is the commonest cancer in women. The latest estimates indicate that one in twelve women will contract breast cancer. There is a one in three or one in two risk for certain women before age fifty.

Risk factors for breast cancer
Close family member (mother or sister) having had breast cancer.
Poverty and poor nutrition.
No children (lack of breast-feeding may be a factor).
Late first pregnancy.
Early menarche.
Late menopause.

There are various types of tumour, and some can spread locally via the lymphatic and blood systems. The cancer may spread to the other breast and can go as far as the lung, liver and other organs. It usually shows as a hard, painless lump often fixed to the skin below, there may be skin changes and a blood-stained discharge from the nipple. Diagnosis is by biopsy and scan to determine if there is any spread of malignancy.

The orthodox treatment is surgical removal of the cancerous tumour. The mastectomy which removes the whole breast has been replaced to some extent by breast conservation surgery (BSC) – either lumpectomy which removes the tumour only, or quadrantectomy which removes part of the breast when the tumour is small and confined to one breast. If there has been spread of malignancy more extensive surgery is often recommended: a radical or modified radical mastectomy removes skin, associated glands under the arm and possibly some of the chest wall.

There has been shown to be no difference in outcome (in terms of recurrence of cancer or length of survival) between the BSC and mastectomy procedures in a number of studies of a simple discrete tumour in one breast. BSC is recommended as the best course of action for women with early stage 1 or 2 breast cancer. This is a far better treatment from the woman's point of view as it is less traumatic psychologically and physically and takes less recovery time. However, you may have to look around for a surgeon willing to perform conservative surgery.

As the loss of a breast is so traumatic psychologically, it is easier if you are informed and in control throughout your treatment. If a biopsy is carried out under anaesthetic, make sure the surgeon will bring you round if he finds cancer so that he can discuss the options, rather than just going on to remove the whole breast.

Lumpectomy is usually followed by a short course of radiotherapy. Other treatment includes use of cytotoxic drugs. These are basically poisonous chemicals that kill the cancer cells that are multiplying fast, and fewer of the normal cells. Side-effects may include fatigue, bleeding, nausea, vomiting and hair loss. Follow-up treatment may include anti-oestrogen drugs if the tumour was shown to be hormone-dependent.

Nowadays there is less fear and more open discussion of breast cancer, and there have been growing complaints from women over the side-effects of cancer treatment: for example, some have found the damage to their arms to prove extensive, varying from unsightly deformity and constant pain to loss of use.

Quality of care varies greatly throughout the UK and there is no consensus on treatment. It seems to be recognized that it is the 'finer tuning' of treatment after surgery that determines whether the cancer will recur. A recent government report states that the best chances for breast cancer patients are in specialist breast care units: there are very few of these at present, and it recommends their extension. Individualization of treatment seems to be the way forward. There has been no unequivocal evidence for the overall effectiveness of either screening or orthodox treatment in terms of incidence or survival in the last twenty years and the record in the UK is the worst in Europe.

Prevention of breast cancer
It is not known what triggers breast cancer. In 1988 a mammogram screening programme was set up

in the UK to screen women between the ages of fifty and sixty-five thought to be high-risk. The aim is to identify tiny cancers before they can be felt as lumps. Out of every 100 women screened one is found to have early cancer. The likelihood of surviving ten years or more is 80–95 per cent following an early treatment. There are pressures to extend the service to younger women in future, although it is not as easy to identify changes in a young woman's breasts as the tissue is much denser.

Many cancers are hormone-dependent, and it is known that hormones affect the progress of cancer. Secretion of adrenaline, as in prolonged stress, exhausts the body and the hormonal system: the toxins that build up as a result of lack of discharge are harmful. Abnormal levels of hormones, especially oestrogen in hormonal contraception, are implicated in cervical cancer, and HRT in menopause with uterine cancer. There is a message here for those women interested in their long-term health.

You can take measures yourself to prevent breast cancer. It is suggested that up to 60 per cent of all cancers may be related to incorrect diet. A vegetarian diet with plenty of fresh food rich in vitamins and minerals is preventive. Eliminate high sugar intake as this has a definite correlation with cancer. There is evidence to show that anti-oxidants Vitamin A, C and E (alpha-tocopherol) protect against cancer. Selenium works in conjunction with Vitamin E to prevent cancer. Omega 3 fatty acids are thought to be preventive of cancer by forming prostaglandins that regulate the functioning of the immune system, so eat plenty of oily fish or take fish oils as supplements; vegetarians should take EFAs in Evening Primrose oil. You should cut down on the overall amount of fat in your diet. Hydrogenated oils, such as in margarine, are now thought to be carcinogenic (see Anti-cancer diet, page 145). Instead use virgin olive oil for cooking and sunflower or safflower for salads. Try to avoid fried foods. If you stir-fry, add a little water to the pan rather than oil. Avoid any foods that are suspected of being carcinogenic. Iodine deficiency and low thyroxine levels may be factors, and taking kelp tablets will supply iodine and other minerals.

Breast-feeding is protective against breast cancer, and the longer it goes on the better the mother's chances of not contracting cancer in later life.

Have yourself checked for heavy metal toxicity via blood or hair sample.

Decrease the levels of environmental toxins to which you are exposed at home and at work: there is a strong connection between environmental pollution and cancer. Look at your life-style – decrease stress levels; get sufficient rest and sleep; avoid overwork for prolonged periods of time. Take aerobic exercise two to three times a week. Work on getting rid of childhood psychological trauma and toxic attitudes.

Treat any existing chronic health problems, especially ALLERGIES.

Try to keep yourself in peak condition. There is no more precious gift from nature than good health.

Cancer self-help

Any complementary medical anti-cancer therapy or herbal treatment should be under the guidance of an experienced practitioner in the field. A cleansing and detoxifying diet may be recommended. Juice fasting (see page 145) may be suitable in the early stages, but not if the patient is too debilitated. General guidance is to stop smoking and drinking alcohol and caffeinated drinks. Do not take sugar. Eat only unadulterated food, to avoid chemical residues, and drink plenty of spring water. Base your diet on wholefoods with just a little poultry, which should be organic. Avoid oestrogen-containing foods such as animal meats, milk and hen's eggs reared on hormone-boosted feed (see Anti-cancer diet, page 145). Avoid foods or additives known to be carcinogenic.

On the supplements side, the work of Dr Linus Pauling has shown improvement in cancer treated with high intakes of Vitamin C, starting at 5g or more daily; this works on the principle that the more seriously ill the patient the more Vitamin C is absorbed from the gut.

Women report that having a diagnosis of breast cancer is like a bereavement and they go through a whole range of emotions; it can be extremely shocking and stressful, and there is no doubt that counselling is very important. Psychotherapeutic methods of treatment are gaining credence as it is recognized that a person's psychological state has an important bearing on their recovery. It is harmful to suggest that there is a cancer 'type' as this can lead a woman to believe that she is to blame for her predicament; on the other hand, there is a definite correlation between passivity and lack of will to live and survival rate. It is often the most awkward patients that beat impossible odds. The Simontons have demonstrated the usefulness of self-suggestion techniques to support the body's ability to heal: these include visualization, where for example you imagine the cancer is being cleared away by beneficial cells. Meditation, yoga, prayer, healing or anything that provides deep relaxation has a place. Studies have also shown that belief in a treatment, whether orthodox or alternative, affects how well a patient does. Bear in mind that it is difficult for anyone to predict how a woman will respond to the challenge of breast cancer, and different methods will work in different ways on different individuals.

It is possible today to take the best that orthodox surgery has to offer, worsen its ill-effects, and supplement it with gentle, positive therapy. (For various accounts of this see Dr Bernie Siegal's *Love, Medicine and Miracles*, Louise Hay's *Heal Yourself* and Beatta Bishop's *A Time To Heal*.) For the Bristol Cancer Diet contact The Bristol Cancer Centre (see page 202).

Supplements

The following supplements are recommended in addition to allopathic treatment of breast cancer, although the use of vitamins and minerals is still seen as an unorthodox way of treating cancer by many specialists.

Vitamin C: 4–5mg daily in divided doses of 1000mcg to start with. It can be increased, but take advice on this.

Vitamin A: 800 IUs daily. To increase the effects of radiation treatment: up to 10,000 IUs daily for a week afterwards. 1600 IUs daily for two to three weeks is protective against some of radiation's harmful side-effects.

Vitamin E: 600–800mcg daily.

Among the minerals zinc and magnesium are most important. 1 multi-vitamin and 1 multi-mineral tablet including trace minerals daily, and potassium iodide 200mcg.

Coenzyme Q is an anti-oxidant and immune-system stimulant which helps heal side-effects of radiation and cytotoxic drugs.

CANCER

See under BREAST PROBLEMS, CERVICAL PROBLEMS, OVARIAN CANCER, UTERUS PROBLEMS.

CANDIDIASIS

Candida, or monilia, commonly known as thrush, is caused by the proliferation of a normally benign fungus, candida albicans, on the mucous membranes of the vagina. It is a parasite that does not normally cause problems – its spores are found wherever there are people. However, if the conditions are right it can proliferate rapidly on the mucous linings of the vagina, bowel, mouth or skin. This causes thrush, a thick, white, cheesy discharge which smells yeasty. White plaques can be seen in the mouth or vagina. In the second stage, the spores multiply and can enter their mycelial or fungus form in which they grow by branching and invade surrounding tissues, causing candidiasis. It is estimated that up to 30 per cent of people are suffering from problems resulting from candida infestation.

Symptoms are burning and irritation of the external genitalia. Scratching can cause vulval soreness and swelling. The vagina and vulva look very red and inflamed. Intercourse is painful or impossible; and in any case is not advisable during candida infection. Urination may cause burning.

It is known that repeated use of antibiotics for urinary or other infections destroys the ecobalance of the flora normally present in the intestinal tract, allowing the yeast to colonize. A lowering of the body's resistance for any reason such as use of steroids, hormonal contraceptives and immunosuppressive drugs allows candida to get a hold. The ecobalance can be changed through use of vaginal hygiene aids and perfumed toiletries. Diabetes is a possible cause of persistent thrush. Stressful life-styles, emotional upsets, lack of sleep and poor diet among other things, may predipsose to the condition.

Candida can affect the bowel and spread throughout the intestines (when symptoms are diarrhoea, distension, wind, nausea) and there is a strong connection between vaginal and intestinal candida. It is thought that in the second stage or mycelial form it can penetrate the intestinal lining, allowing a portal of entry for incompletely digested food particles to enter the bloodstream. (This may cause an assault on the immune system and be responsible for food sensitivities or ALLERGIES.) Toxic waste is produced by candida activity and can also be absorbed into the blood, particularly affecting the brain.

Many symptoms have been attributed to chronic candida infestation including the following:

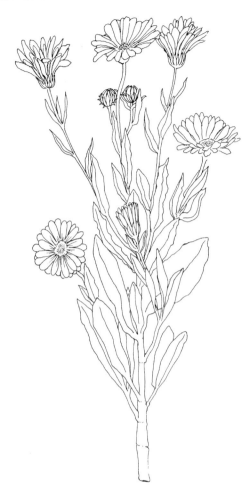

Marigold *(Calendula officinalis)*

depression, anxiety, irritability, heartburn, lethargy, food and environmental ALLERGIES especially yeast-related, acne, migraine, sore joints, recurring CYSTITIS, painful periods (see page 22), PMS (see page 16) and recurrent VAGINITIS. It is thought to be a causal factor in gynaecological diseases such as Endometriosis (see page 24) and can worsen menopausal symptoms (see page 85). Linked to poor immunity, it is implicated in many cases of Chronic fatigue syndrome (see page 108). A further constellation of allergy symptoms makes the situation much worse. (The connection between many of these symptoms and candida is borne out in practice but orthodox medical opinion is still reserving judgement.)

Candida can be very stubborn to treat and often recurs. If it becomes widespread in the body it is known as systemic candidiasis and represents a severe breakdown of immunity. This is a rare condition and hospitalization is imperative. It is often a complication of AIDS.

Diagnosis of candida relies on vaginal swab or stool culture. (*Note:* Candida is not always found in the bowel unless it is in its second, overgrowth stage). The diagnosis of candidiasis relies on case history and the result of treatment. (*Note:* Candida may be present without causing symptoms.) Orthodox treatment includes anti-fungals such as Nystatin and Canestan applied to the vagina. Nystatin and a stronger-anti fungal, Diflucan, is also given internally, often for several months. But it is not recommended for long periods of time because of the possibility of liver damage. These anti-fungals are effective, but if the underlying causes have not been dealt with or the condition is deeply entrenched, thrush will come back quickly. It is essential to adjust diet and rebalance the flora in the gut and vagina (see below). This may take several months too, but is longer-lasting.

Self-help
Candida thrives on sugar- and yeast-containing foods in an alkaline environment, and clinical experience shows that avoidance of these can vastly improve and in many cases cure the condition. (See Anti-candida diet, page 139.) Often there are cravings for those foods that make the problem worse, such as bread, sugar, cheese and alcohol, which make the sufferer feel better initially but then lead to a low. A higher than normal fibre diet using oat bran fibre is recommended to speed transit time through the gut.

Anti-yeast medications can be avoided by reinoculating the bowel or vagina with bio-cultures of lactobacillus, as found in natural live yoghurt. These provide symbiotic, good acid-promoting bacteria to counter the parasite invasion. *Note:* If you are going to apply yoghurt internally, ideally do it *after* a herbal douche, so that the lactobacillus can recolonize the vagina. The yoghurt can be applied with a finger or spoon (a bit messy) or an applicator used for vaginal creams, or it can be diluted with boiled water and used as a douche.

Avoid nylon underwear and tight-fitting clothing that encourages the sort of warm, damp environment in which candida thrives. As it can be passed back and forth between you and your partner, he should be treated as well, even if he has no symptoms, using an external application. Using a condom protects against this to some extent. It is important to have a smear test a week after finishing treatment to see that it has gone.

Raise your general level of health to improve your immunity. Deal with ALLERGY if necessary. As candida in the bowel is connected with toxicity and poor elimination, Colon cleansing is recommended in stubborn cases.

Herbal treatment
The aim initially is to return candida to its first, non-invasive stage. It is then necessary to take a whole-person approach with herbs to clear the condition completely. Those recommended include: Red Clover, Echinacea, Usnea (Bear's Lichen), Golden Seal, Garlic, Burdock, Dandelion Root, as dried herbs combined in infusion/decoction. Dose: 100g a week, 1 cup three to four times daily. It is best to avoid alcoholic tinctures in this condition. Some of these herbs are available separately as tablets. It may take from one to six months for the candida to clear, depending on how long it has been a problem.

For further information see Directions for use of herbs in chronic fatigue syndrome (page 118).

Douches:
For local treatment try a lemon juice douche first to alter the pH of the vagina; this will sometimes control a mild infection. Add 10ml lemon juice to ½ litre water. Still use lactobacillus treatment afterwards. If this does not work, use herbal douches or herbal pessaries: you can use dried herb or tincture to make douches, powdered herb or tincture for pessaries (see pages 12 and 10).

Douche with equal parts of Chamomile, Marigold, Golden Seal and Thyme tincture plus 1 drop of Tea Tree essential oil diluted with fifteen parts water (it may nip to start with but this soon wears off). If using dried herbs, combine to make an infusion, then add Tea Tree oil. Use once or twice daily, depending on severity, until the condition clears – usually two weeks.

Pessaries
These are made with Chamomile, Marigold, Thyme and Tea Tree oil added to a cocoa butter base (see page 10). They melt inside the vagina, gradually releasing the beneficial herbs, and are best used at night. Marigold ointment with Tea Tree oil added, 5 drops to 50g, is anti-fungal and soothing used locally. Apply two to three times daily.

(Proprietary-brand pessaries and cream containing Tea Tree oil can be purchased over the counter.)

Note: Essential oils are highly effective in small doses and so should always be less than 1 per cent of a dilution, to avoid burning the delicate membranes.

Supplements
Make sure supplements are hypoallergenic and yeast-free.
Vitamin C: 500mg daily for one to six weeks or until the condition clears up.
Vitamin B complex: 50mg daily, including Vitamin B₅ (pantothenic acid): 200mg daily.
Vitamin E: 400 IUs daily.
Vitamin A as beta-carotene: 10,000 IUs or 6mg daily.
Biotin: 200mcg daily (conversion to candida second stage depends on deficiency of this).
Zinc: 30mg daily.
Garlic: 1 capsule or tablet daily.
Probiotics or lactobacilli (acidophilus) as capsules or powder: 1 capsule or 1g three times daily, or eat one large tub of live yoghurt. (Lactobacilli can also be bought in ready-made pessaries.)

Note: After a course of douching always take lactobacilli for one to two weeks to restore natural bowel flora.

Caprylic acid, a derivative of coconut oil, is sometimes used in stubborn cases. Take advice as regards dosage. It should be taken with a daily multi-vitamin and multi-mineral.

Try supplements for four to six weeks and continue for longer if thrush is recurrent, or if you have had a candida problem for a long time.

Enzyme-potentiated desensitization
If these natural measures are not effective, EPD is sometimes appropriate, especially if there are multiple allergies involved. The enzyme complex is there to potentiate it; the effect is to galvanize the immune system into action. A very dilute amount of the substance is injected under the skin and many sufferers report relief. Desensitization can also be accomplished homoeopathically with a very dilute, potentized oral dose of candida, and then the programme of supplements above followed. (For information see Institute of Allergy Therapists, page 202.)

CERVICAL PROBLEMS

Diseases affecting the cervix, or opening of the uterus to the vagina, include inflammation or cervicitis, cervical erosion, dysplasia of the cervical cells, and cervical cancer. Up to 2000 women a year die of invasive cervical cancer in the UK and many of these mortalities could have been prevented.

Symptoms are few or none except in the later stages of cancer so it is imperative to have regular tests to detect any changes early. In the vaginal smear or pap test a sample of cells is scraped from the cervix and examined under a microscope. It may be a little uncomfortable but should not be painful. You may have to wait several weeks for the result. Because of the high degree of anxiety that it provokes, many health authorities now provide information on the test and results.

A massive cervical screening programme has been instituted in the UK. In other countries it has been demonstrated that intensive cancer screening has reduced incidence and mortality from cervical carcinoma. Those women aged thirty to fifty should have a smear every three years and then yearly from age fifty to sixty-five. Following an abnormal result the test is done at six months initially, then yearly for two years.

As the orthodox approach in the early stages consists only of surgical removal of the offending cells, herbal treatment and vitamin therapy used in conjunction have a lot to offer.

Common benign conditions of the cervix like cervicitis, cervical erosion, cervical polyps and cysts all respond well to herbs, particularly applied locally as douches, pessaries, etc.

Cervicitis

Cervicitis is an infection of the cervix and is a common gynaecological problem. Symptoms include a thick, yellowish-white discharge, with or without traces of blood. Making love may be painful. There may be aching lower abdominal pain and pain on passing water. It is usually diagnosed during a vaginal examination by speculum. The cells of the mouth and neck of the uterus appear red and inflamed, usually as the result of infection. If the glandular cells inside the cervical canal are turned to the outside (called an ectropion), they are unprotected and prone to infection. The vagina is not a sterile environment, but the proliferation of germs occurs if its flora are disturbed in some way, or if general health is poor. Chlamydia infection is a frequent cause of bacterial vaginitis, cervicitis and urethritis. Young women and those on the contraceptive pill are most at risk. Herpes virus, abortion, childbirth and the IUD are all possible causes. It is important to get treatment as PELVIC INFLAMMATORY DISEASE, sterility and difficulties in pregnancy and childbirth can result if untreated.

Cervicitis is also caused less commonly by a gonococcal venereal infection and in this case should only be treated by a medical practitioner.

Orthodox treatment is with antibiotics – several courses may be needed. Surgical treatments include cauterization by freezing or laser. Cervicitis can be successfully treated herbally but it is best to take advice from a medical herbalist skilled in this field, following tests for bacteria. It may take several treatments over a period of weeks, stopping for periods, combining herbs to take with douches of anti-bacterials and essential oils applied internally.

Herbal treatment

Antibiotic herbs to take internally: Echinacea, most effective for purulent infections, initially 20–40 drops of tincture diluted, every half hour until symptoms improve, then three times daily. Usnea (Bear's Lichen) is an important alternative antibiotic herb.

Treating the whole person is important, and a herbalist would use remedies such as Dandelion, Burdock, Garlic, Cleavers, Parsley Piert and Sweet Violet. Herbal analgesics for pain and discomfort can be added in as needed.

Useful herbs for douches include Barberry, Myrrh, Golden Seal and Echinacea, diluted one part to fifteen parts water. Cocoa butter suppositories can include one drop of essential oil of either Lemon, Oregano, Garlic, Thuja or Cypress (see pages 12 and 10 for douches and pessaries). These can also be applied very dilute on a home-made tampon of sterile gauze.

Note: Essential oils are highly effective in small doses and should not be more than 1 per cent of a dilution, to avoid burning the delicate cervix.

Self-help

Make life-style changes – take more exercise, relax more, stop smoking, drink less alcohol. Promote general health. Cold sitz baths (see page 12) to get circulation to the area going with water up to your hips are invigorating. Start with a few minutes and work up to ten minutes daily. Try Abdominal and pelvic exercises as well to improve circulation (see page 195).

Supplements

Take supplements for one to two months or until the condition clears.
Vitamin C: 1000–2000mg daily.
Vitamin A as beta-carotene: 6mg daily.
Vitamin E: 600 IUs daily.
Zinc: 30mg daily plus 1 multi-mineral tablet daily. Locally, Vitamin E from a capsule broken open and applied to the cervix with a clean finger every night until the condition clears.

Cervical polyps and cysts

Polyps are harmless and do not require treatment unless they become very large. Usually inside the uterus, they are fragile and may bleed if they protrude from the cervix. Orthodox treatment is surgical removal.

A retention or Nabothian cyst is caused when a gland in the cervix becomes blocked during erosion. It may feel like a small pea on the rim of the cervix and is harmless.

Herbal treatment

Follow guidelines for treating the whole person (see Dysplasia, below) and in addition try douching with equal parts of Cranesbill, Witch Hazel, Birth Root and Golden Seal, diluted one part to fifteen parts water, for one to two months if you want to shrink a cyst or polyp (hold in for at least ten minutes). (See also uterine FIBROIDS for treatment that may help polyps.)

Cervical erosion or eversion

The outside of the cervix – the part that extends into the vagina – is lined with a type of horny cell found on the outside skin of the body, to protect the entrance to the uterus. The mucus-producing cells in the cervical canal are much more sensitive. If these cells start to appear outside the canal in place of the tougher cells it is termed an eversion. The cells are then at risk of damage or erosion. Eversion can occur during pregnancy or puberty or under influence of hormones. Women on the contraceptive pill are more at risk.

There are not necessarily any symptoms although there may be a discharge, possibly infected. It is usually diagnosed after a visual vaginal examination. As this is the area where cervical cancer develops, care must be taken. Orthodox treatment is to remove the cells by cryosurgery (freezing) if it is extensive or if dysplasia is suspected. Erosion that does not reverse can lead to cervical dysplasia and cancer. However, it is estimated that 95 per cent of women suffer it at one time or other in their lives, and it usually reverts to normal.

Herbal treatment

Follow advice to strengthen immunity. Take the herbs and supplements suggested for Dysplasia below for a month, or until you have the results of the next smear test. In addition you can use a douche composed of the following: equal parts tincture of Thuja, Golden Seal, Marigold, Witch Hazel and Marshmallow, diluted one part to fifteen parts water once daily for two months or until the test result shows the condition has cleared (see page 12 for directions).

Dysplasia or cervical pre-cancerous changes

Dysplasia means growth of abnormal cells as their shape or organization changes. It is diagnosed following a vaginal smear or pap test and examination. It is often the result of untreated cervical erosion. Three transitional pre-cancerous stages are universally recognized within the general heading of cervical intraepithelial neoplasia (CIN).

In the early stages dysplasia is a benign condition. Although a positive smear test result is alarming, often it only means cervical erosion or inflammation, or it may be early metaplasia which is a transformation to a horny or defensive type of cell. This is harmless and reversible when the irritation goes. *Note:* A request for a second smear may be made if not enough cells were obtained at the first one. Ask to be given as much information as possible.

Invasive carcinoma is usually preceded by a long period of dysplasia and it is this that the smear test is seeking to find. If you have an abnormal test result you may be recalled for another test, called a colposcopy, when the cells will be examined through a high-powered binocular microscope – it is not painful. Sometimes a biopsy of a small section of the mouth of the cervix will be taken for examination, for which there should be a local anaesthetic.

Treatment of pre-invasive lesions is by cauterization, usually laser these days, or by cryosurgery (freezing), for which there should be a local anaesthetic. In cases where there is widespread local moderate to severe dysplasia, treatment may be a cone biopsy that removes a cone-shaped section of the cervix. This is examined to determine if it is invasive. As this is a fairly major surgical procedure and can cause problems in any future pregnancy as it affects dilation of the cervix, it should not be done unless absolutely necessary.

Spontaneous regression of the cells from dysplastic back to normal does occur without treatment, although it is also believed that it can progress rapidly to cancer in some cases.

Some authorities now see cervical dysplasia as a sexually transmitted disease related to infection, particularly with the human papilloma virus (HPV) that causes genital warts (Condylomata) in women and men. Safe sex, using a condom, may well be preventive.

Two clear repeat smears after an abnormal one are the indication to go back to a smear every two years.

Self-help

Dysplasia may be due to a defect of the immune system and repeated exposure to irritations from substances introduced to the vagina, or to infection, so take action to increase your immunity. If you or your partner have genital warts they can be locally removed by freezing. Genital herpes should also be treated if you have a recurring problem.

After a dysplasia result, take vitamins and mineral supplements and herbal remedies while you wait for a follow-up test. In some cases where this has been done the next test has proved normal. Vitamin A particularly is known to affect cellular differentiation and prevent malignant transformation. The aim is to raise your general level of health, as dysplasia reflects a generally low level.

Life-style changes are also advised: stop smoking, discontinue the contraceptive pill or HRT, start a diet aimed at maximum immune system support, based on fresh whole foods, low in fat and sugar, and high in fibre. Take no stimulants or recreational drugs and eat no refined foods (see Healthy wholefood diet, page 126). Avoid foods or additives known to be carcinogenic. Avoid oestrogen-containing foods such as animal meats, milk and hen's eggs reared on hormone-boosted feed.

A complementary medicine practitioner could look at whether you have a possible tendency to cancer and suggest corrective measures.

Herbal treatment

Self-help measures should be used *in addition* to any orthodox treatment recommended. Consult a medical herbalist skilled in this field if you are diagnosed with moderate to severe dysplasia, classified as CIN 2–3. The following is *only* for early dysplasia or CIN 1.

Follow the rule of treating the whole person. Try a two-month programme of herbs and supplements. Herbal remedies that have been found useful in treating dysplasia are Red Clover, Liquorice, Golden Seal and Dandelion Root. Take in equal parts as tinctures or teas, 2.5ml or 1 cup three times daily for eight weeks. In addition the following remedies should be applied.

First week: Apply Vitamin A (as retinol, 25,000 IUs) on a tampon nightly. Try to place as high as possible to reach the cervix. (Vitamin A as a cream is difficult to get in the UK, so break open a capsule.)

Second week: Use a pessary nightly made up of Myrrh, Marigold, Golden Seal, Marshmallow and Cranesbill, tinctures ½ml each with 1 drop of each of Thuja and Cypress essential oils in a cocoa butter base: this quantity makes five pessaries (see page 10 for directions). If you don't want to make a pessary, soak a home-made tampon of gauze in an infusion of the herbs, remembering to tie on a piece of cotton to remove it with.

Third and fourth weeks: Repeat weeks one and two.

Note: Do not exceed the amount of essential oils as they can burn the delicate cervix.

Supplements

Take supplements for two months to start with, or longer depending on results of follow-up test.

Vitamin C: 5000mg daily (food sources: all fruits and vegetables, especially blackcurrants, citrus fruits, rosehips, broccoli, green peppers).

Vitamin A as beta-carotene: 6mg daily or 10,000 IUs (food sources: green leafy vegetables, carrots and other orange vegetables).

Folic acid: 5mg daily.

Vitamin B complex: 50–100mg daily (food source: brewer's yeast).

Vitamin E: 600 IUs daily (food sources: cold-pressed vegetable oils).

Multi-mineral: 1 daily.
Potassium iodide (food sources: shellfish and other foods rich in iodine).

Cervical cancer

Cervical cancer is most common in the forty-five to seventy-five age group. The lowest-risk group is under thirty-five. The number of younger women affected seems to be on the increase, however. (Cervical cancer appears to be connected to hormone levels, especially oestrogen; more widespread use of the contraceptive pill may be a cause.)

Risk factors for cervical cancer
First intercourse at early age.
Multiple sexual partners through life.
Sexual exposure to men who have many sexual partners (more likely to have contact with a woman with cervical dysplasia).
Contracting a sexually transmitted disease, especially HPV.
Sexual exposure to men of low socioeconomic status.
Being a heavy smoker (two to three times incidence).
Three or more children.
Poor diet.
Long-term hormonal contraceptive use.
Chronic cervicitis.
Contracting genital herpes virus infection.
Exposure to environmental carcinogens.

Cervical cancer is diagnosed when a colposcopy or biopsy finds invasive carcinoma, in other words it has spread beyond the immediate cells at the mouth of the cervix. It may have spread locally or further via the lymph system. Cervical cancer is classified in four stages, depending on severity.

There are often no symptoms of cervical cancer. Sometimes there may be a bloodstained discharge or slight vaginal bleeding in between periods, during defecation or after intercourse in a menstruating woman. After menopause any bleeding should be examined seriously. In the later stages there may be an infected foul-smelling vaginal discharge. Treatment depends on the cancer stage that is diagnosed, whether it is confined to the uterus or has spread. Orthodox treatment is by radiotherapy via the vagina and/or externally and hysterectomy if necessary. Treatment may include chemotherapy.

Self-help
Stop taking the contraceptive pill or HRT. Lose weight if overweight, lower blood pressure if it is high. Change diet to an optimally healthy one – low-fat, high-fibre, no caffeine, no meat, a little fish or chicken, all organically grown or reared. Avoid foods or additives known to be carcinogenic. Avoid oestrogen-containing foods such as animal meats, milk and hen's eggs reared on hormone-boosted feed (see Anti-cancer diet, page 145). Take a serious look at your life-style, making any changes that are necessary. Lower stress levels particularly. Learn self-suggestion techniques. Contact Bristol Cancer Care Centre for advice, see page 202. Ask for counselling if you need it. (See also Cancer self-help, page 164).

Herbal treatment
Any complementary medical anti-cancer therapy or herbal treatment should be under the guidance of a practitioner skilled in the field and in conjunction with surgery if necessary. A cleansing or detoxifying diet may be suggested to start with.

Supplements
Take the following until you have a clean bill of health.
Vitamin C: from 5000–10,000mg daily, using the bowel tolerance rule. (Start at 1000mg daily and increase intake gradually by 1000mg daily until it causes loose bowel motions, then cut back by 1000mg.) Food sources: all fruits and vegetables, especially blackcurrants, citrus fruits, rosehips, broccoli, green peppers.
Vitamin A as beta-carotene: 12mg daily or 20,000 IUs. (Food sources: green leafy vegetables, carrots, and other orange vegetables.)
Folic acid: 5mg daily.
Vitamin E: 600 IUs daily. (Food sources: cold-pressed vegetable oils.)
Multi-mineral: 1 daily.
Zinc: 50mg daily.
Selenium: 200mcg daily.
Potassium iodide (food sources: shellfish and other foods rich in iodine).
Multi-vitamin: 1 daily.

Prevention of cervical cancer
Following treatment of any dysplasia it is wise to follow a long-term immune system support diet. Make eating really healthily a priority in your life. Give up smoking permanently and reserve alcoholic drinks for special occasions. Take appropri-

ate supplements daily, such as a multi-vitamin or multi-mineral.

Have regular cervical smears. It is safer if your partner uses a condom, or thoroughly washes his penis before intercourse. Treat any vaginal infections as soon as they occur. Avoid hormonal contraceptives.

Think about your life-style and make improvements in the quality of your life where possible. Learn to cope with stress as it is an integral part of modern life, but cut back if you suffer from the cult of busyness. Some women literally never have a minute to themselves, apart from when asleep! Learn to relax properly and give your attention to solving any emotional problems; some cancers follow bereavement, separation, divorce or other loss.

CONSTIPATION

See under BOWEL PROBLEMS.

CYSTITIS

See under URINARY PROBLEMS.

DIARRHOEA

See under BOWEL PROBLEMS.

DIVERTICULITIS

See under BOWEL PROBLEMS.

DRY VAGINA

See under VAGINAL PROBLEMS.

EMOTIONAL PROBLEMS

Emotional and mental problems are inextricably tied up with the physical. The concept of psychosomatic illness, that is, the power of mind to affect the physical functions of the body, is not a new one, and has been used in the past as an explanation for some unexplained disease symptoms. Today it is becoming much more widely recognized. A branch of medicine called Neuro-

Immunology is studying the connection between the brain and the immune system. A newly named illness, post-traumatic stress disorder, recognizes the specific effects trauma can have on the mind and body.

The affect of prolonged stress, such as overwork, over-responsibility, or worry, is potentially physically harmful. (See also Fatigue and Chronic Fatigue Syndrome, pages 107–21.) A certain amount of stress makes for good performance, but as Dr Hans Selye in his book *The Stress of Life* shows, after a while 'general adaptation syndrome' comes into play to allow the body to continue under this pressure, and if it goes on for too long then health breakdown begins.

Mental health is subjective: who is to say one person is healthier in their mind than another? It is only when symptoms cause someone to seek help, or their behaviour becomes anti-social and is perceived as a problem by family and society that it is labelled mental illness. Psychiatric terminology, while useful for diagnosis, results in putting emotional and mental states into neatly labelled boxes where they do not easily fit. Unfortunately it is beyond the scope of this book to deal with the various manifestations of mental illness. Much, however, can be done to help, and a visit to a qualified practitioner is recommended.

It is important to remember that some negative emotions are appropriate to certain situations, such as depression after loss of a loved one, but this should gradually lift in time. Loss of a partner, divorce, or loss of job are obvious causes of distress. Major life-changes often precipitate emotional upheaval, even happy events such as marriage and the birth of children. Emotions are there to help us come to terms with new situations and should not be denied or suppressed. Tranquilliser drugs prescribed for unhappy occasions should be taken on a very temporary basis as they mask the problem, leading to addiction in many cases, the person being unable to come to terms with the original situation.

In a world where the main focus is on having and doing rather than being, true inner contentment essential to mental and emotional well-being is hard to find. There are many techniques for accessing this state, including deep relaxation, meditation, prayer, communing with nature, etc. What works for you is the important thing; only your own experience can ascertain the real and lasting value of a deeply meaningful practice. Meditation, once considered unusual, is now almost universally recognized as a beneficial therapeutic exercise.

Herbal treatment is used to relieve symptoms by calming mind and body. It alleviates anxiety and by nourishing the nervous system can ease depression; it is gentler and takes longer than orthodox drugs to work but has no side-effects. Herbs and Dr Bach's Flower Remedies need to be seen as part of a 'whole person' approach in conjunction with counselling or psychotherapy.

Depression

For specific treatments see Post-natal depression (page 66), Emotional problems in pregnancy (page 46), Menopausal depression (page 90).

Depression covers a wide range of negative experience from feeling down and 'blue' to clinically diagnosed depression with a host of possible physical as well as mental symptoms. Two main types in women are recognized: reactive depression, in response to adversity or traumatic life events by women vulnerable to stress, which is usually temporary. In contrast, endogenous depression, with recurring depressive episodes where no precipitating factors are found, is usually blamed on hormonal or biochemical imbalances. This type of depression is established over a period of time and symptoms include sleep problems, weight loss or gain, exhaustion, loss of concentration and enjoyment, and sometimes despair and loss of sense of any meaning to life. Suicidal thoughts are common and actual suicide does occur among this group more frequently than with any other illness. If you start to think in this way, get help quickly.

Orthodox treatment is by anti-depressant drugs.

Herbal treatment

Nourishing tonics (trophorestoratives): Lemon Balm, Oat, Vervain, St John's Wort, Skullcap. Total: 100ml/g a week. Dose: tincture, 5ml three times daily, or infusion/decoction of dried herb in equal parts, 1 cup three times daily.
Adaptogens: Ginseng Root or Siberian Ginseng, 5ml twice daily.
Nervous system stimulants: Rosemary or Damiana, 50ml/g a week.

Try the nourishing tonics in the early stages for six to eight weeks, then add stronger herbs as improvement takes place.

See also Dr Bach's Flower Remedies, Gorse, Mustard, Sweet Chestnut (see page 174).

Anxiety

For specific treatments see Emotional problems during pregnancy (page 40), Emotional problems of menopause (page 90).

Anxiety is a normal feeling and is constructive in some situations. Anxiety neurosis occurs when the anxiety is out of all proportion to the situation. It may be caused by fear and stress of various sorts or may result from specific events or childhood experiences. Women who have a lifelong pattern of vulnerability to stress are more likely to suffer from it. It may be all-pervasive or occur in certain situations only. Agoraphobia or fear of wide-open spaces is an extreme form.

Symptoms are often temporary but can make life very difficult for some, varying from nervousness with shaking and sweating in certain situations, to heart palpitations and panic attacks when the person fears she is losing control. Talking yourself down is possible and various coping techniques such as creative visualization, once well established, can help even in the worst situations. Counselling or psychotherapy may be needed. Orthodox treatment is by tranquillizer-type drugs, although these are more restricted nowadays because of the danger of addiction. Herbal medicine is very effective in helping women come off these drugs.

Herbal treatment

Anxiolytics (in order of strength): Lime Flowers, Chamomile, Betony, Hyssop, Valerian in equal parts. Total: 100ml/g a week. Dose: tincture, 5ml three times daily, or infusion/decoction of dried herb in equal parts, 1 cup three times daily. Add Hops where there is tension, 40ml/g per week.
Nourishing tonics: Skullcap and Oats in equal parts. Dose: 50–100ml/g a week as tincture or infusion.

Stress and nervous tension

Stress is probably one of the major causes of people's problems today. The pressure experienced by time-tabling everything extends from the workplace into the home until it may seem there is no place to relax. The body is constantly in a state of alarm. Women especially are at risk if they are working mothers and wives. Stress is blamed for many physical ailments including IRRITABLE BOWEL SYNDROME, ulcers and other digestive problems; high blood pressure, hardening of the arteries and strokes; anxiety, irritability, hormonal problems and insomnia among others. It reduces resistance to disease. The body systems most affected by general adaptation syndrome are the nervous system and endocrine system. Symptoms of their over-activity are exhaustion, irritability, feeling jittery and anxious. (See also Tiredness and Chronic fatigue syndrome, pages 107 and 108.)

Self-help

Many women are unwilling or unable to make the life-style changes necessary to alleviate stress. Try to make any changes you can to allow a slower pace. Meditation twice a day may be an effective method of coping; there are different techniques but all bring about beneficial physical changes, including slow alpha brain waves equated with deep relaxation, lowering of heart and breathing rates and increased skin electrical resistance show-

ing improved body functioning. It is a discipline that needs regular practice for maximum effect but is well worth it.

Herbal treatment

While not being a substitute for relaxation, the formula below has been helpful in many cases.

Valerian	30 per cent
Skullcap	30 per cent
Hops	20 per cent
Vervain	20 per cent

Total: 100ml/g a week. Dose: tincture, 5ml three times daily, or infusion/decoction of dried herb in equal parts, 1 cup three times a day.

There are many proprietary herbal brands available on the market. Check constituents before buying.

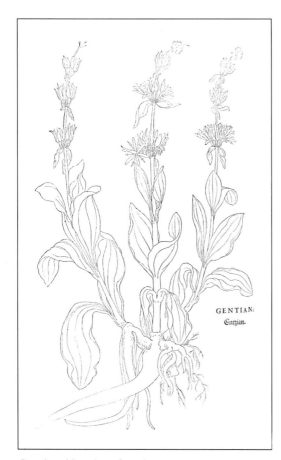

Gentian (*Gentiana lutea*)

Dr Bach's Flower Remedies

(Reproduced with the kind permission of The Dr Edward E. Bach Centre)

General indications for use for emotional problems

1 *Agrimony.* Hiding worries behind a brave face.

2 *Aspen.* Apprehension for no known reason.

3 *Beech.* Criticism and intolerance of others.

4 *Centaury.* Weak will; exploited or imposed upon.

5 *Cerato.* Doubting own judgement, seeking confirmation of others.

6 *Cherry Plum.* Uncontrolled irrational thoughts.

7 *Chestnut Bud.* Refusal to learn by experience, continual repetition of same mistakes.

8 *Chicory.* Over-possessiveness – self-centredness, clinging and over-protectiveness, especially of loved ones.

9 *Clematis.* Inattentiveness, dreaminess, absent-mindedness, mental escapism.

10 *Crab Apple.* The 'Cleanser'. Self-disgust/detestation. Feeling ashamed of ailments.

11 *Elm.* Sense of being overwhelmed by inadequacy and responsibility.

12 *Gentian.* Despondency.

13 *Gorse.* Pessimism, defeatism.

14 *Heather.* Talkativeness, obsession with own troubles and experiences.

15 *Holly.* Hatred, envy, jealousy, suspicion.

16 *Honeysuckle.* Living in the past, nostalgia. Homesickness.

17 *Hornbeam.* Monday morning feeling, procrastination.

18 *Impatiens*. Impatience, irritability.

19 *Larch*. Lack of self-confidence, feelings of inferiority. Fear of failure.

20 *Mimulus*. Fear of *known* things. Shyness. Timidity.

21 *Mustard*. Dark cloud that descends, making sufferer saddened and low for no known reason.

22 *Oak*. Inability to struggle bravely against illness or adversity in sufferer who is normally courageous/strong.

23 *Olive* . Fatigue, loss of energy.

24 *Pine*. Guilt complex, self-reproach even for mistakes of others. Constant apologizing.

25 *Red Chestnut*. Obsessive care and concern for others.

26 *Rock Rose*. Sudden alarm, scared, panicky feeling.

27 *Rock Water*. Rigid-mindedness, self-denial.

28 *Scleranthus*. Uncertainty, indecision, vacillation. Fluctuating moods.

29 *Star of Bethlehem*. For all the effects of serious news, or fright following an accident, etc.

30 *Sweet Chestnut*. Utter dejection, bleak outlook.

31 *Vervain*. Over-enthusiasm, fanatical beliefs.

32 *Vine*. Dominating/inflexible/tyrannical/autocratic/arrogant characteristics. Usually good sense of leadership.

33 *Walnut*. Assists in adjustment to transition or change, e.g. puberty, menopause, divorce, new surroundings.

34 *Water Violet*. Pride, reserve, enjoyment of being alone.

35 *White Chestnut*. Persistent unwanted thoughts. Preoccupation with some worry or episode. Mental arguments.

36 *Wild Oat*. Helps determine intended path in life.

37 *Wild Rose*. Resignation. Apathy.

38 *Willow*. Resentment, embitterment, self-pity.

39 *Rescue Remedy*. A combination remedy. All-purpose emergency composite for the effects of anguish, stress of examinations, etc. Comforting, calming and reassuring to those distressed by startling experiences.

ENDOMETRIAL CANCER

See under UTERUS PROBLEMS.

ENDOMETRIOSIS

See Menstrual Problems (page 24).

ENDOMETRITIS

See under UTERUS PROBLEMS.

FIBROIDS

Uterine fibroids are benign growths that are very common, especially in women aged between thirty-five and forty. They range in size from very small to sometimes very large. One type grows on a stalk outside the uterus in the pelvic cavity, another grows inside the wall of the uterus. They take several years to develop and there is often more than one. Fibroids are three times as common in women with no children. Their development is related to oestrogen stimulation and they may grow considerably in pregnancy. The contraceptive pill is a possible culprit. They may lead to infertility and miscarriage and a large fibroid is considered a reason for caesarian delivery.

There are often no symptoms except possibly a dragging feeling in the lower abdomen, but they may cause heavy or prolonged periods if they are large (see Menstrual problems, page 20), or CYSTITIS and painful intercourse due to pressure from the fibroid. Anaemia may be caused by heavy periods. Pain is rare. Acute pain in the lower abdomen is caused by the twisting round of a stalk. The growth may become infected or degenerate in some other way. The only orthodox treatment is surgery, which is not necessary if the fibroids are small or untroublesome. Depending on age, either a D&C and myomectomy (removal of fibroid only), or sometimes hysterectomy is suggested. Some times a myomectomy is not possible as the growth is inside the uterine wall. Myomectomy often needs to be repeated several times unless the whole person is treated.

Self-help

As with any abnormal growth, fibroids may be caused at least in part by a reaction to toxicity, and dietary over-load. Make your diet optimally healthy – low-fat, high-fibre (see Healthy wholefood diet, page 126). Measures such as Colon cleansing (see page 146) are recommended. Fasting (see page 144) is corrective of underlying imbalance: three to seven days at the beginning of treatment and then a day a week will be very helpful in clearing this condition. The body is probably finding it difficult to eliminate wastes and the liver to deal with breakdown of hormones. There may be constipation. Cut out any hormonal contraceptives immediately and review any steroidal drugs you are currently taking with your doctor. Avoid oestrogen-containing foods from commercially farmed animals. Pelvic congestion of the type seen in congestive period pain (see page 22) is a contributory factor. A remedy is a sitz bath (see page 12), a short, sharp treatment – sitting with your rear in cold water for a few minutes each morning – this really stimulates the circulation. Pelvic exercises such as the pelvic rock are also beneficial (see Abdominal and pelvic exercises, page 195). Both these treatments need to be regular for at least six months to show real benefit.

Herbal treatment
Circulatory herbs: Hawthorn Flowers, Horse Chestnut, Yarrow.
Eliminatory herbs: Dandelion Leaf, Burdock, Cleavers.
Hormonal balancers: Chaste Berry, Raspberry Leaf, Lady's Mantle, Wild Yam, Motherwort, Liquorice.
Herbs for bleeding: Birth Root, Golden Seal, Greater Periwinkle.
(For further information see Directions for use of herbs in menopause, page 101.)

Formula for fibroids

Greater Periwinkle	40 per cent
Dandelion	20 per cent
Cleavers	20 per cent
Lady's mantle	10 per cent
Chaste Berry	10 per cent

Total: 100ml/g a week. Dose: tincture, 5ml three times daily, or infusion/decoction of dried herb, 1 cup three times daily. In addition you may need to take a separate formula composed of herbs for heavy bleeding for one to two weeks before and during a period.

Six months of treatment depending on the size/number of fibroid/s usually produces improvement. If you have had fibroids removed it will prevent them coming back. Very large fibroids may have to be removed; do take professional advice if you have very heavy bleeding and remember that these treatments do not start to work within only a few weeks.

HEAD PAINS
Headache

This is a common symptom but is rarely a signal of a serious problem. The commonest reason for a headache is muscle tension caused by stress. Among other frequent causes are migraine, ANXIETY, insomnia, ALLERGY, HYPOGLYCAEMIA, CONSTIPATION, sinusitis and Pre-menstrual syndrome (see page 16).

Chronic or recurrent headache that has started recently should be referred to a doctor for further tests. More serious causes are high blood pressure, concussion following head injury or damage to blood vessels in the brain, which may lead to haemorrhage or a stroke. Call an ambulance immediately if accompanied by symptoms of nausea, vomiting, drowsiness, confusion and light intolerance (if you are not subject to migraines).

Headaches result from pressure on the pain-sensitive structures of the head or the cranial nerves in the neck; dilation or contraction of blood vessels stimulates nerve endings, causing pain. Headache may be due to the neck vertebrae bones being out of alignment, which an osteopath should be able to correct.

Note that headache can be caused by withdrawal from foods to which one is allergic and in this case should pass within three to four days. Headaches due to HYPOGLYCAEMIA are accompanied by fatigue, dizziness and hunger.

Orthodox treatment, besides attention to the cause, is symptomatic pain relief.

Migraine

Sometimes any severe head pain is called a migraine but a true migraine is probably caused by alterations in blood flow to the brain due to expansion of the arteries, known to accompany the migraine attack. There is usually a preceding phase of depression or irritability, visual disturbance and lack of appetite. The pain may be one-sided or generalized over the whole head and is often accompanied by nausea and/or vomiting. Attacks may recur very frequently (when they are known as 'cluster headaches'), then not for a while or they may have a regular pattern such as once a month. Untreated, they may last for hours or days. Triggers are often stress of any sort, bright or fluorescent lights or VDUs.

Migraine happens more often in women than in men, starting between the ages of ten and thirty. More than 50 per cent of women affected have a family history of migraine. They often stop after the age of fifty.

Orthodox treatment is by drugs such as Propanalol. Counselling is sometimes used. Biofeedback has been used with some success to teach sufferers to control blood vessel spasm.

Self-help

Life-style changes are important, including more relaxation if due to stress and tension. Any of the following should help: regular massage or yoga, meditation, or Alexander Technique if migraine is due to postural problems.

Attention to diet can be preventive of headache and migraine, depending on the type of headache and the causes, which range from ALLERGIES to food or environmental pollutants, toxins in food, HYPOGLYCAEMIA, CONSTIPATION, and tension.

Migraine headaches: caused by foods containing tyramine, such as ripe cheese; nitrates in food and water, monosodium glutamate (flavour enhancer), caffeine in coffee, tea and chocolate, and alcohol (sherry, red wine and beer).

Food allergies: caused by all the above plus commonly wheat, all dairy products, eggs, meat extracts and preserved meats, yeast, in fact anything to which the person is sensitive (see ALLERGY and Elimination diet (page 137) to identify food sensitivity).

Toxins: many chemical food additives, preservatives, and flavourings. Traces of pesticides and fertilizers in food. Traces of hormones and antibiotics given to animals. Heavy metals: lead, cadmium; aluminium and copper from cooking utensils.

A good-quality wholefood diet avoiding processed food and high in protein, not necessarily animal, is recommended.

Supplements

Vitamin B complex with extra Vitamin B_5 (pantothenic acid): 500mg daily, and Vitamin B_6: 50mg daily for a month to see if it helps.
Vitamin C: 500mg daily.
Multi-mineral including calcium, potassium, zinc and selenium.

Herbal treatment

Any treatment for stress and nervous tension needs to be long-term. Try including the following (all doses are for tincture three times daily, or infusion/decoction of dried herb, 1 cup three times daily; herbs underlined are first choice).

Sedatives: Wood Betony or Lemon Balm, 5ml/g, or Valerian, 3ml/g, or Skullcap, 2ml/g.

For headache: Crampbark, 5–10ml or Valerian, 2–5ml tincture every two hours.

Local application: During a headache lie down with a compress on the forehead wrung out in ice water with 2 drops Peppermint or Lavender essential oil added.

For migraine headache: For long-term treatment try Feverfew. It must be fresh, either as specific tincture 5ml daily or freeze-dried in capsules, 3 daily or as fresh leaf from the garden. This can be taken in a sandwich, a leaf once a day. Some women report that two to three months of this has decreased the incidence and severity of migraine considerably. Treatment of nervous tension is also often appropriate. For treatment during an attack see Headache, above.

Other herbs that may be useful: Chamomile or Rosemary, 2–5ml, or Lime Flowers, 8–10ml, or Jamaican Dogwood, 2–8ml.

HYPOGLYCAEMIA

This is a condition of low blood sugar (glucose) which can lead to a variety of physical and mental symptoms. All the cells in the body require glucose for their functioning, especially the brain, hence if it is lacking the effects are widespread.

Hypoglycaemia is common in insulin-dependent diabetics as a result of taking too much insulin. Emergency treatment is glucagon (a hormone) or glucose by injection.

In adults, late-onset diabetes is often a result of life-long over-consumption of refined carbohydrates such as white bread, white flour products and white rice, and sugars. When refined carbohydrates and sugar are eaten they are swiftly digested and absorbed and cause a rapid rise in blood sugar. This enhances the production and secretion of the hormone insulin from the pancreas which acts to lower the blood sugar again. The drop in blood sugar is often extreme, and affects other hormones such as adrenaline, the over-production of which causes some of the worst symptoms.

Hypoglycaemia is diagnosed by a blood test known as the fasting glucose tolerance test. Samples are taken over a period of several hours looking for blood sugar to fall below a certain level.

A further condition, known as reactive hypoglycaemia, is recognized by naturopaths and other natural therapy practitioners, but the phenomenon is not generally accepted by the orthodox medical profession. In this case, in the absence of diabetes, blood-sugar levels appear to be normal but women still experience similar unpleasant symptoms. It is suggested that their blood glucose levels fluctuate more than usual within a narrow range; but unless a blood test is actually taken at the time of the drop, it will not show. It is suggested that stress, over-consumption of carbohydrate or caffeine, food allergies and smoking are all contributory causes.

The hypolgycaemic woman may have some or many of the symptoms listed below. They are often of sudden onset and usually occur before breakfast, a few hours after eating, after exercise or after emotional stress.

Intellectual symptoms: Confusion, forgetfulness, loss of concentration.

Emotional symptoms: Impatience, irritability, bad temper, crying, depression, anxiety, phobias, suicidal feelings, loss of purpose or sense of meaning in life.

Nervous symptoms: Headaches, dizziness, trembling, numbness, fainting, blurred vision, twitching of muscles, sensitivity to light.

Bodily symptoms: Fatigue or exhaustion, bloating, abdominal pain, muscle and joint pain, insomnia, backache, diarrhoea, cold sweats, palpitations, hunger.

Pre-menstrual symptoms (see page 16) and hot flushes in menopause (see page 87) are sometimes associated with hypoglycaemia.

Self-help

Avoid stress and exhaustion. Practise relaxation techniques. Get plenty of sleep and take exercise regularly but not to the point of exhaustion.

The main treatment is dietary. Be sure to eat something every two hours. Keep glucose tablets with you for use in an emergency. See Hypoglycaemic diet (page 143), and keep to the dietary recommendations to normalize blood-sugar levels. Supplements that help include Vitamins C and B complex, and multi-minerals with extra chromium and zinc.

Herbal treatment

Herbs should be taken in conjunction with dietary correction, and a whole-person approach is needed for recovery. A medical herbalist would be able to advise on this; in the meantime you could try the following:

Nervines and sedatives for stress: As fresh juice or tablets take Valerian, Skullcap or Oats. Avoid alcohol.

Tonics for adrenal support: Panax Ginseng or Siberian Ginseng, 5ml elixir three times a day of either.

Nettles are often used in treatment as tea, 1 cup three times daily or juice, 1 tablespoon twice daily. Chinese Liquorice (Gan Cao) is reputed to rebalance hormone levels and is a useful addition to a formula.

Goat's Rue has a reputation for rebalancing insulin levels.

HYSTERECTOMY

Surgical removal of the uterus; complete hysterectomy includes the ovaries as well. It is a major operation and recovery takes at least six to eight weeks. Reasons for hysterectomy include FIBROIDS if large and troublesome (but myomectomy or removal of fibroid only should be tried first), CERVICAL or OVARIAN CANCER, CANCER OF THE UTERUS, and complete uterine prolapse. Hysterectomy should only be performed if absolutely necessary, it is no longer routinely performed because of heavy bleeding. Bear in mind that your periods will stop immediately and early menopause begin following hysterectomy, but if the ovaries are not removed you may still experience the hormonal swings of a menstrual cycle. HRT is usually prescribed for a period of time for a woman who is not of menopausal age after complete hysterectomy.

See Herbal treatment of menopausal symptoms (page 89) for help.

IRRITABLE BOWEL SYNDROME

See under BOWEL PROBLEMS.

OVARIAN CANCER

This mainly affects women in the fifty to seventy age bracket. In the USA screening by ultrasound is common in private gynaecological practice for women over fifty but is not routine in the UK. There is a lobby to change this. Candidates for screening should be those women who have a close relative who had ovarian cancer, or who have had endometrial or breast cancer themselves. Ovarian cancer is associated with having no children, few children or children late in life. A diet high in fat is implicated, as are high oestrogen levels. Environmental factors are thought to play a major part in causation. A depressed immune system for any reason may be a trigger; elderly women who have been recently bereaved seem to be particularly at risk.

Any or all of the symptoms of cancer may be present at an advanced stage, including pain, loss of weight and post-menopausal bleeding. Usually the ovary is removed and sometimes the uterus as well (see HYSTERECTOMY) with chemotherapy and radiotherapy as back-up; following diagnosis in the early stages the chances of complete recovery are good.

Self-help
Changes in diet, taking supplements and dealing with any existing emotional trauma will help recovery. Any complementary medical anti-cancer therapy or herbal treatment should be under the guidance of an experienced practitioner in the field. Treating the whole person can take place in conjunction with orthodox treatment (see also Cancer self-help, page 164).

Supplements
Vitamin A as beta-carotene: 10,000 IUs daily.
Vitamin C: to bowel tolerance levels daily.
Vitamin E: 800 IUs daily.
Essential fatty acids (EFAs) as Evening Primrose oil: 1000mg twice daily.
Selenium: 200mcg daily.
Multi-mineral including trace elements vanadium and molybdenum.

OVARIAN CYSTS

Most tumours in the ovary are benign (94 per cent), and there are different types. Cysts are usually fluid-filled. They do not generally present a problem unless they produce abnormal quantities of sex hormones or become exceptionally large. In this case they may twist or rupture causing bleeding and pain. Symptoms are vague – a slightly swollen abdomen, discomfort but no real pain; the bladder

is only affected by pressure if the cyst is large. Often there are no symptoms and a cyst is only diagnosed during a routine pelvic examination.

Polycystic ovaries are connected with infertility problems where hormone levels are abnormal.

Orthodox treatment is surgery for cysts over a certain size, or in an emergency such as rupture and haemorrhage (symptoms are severe pain, vomiting and collapse). Sometimes the ovary is removed as well. Although the chance of ovarian cancer is only 6 per cent, most surgeons prefer to err on the safe side.

Self-help
Ovarian cysts probably originate with an imbalanced hormonal pattern and sluggish metabolism as with many other problems in the pelvic area.

Chaste Berry is specific for treatment. It brakes hyperfolliculaemia in the ovary, which is the probable cause of cysts. Take 2ml daily on rising, while on treatment. Also follow suggestions for eliminatory herbs under FIBROIDS. Detoxification is often indicated (see Colon cleansing, page 146) and dietary change. See also self-help for fibroids.

There is a suggestion that cysts are connected with environmental pollution.

Supplements
Vitamin E: 800 IUs daily.
Vitamin B complex: 50–100mg daily.
Pituitary glandular extract (available only from practitioners).
Essential fatty acids (EFAs) as Evening Primrose oil: 500mg twice daily.

PELVIC INFLAMMATORY DISEASE (PID), OR SALPINGITIS

PID is a general inflammation of the pelvic organs. It is usually caused by bacterial infection rising from the uterus (see Endometritis, under UTERUS PROBLEMS, and Cervicitis, under CERVICAL PROBLEMS), infecting the Fallopian tubes and ovaries. It is relatively common and if not treated can become chronic. It is more likely after the cervix has been opened by abortion, miscarriage, infection following childbirth or insertion of an IUD. Women with many sexual partners are more prone because of their exposure to more sources of infection.

Symptoms range from mild to severe, developing gradually or coming on suddenly. In the latter case there will be lower abdominal pain, tender to the touch, accompanied by a fever and possibly a vaginal discharge which smells unpleasant and contains pus. In the long term periods become heavy and painful and intercourse may be painful. There may be pain on passing water or opening the bowels. If the condition is not treated it can lead to scarring of the tubes, abscesses and possible infertility. Chronic PID leads to general ill-health. Orthodox treatment is by broad-spectrum antibiotics for several weeks, but this often is not 100 per cent successful and has to be repeated. Abcesses are often inaccessible to antibiotic treatment and they need to be drained by surgery.

Herbal treatment
Hot poultices of an anti-inflammatory and analgesic herb such as Chamomile over the abdomen, replaced frequently, or clay poultices once a day while PID is acute are recommended. While taking professional advice, the following may be tried in conjunction with any other treatment (those underlined are the herbs of choice).
To take internally as an anti-microbial and to aid the immune system: Echinacea, most effective for purulent infections, initially 20–40 drops of tincture diluted every half-hour until symptoms improve, then three times daily. Usnea (Bear's Lichen) is an important alterative antibiotic herb. One or two of the following herbs from each category.
Antiseptic and anti-microbial: Garlic and Golden Seal, or Marigold or Rosemary.
Anti-spasmodic and analgesic for pelvic area: Black Haw, or Pulsatilla, or Wild Yam, or Valerian.
Uterine tonic: False Unicorn Root, combines well with Echinacea.
Lymphatic drainer: Cleavers, Blue Flag, Parsley Piert.
(The above herbs may need to be taken for six to eight weeks and until it is confirmed the condition has cleared.)
(For further information see Directions for use of herbs in menstrual problems, page 26.)

Self-help
Bed-rest is essential in the acute stage, with a light diet and plenty of fluids including herbal infusions. Take Vitamin C to bowel tolerance levels.

SEXUALLY TRANSMITTED DISEASES (VENEREAL INFECTIONS)

Gonorrhoea (clap) causes copious discharge with frequency of painful urination in men. In women there may be no symptoms. Gonococcus bacteria can cause acute cervicitis. Infection with the Chlamydia virus is the main cause of non-specific urethritis (NSU) in women with or without discharge; it may cause pain but often is symptomless and may lead to PELVIC INFLAMMATORY DISEASE. It is very important therefore that men tell their partners if they have a discharge and, if you suspect something is wrong, to have it investigated. STDs are associated with many sexual partners. Venereal infection should be treated by a specialist: there are special clinics set up for the purpose in every health authority in the UK and you may remain anonymous if you prefer. Diagnosis is by urine test and swab culture, followed by treatment with various combinations of antibiotics. You can help recovery by raising your general level of health – a course of Vitamins A, C, D and E will help. A herbalist will be able to help with general constitutional support. Any sexual contacts should be told so that they can be treated. Do not have intercourse until you are clear of infection. Remember that NSU is frequently spread back and forth between partners.

AIDS or acquired immune deficiency syndrome is the biggest worry today among the diseases spread by sexual contact. It is transmitted via fluids, including blood and semen. It is caused by human immunodeficiency virus (HIV) and the effects of full-blown AIDS are severe, destroying the immune system, and the condition is eventually fatal. It affects mainly males who are homosexual, haemophiliacs through blood transfusion and drug-users who share needles. There is evidence, however, that incidence is growing in the heterosexual population, and more women are becoming the passive victims of HIV positive men who knowingly or unknowingly pass it on. Being HIV positive is not the same as having AIDS. It cannot be stressed too often that getting your partner always to wear a condom is effective against the spread of sexually transmitted disease. There is to date no successful orthodox treatment for AIDS. A number of herbs have been explored, and can provide immune-system support; for further information consult a medical herbalist skilled in this field.

SKIN AND HAIR PROBLEMS

Many women visit herbalists for all types of skin difficulty. Nature provides many wonderfully effective herbs to clear and beautify the skin. Herbalists see skin as reflecting very much the internal state of the body and mind, and it is one of the body's escape routes for releasing unwanted or harmful substances, for example toxicity due to unsuitable diet or emotional imbalance. Treatment is based on internal taking of herbs as much as external applications to heal the skin. In this type of condition a whole-person approach is particularly important. A medical herbalist would consider all aspects of your constitution and personality to decide what to prescribe.

The skin conditions that a herbalist sees most often are probably acne, eczema and psoriasis. A more generalized condition known as dermatitis, meaning irritation of the skin, also often responds well to herbs. As treatment is individual only an outline can be given here. If these suggestions do not help within two months, visit a medical herbalist.

Eczema

This uncomfortable problem is characterized by an itching, red, patchy rash appearing on the inside of arms and legs, especially behind the knees and inside wrists, but it can spread anywhere on the body. At its worst, when inflamed, it can be so dry that it cracks and bleeds or may exude fluid. It can come and go, sometimes reappearing after years. Allergic dermatitis is a type of eczema due to skin sensitivity to some external factor, often detergent; eliminating the cause gets rid of the eczema.

A number of different types of eczema are recognized. It is beyond the scope of this book to go into all of them, and treatment of the commonest type only is discussed. For successful treatment it is essential to treat the root cause. In the meantime you could try the formulas below, or the external applications which will all soothe and relieve in some measure.

Eczema is a genetic problem if it starts in early childhood, or if there is a family history (individuals in this category are known as atopic and may develop other symptoms later on such as ASTHMA). It may be due to an allergic reaction, especially to dairy products, house-dust mites or other environmental factors (see ALLERGY). It is suggested that early weaning is a causative factor and that if eczema is in the family, the longer you breast-feed the better chance your child has of avoiding it.

Self-help
Starting in later life it may be due to an allergic reaction. It is always worth trying a dairy-free diet for four to six weeks, whatever your history, as in many cases this does clear up eczema. There must be total exclusion of all bovine products, including beef (see Milk-free diet, page 141). Other foods to watch are sugar, chocolate, all pork products and shellfish. Beware of certain food additives; E numbers that are contra-indicated for children's food may cause or worsen eczema in adults.

Sometimes eczema is a psychological reaction. Emotional factors and stress usually make the problem worse for sufferers. A herbalist would usually include herbal nervines or sedatives in any prescription; in some cases tranquillizing herbs are sufficient to clear the problem. More relaxation in this case goes without saying.

Treatment depends on the stage of eczema, being different for when it is dry and when inflamed or weeping fluid. In Western herbalism the term depurative or alterative is used to describe the action of blood-clearing or cleansing in relation to skin; this oftens throws out more before it improves matters. In the author's experience, depuratives should only be used when the condition is chronic and cold. In Chinese herbalism the terms heat or wind in the blood describe similar conditions and Chinese herbs are said to have a cooling and calming action; applied to Western herbs, this theory provides effective treatment in many cases. As a general rule, don't stir up the condition when it is inflamed.

Herbal treatment
Try a combination of these in equal parts as a standard infusion or see formula below.
Alteratives: Red Clover, Burdock, Yellow Dock, Oregon Grape, Fumitory or Echinacea.
Herbs with a cooling nature: Nettles, Heartsease Pansy, Catnip, Lemon Balm or Cleavers.

Nervines: Lemon Balm, Oats, Vervain (as above).

Sedatives: Skullcap, Lavender or Chamomile (as above)

Total: 100ml/g a week. Dose: tincture, 5ml three times daily, or infusion/decoction of dried herb in equal parts, 1 cup three times daily.

(See also EMOTIONAL PROBLEMS.)

Formula for chronic eczema

Red Clover	20 per cent
Cleavers	20 per cent
Echinacea	20 per cent
Yellow Dock	20 per cent
Chamomile	20 per cent

Total: 100ml/g a week. Dose: tincture 5ml three times daily, or infusion/decoction of dried herb in equal parts, 1 cup three times daily.

Topical applications

- Chickweed cream (for itching) and Comfrey cream (soothing and healing) with essential oils added – 2 drops of any of the following:
- Chamomile oil for an allergic skin response.
- Peppermint oil for irritation.
- Lavender oil for inflammation.
- Tea Tree oil or Myrrh oil, 1–2 drops if there is infection
- Evening Primrose oil, 2–5ml to 50g of cream or can be used neat in an emergency. (This is a healing and anti-inflammatory cold-pressed oil.)

Note: When there is bleeding beware of infection – add anti-bacterial oils. You may have to astringe the skin with Witch Hazel before returning to the dry skin treatment.

- Infusions of Chamomile Flowers or Chickweed added to bath-water for a long soak stop itching. (Excellent too for the rash of measles or chickenpox.)

For acute (wet) eczema

In this acute stage when there may be bleeding as well, careful attention is needed. Cream should not be used but rather herbal infusions to wash skin frequently or applied as herbal compresses: soaking a whole limb in cloths wrung out in infusion may be necessary for two to three days. In addition bed-rest and light diet should be followed if the eczema covers a large body area. Bruised fresh leaves of Plantain applied to skin are a traditional remedy.

Local applications: Ribwort Plantain or Witch Hazel (to astringe) and Marigold or Chamomile (for inflammation) as infusions. Add essential oils of Myrrh or Thyme or Lemon for infection, 1 drop per litre of infusion, agitate well to disperse. When skin starts to improve, instead of astringents substitute Marshmallow or Comfrey to complete the healing process.

To take: Herbs with a cooling nature above, and drink Cleavers tea: 1 litre daily will stop the weeping.

Psoriasis

An angry condition characterized by very red discrete patches or plaques of skin that start coin-sized and enlarge to cover quite large areas in the worst cases. It is due in fact to skin cells reproducing about five times faster than normal, so an enormous amount are shed every day: This causes a whitish/silver coloration over the lesions when they are active. In time they can become quite tough and leathery. It usually starts on the outside surfaces of the limbs, on knees and elbows

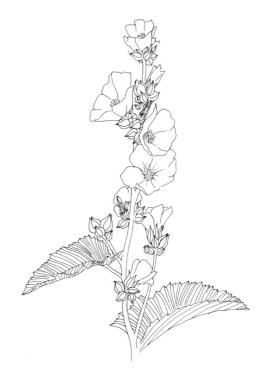

Marshmallow (*Althea officinalis*)

especially, although it can spread anywhere on the body. It can be extremely itchy when active.

There is usually a family history of psoriasis, although this may not appear until later life. Herbalists believe that toxicity in the body from years of incorrect living and diet can trigger it, as well as/or emotional factors such as bereavement or prolonged stress. Skin trauma or injury can precipitate psoriasis in the area if already prone to it. The same principles as those for eczema apply when the skin is acutely inflamed and lesions are active; however, initial treatment does need to clean the blood to clear the skin and depuratives/alteratives are generally used.

Herbal treatment

Combine from the following or see formula below:

Alteratives: Figwort, Burdock, Sarsaparilla or Oregon Grape.
Hepatics or liver herbs: Dandelion or Barberry.
Lymphatic herbs: Cleavers or Blue Flag.
Sedatives and nervines: Valerian and Hops.
Total: 100ml/g a week. Dose: tincture, 5ml three times daily, or infusion/decoction of dried herb in equal parts, 1 cup three times daily.
See also under Eczema (page 181).

Note: Maximum dose of tincture should not exceed 20ml daily (140ml a week).

Formula for chronic psoriasis
Sarsaparilla	25 per cent
Figwort	25 per cent
Barberry	25 per cent
Cleavers	25 per cent

Total: 100ml/g a week. Dose: tincture, 5ml three times daily, or infusion/decoction of dried herb in equal parts, 1 cup three times daily.

Topical applications
• Marigold cream with 1–2 drops of essential oils of Chamomile and African Marigold (Tagetes). The latter slows down the rate of cell reproduction.
• Chickweed cream for itching.
• Essential oil of Peppermint for itching.
• Cleavers as a wash, or poultice of fresh plant.
Compresses of herbal infusions (see ECZEMA) may be needed if the skin is badly inflamed, very red and itchy. See page 11 for directions.

Self-help

Diet is very important, and drinking sufficient water is a must, as is taking enough exercise, to stimulate and clean the system. Foods that people have found to worsen psoriasis include simple carbohydrates, especially sugar, alcohol, spices and acid foods – vinegar, citrus fruits – also dairy produce in some cases. Try an optimally healthy diet (see Healthy wholefood diet, page 126) with these measures, which should produce improvement. In addition the following supplements may help.

Supplements

Vitamins A, C, and E combined.
Vitamin B_6: 25–50mg daily.
Zinc: 25–50mg daily.
Flaxseed (Linseed) oil, high in EFAs: 2–4 teaspoons or 2–4 capsules daily, or Evening Primrose or Borage (Starflower) oil: 500mg capsules, 4–6 daily depending on severity, cut down as condition improves.

Abscesses and boils

An abscess is a large, painful, hot swelling containing pus. It is usually due to a hair follicle infection in the groin, around the anus or under the arms and generally occurs in those who are debilitated. If the lump is painless expert help should be sought. Deep internal abscesses are removed by surgery if antibiotics don't work. These may be seen as the body's attempt to rid itself of various toxins by producing a focus of infection and this elimination should be encouraged rather than suppressed.

Abscesses that are just below the skin and boils on the surface (furunculosis) can be dealt with quite effectively with local treatment. They should be encouraged to come to a head, burst and discharge their contents, in antiseptic surroundings – they should not be picked at. Traditional treatments are very effective and have only been superseded by broad-spectrum antibiotics in recent years, but with diminishing returns.

Self-help

A crop of boils is usually a sign of being run down. Think about your life-style and nutrition. Diet should be reviewed, and plenty of raw fruit and vegetables, especially Garlic, included, as well as sufficient protein. Take 1000mg of Vitamin C daily and 25mg of zinc until the boils clear. If they are persistent, see a medical herbalist for constitutional treatment.

Herbal treatment

Bathe the affected area with an infusion of herbs and essential oils. For the genital area make a sitz bath (see page 12 for directions).

- Infusion of Marigold Flowers, cooled and strained. For a sitz bath, 600ml to enough warm water to fill a large shallow plastic bowl, adding 2 drops each of essential oils of Lavender and Thyme. Sit in the bath for ten to fifteen minutes twice a day, repeating for several days if necessary, until the abscess or boil comes to a head and discharges.
- An abscess may need a poultice of Slippery Elm and Marshmallow powder applied, to draw it, in which case moisten the powder with enough boiling water to make a paste to cover a pad of lint and hold in place securely over the affected area for a day, renewing if necessary. One drop of essential oil of Thyme or Lemon may be added for its anti-bacterial action. An ointment of the above can be purchased over the counter.
- Internally, tincture of Echinacea, 5–10ml three times daily, and Burdock, 5ml three times daily, should be taken until the condition clears up. (Both can also be purchased as proprietary tablets, in which case 2–3 three times daily or follow directions.)

Acne

Acne vulgaris

Facial acne commonly occurs in girls aged twelve to twenty and is associated with hormonal imbalance, especially in the pre-mentrual phase. Skin is often oily or greasy, sometimes in a central facial panel. It may also appear on neck, shoulders or back. Raised painful pustules come to a head and may discharge, leaving scarring.

Self-help

The problem of adolescent acne is often compounded by bad eating habits. Plenty of fresh raw salads should be included in the diet, and sugary and fried foods avoided. Wholegrains should replace white refined products, and some fresh fruit be taken every day. Plenty of exercise in fresh air is essential and careful exposure to sunshine can work wonders.

Herbal treatment

- Infusion of Echinacea, Burdock, or Yellow Dock. Total: 100ml/g a week. Dose: tincture,

5ml three times daily, or infusion/decoction of dried herb in equal parts, 1 cup three times daily. It will take up to two or three menstrual cycles to see real improvement.

- Chaste Berry, tincture 2.5ml on rising in the morning from mid-cycle to period for hormonal disturbance. Alternatively, proprietary Vitex tablets are available over the counter.
- Locally, a facial application of Marigold tincture diluted 50 per cent with warm water applied at night will heal the lesions. Add 2 drops of essential oil of Tea Tree for its antiseptic and anti-bacterial action; or astringent oil of Lemon if skin is oily or Chamomile oil for scarring, 2 drops to a basinful of water.

Supplements

Vitamin C: 1000mg daily.
Vitamin E: 400–600 IUs daily.
Zinc: 50mg daily.
Vitamin A as beta-carotene: 4mg daily until it clears.

Acne rosacea

This looks similar to acne vulgaris but occurs in older women, often during or after the menopause. It often appears as a very red rash in a butterfly shape, over the nose and cheeks. It is caused by hormonal changes affecting the sebaceous glands. Stress can sometimes be a factor.

Self-help

A good wholefood diet and no stimulants such as tea, coffee or alcohol. No yeast, as the acne may be a complication of CANDIDIASIS (see Anti-candida diet, page 139). Consider this if you are suffering from a vaginal discharge and general debility.

Herbal treatment

Similar to that for Acne vulgaris above, but add Lady's Mantle and Red Clover to the infusions.

- Facial application of 50 per cent Marigold and 50 per cent Myrrh tincture, diluted as before and dabbed on several times a day, will be antiseptic and soothing. In addition add essential oils of Lemon, Tea Tree, Chamomile and Bergamot, 2 drops of each to 100ml of tincture and shaken well before dilution.

Supplements
As above for Acne vulgaris.

Alopecia

Partial or complete loss of hair in women may be caused by certain hormonal diseases such as myxodema, after severe feverish illness, or after pregnancy. It is usually temporary. Alopecia areata is sudden patchy hair loss in certain areas, usually the scalp, with no obvious cause. It usually reverses in a few months, unless it is very extensive in which case new patches may keep appearing. Alopecia nervosa is diagnosed when there appears to be a psychological cause such as a great shock or other emotional trauma; even prolonged stress. It may be accompanied by a feeling of great fatigue. The contraceptive pill, cytotoxic or antimitotic drugs, or too much Vitamin A, may cause hair loss. If the loss is due to scarring after injury, little regrowth is seen.

Traditionally there are herbs that can be applied locally to improve circulation to the scalp and encourage hair growth. However, it is more likely to clear up after taking a whole-person approach dealing with the underlying cause as well. Vitamin and minerals status will also affect the growth and quality of hair. A hair mineral analysis test is recommended (obtainable from Larkhall Natural Health; see page 203).

Herbal treatment
Externally
Scalp preparation containing the following: Rosemary, Burdock, Nettles and Birch Leaves as tincture. Combine all together in equal parts. This should be painted on, left overnight and washed off the next morning using a Rosemary, Nettle or Birch shampoo, or a very mild proprietary shampoo. Finish with a rinse of diluted Rosemary or Nettle.

Essential oils of Rosemary, Burdock, Lavender and Calamus, 1 drop of each in 50ml almond or avocado oil massaged into the scalp and left on for several hours, wrapped in a warm towel. Do this once a week. The massage itself is important to increase circulation, and should be performed in a circular motion all over the head.

Nerve tonic
Oats, 2.5ml fluid extract or 5ml tincture three times daily, or St John's Wort, 4ml tincture or 2–4g as tea three times daily.

See also EMOTIONAL PROBLEMS.

Circulatory herbs
Prickly Ash, 2ml three times daily, or Ginger, ½ml three times daily, or Rosemary, 4ml three times daily.

Burdock as an excellent blood-cleanser in addition, 1–2ml three times daily.

Self-help
Nutrition is very important, as poor diet is often reflected in poor hair condition. A good, balanced diet based on wholefoods and raw foods and containing sufficient protein is nutritive for the hair, as is avoiding tea, coffee and alcohol which may deplete essential minerals.

Some practitioners of nutritional medicine recommend large doses of vitamins and minerals to correct the condition, and these should only be taken under supervision. However, smaller doses taken over a period of time in conjunction with herbs will help if there are deficiencies.

Essential for healthy hair are the following:
Zinc: 9–15mg daily.
Iron: 15mg daily.
B Vitamins: 25–50mg daily.
Biotin (part of B complex): 200mcg daily.
Beta-carotene (proVitamin A): 4mg daily.
Vitamin C: 500mg daily.
Vitamin E: 400–800 IUs daily may also help as it benefits hormone production.

TRICHOMONAS

See under VAGINAL PROBLEMS.

ULCERATIVE COLITIS

See under BOWEL PROBLEMS.

URINARY PROBLEMS

Conditions that affect a woman's bladder most frequently are cystitis, urinary incontinence and prolapse of uterus.

Cystitis

Symptoms of cystitis of the bladder are increased frequency of passing water, pain on passing water likened to a needling sensation, and sensation of pressure as if desperate to go to the toilet even when there is nothing to pass. There may be aching tenderness over the pubic area.

Other causes of urinary frequency are pregnancy (see Urinary problems of pregnancy, page 53), pelvic tumour pressing on the bladder, uterine and vaginal prolapse, pelvic operations or radiotherapy, and urethritis. Because of the proximity of the bladder to other organs of the pelvis, urinary symptoms may herald other gynaecological problems.

Cystitis is usually caused by a urinary tract infection, often due to bacteria that invade the urinary passage or urethra and ascend to the bladder. The urethra is very short in women and hence is more prone to infection. Germs may be transferred from the vagina or anus during sexual intercourse, although there may be other factors. If inflammation is severe there may be blood in the urine and slight fever. Orthodox treatment is by antibiotics and anti-inflammatory drugs following a urine test to see if a specific bacterium can be cultured: *E. coli* is commonly found.

Self-help
Chronic or frequently recurring cystitis may be due to a small perineum (the area between the anus and vagina) or a habit of wiping from back to front after using the toilet. Be scrupulously clean at all times: if you have a small perineum washing with a mild disinfectant in water after each bowel movement and before and after intercourse may prevent spread of infection – use a shower head or clean cotton wool rather than a flannel. Urinate immediately after making love to flush out any bacteria. Wear cotton underwear; sensitivity to nylon underwear, tights or soap may cause or worsen cystitis.

The pH or acidity/alkalinity of the body as reflected in a urine test is important. It should be pH 7 or 7.5 but becomes acid at pH 5, as the body tries to rid itself of excess acidity, and this is usually the case with cystitis. To correct, take some exercise in the fresh air every day, especially if you have a sedentary job, and practise breathing deeply. Drink plenty of water as it is important to keep up fluid intake. In some cases the urine is alkaline in cystitis, when the body cannot rid itself of acid, but this is more unusual: in such a case acids like citric acid or cranberry juice will help initially.

See Alkaline diet (page 142). Avoid acid-producing foods such as meat, tomatoes, white flour and white sugar. When you have an attack of cystitis, fast on vegetable juices and barley water, not fruit juices. Take a pinch of bicarbonate of soda in a glass of apple juice to start with, to alkalinize the urine if acid. Remember that a food allergy can cause chronic cystitis.

Psychological factors may play a part in chronic cystitis, such as a feeling of not being clean 'down there'. Dr Bach's Flower Remedies are excellent in this case, especially Heather (see EMOTIONAL PROBLEMS). Emotional distress of any sort can of course lower the health sufficiently to allow a bacterial infection to take hold.

Herbal treatment
(Herbs of first choice are underlined.)
Urine pH high (alkaline): Cranberry juice, 1 cup three to four times daily. Drink plenty of water with lemon juice added. Take Garlic, 1 chopped clove or 1–2 strong capsules daily. Combine herbs below.
Urine pH low (acid): Try the following, which work well as teas:
Anti-microbials (for infection): <u>Bearberry</u>, Buchu, Parsley Piert tincture, equal parts, 5ml three to five times daily, or as decoction, equal parts, 5g per cup, three to five times daily.
Demulcent (to soothe membranes): <u>Marshmallow</u> Leaf or Cornsilk, as infusion, 5g per cup three to five times daily (add to above).
Diuretics and anti-inflammatory (for irritation): <u>Couchgrass</u>, 6g *or* Celery seed, 2g per cup, three to five times daily (add to above).

The cystitis should start to clear up within a day or so, but continue treatment for a week to ten days to make sure. Be aware that infection can ascend to the kidney causing pyelonephritis. The symptoms are the same as cystitis but with pain in the kidney area, high fever and vomiting. See your doctor if in any doubt.

Urethritis

Urinary tract infections can cause inflammation of the urethra (urinary passage from the bladder) with frequency and pain. Treatment is the same as for CYSTITIS. It may be caused by trauma such as bruising after sexual intercourse.

Urinary incontinence

Stress incontinence: this is due to lack of control of the neck of the bladder. Small quantities of urine are passed on coughing, laughing or sneezing because of pressure on the bladder, as the result of being pregnant or very overweight, or by prolapse of the bladder or uterus. It is a reversible condition that often happens during pregnancy due to hormonal changes or after Childbirth (see page 63) when the muscles of the pelvic floor are weakened. Lower oestrogen levels following Menopause (see page 87) can build on already weakened muscles so that they become lax, allowing dribbling of urine. It is thought that up to 30 per cent of women aged fifty to seventy-five suffer with it. To correct, practise PC muscle exercise, which retrains the muscle controlling outflow (see Abdominal and pelvic exercises, page 195).

Urge incontinence: this means having to go to the toilet immediately, and the stream is unstoppable. It can happen in acute cystitis or with stress incontinence. PC exercise (see page 195) is corrective in many cases, especially after menopause; after improvement you may need to keep it up twice daily. It may also be a result of hyper-sensitivity of the nerves supplying the bladder. Orthodox treatment uses drugs to reduce sensitivity. Emptying the bladder frequently before it becomes full is imperative. If the PC exercise does not work, retraining bladder control may improve matters, and this is done by gradually increasing the amount of urine that you can hold before passing it; ask your doctor for referral to a physiotherapist.

Herbal treatment

Treat CYSTITIS if symptoms of pain or discomfort are present on passing water. If due to hyper-sensitivity a herbalist would treat by using nervines and anti-spasmodics for the pelvic area as well as the following: Agrimony, Horsetail or Sweet Sumach. Any successful treatment would need to be part of a whole-person approach and it is advisable to seek good advice in this case.

UTERUS PROBLEMS

The main problems affecting the uterus include endometritis, endometriosis (see Menstrual problems, page 24), uterine prolapse, uterine cancer and benign tumours (see FIBROIDS).

Endometritis

This is inflammation of the lining of the uterus. It may be caused by infection and can be acutely painful, as after childbirth or abortion, or it may follow atrophic changes to the uterus during menopause. Or it may be due to infection with Gonococcus (see SEXUALLY TRANSMITTED DISEASES). Symptoms are dull or sharp pain over the pubic area, aching in the groin, and discharge which may be pus-stained. It can develop into PELVIC INFLAMMATORY DISEASE if it spreads. Orthodox treatment is by antibiotics. It is not advisable to treat this yourself, but if it is a chronic condition a medical herbalist can help. Any self-help measures would include raising your general level of health.

Cancer of the uterus

The most common type is that of the lining of the uterus, or endometrial cancer. The usual symptom is abnormal bleeding. It is more common after menopause, and the danger signs are any bleeding after periods have stopped for six months or more. (Cancer is not the only reason for post-menopausal bleeding, but if it occurs it is essential to get an immediate, thorough medical check-up.) Other symptoms are bleeding in between periods or prolonged or heavy bleeding if still menstruating. There may be a watery discharge from the vagina. Diagnosis is by a D & C or biopsy of the uterine lining.

Unopposed oestrogen therapy after menopause is known to cause endometrial cancer and for this reason HRT (see page 99) now includes progesterone to modify the effects on the uterus. Hormone imbalance is therefore a factor, and women at highest risk are those with a late menopause, or women who have few or no children, who have had more years of oestrogen stimulation, and women who are very overweight and have more oestrogen stores. Other risk factors are diabetes mellitus, high blood pressure, polycystic ovaries or CANCER OF BREAST, CANCER OF OVARIES or of colon. It is sometimes found in association with uterine FIBROIDS.

Orthodox treatment depends on age, usually consisting of a combination of surgery and radiation, with chemotherapy used to back up other treatment. Hormonal treatment with progesterone may cause tumours to shrink. The chances of complete recovery are very good if endometrial cancer is treated in the early stages.

Self-help

Nutritional deficiencies associated with development of uterine cancer are a diet with a high proportion of fatty foods and not enough fresh green vegetables, fruit and unrefined cereals, leading to deficiency of beta-carotene, Vitamin E and minerals, particularly selenium.

Any complementary medical anti-cancer therapy or herbal treatment should be followed under the guidance of an experienced medical practitioner in the field. Treating the whole person can take place in conjunction with orthodox treatment (see also Cancer self-help, page 164).

Supplements

Vitamin A as beta-carotene: 10,000 IUs or 6mg daily.
Vitamin C: to bowel tolerance levels.
Vitamin E: 800 IUs daily.
1 multi-vitamin daily.
Multi-minerals including selenium, 200mcg daily, and trace minerals manganese and vanadium.

Uterine and vaginal prolapse

Caused in almost all cases by laxity of the ligaments and pelvic floor muscles holding the uterus in place following childbirth, especially after three or more children. The uterus or vaginal walls fall downwards and may appear at the opening to the vagina, depending on the extent of the prolapse. The cervix may appear at the opening on coughing or sneezing. Symptoms depend on which organs are being pressed on. There may be dragging-down sensations, backache, urinary frequency, stress incontinence and tiredness.

Orthodox surgical treatment to repair the damage is often effective, but is unsuitable for a woman who wants more children. Treatment sometimes has to be repeated. Worth trying first is a specially designed plastic ring inserted in the vagina to hold everything up. It should be measured and fitted, its use monitored, and it should be changed every three months if necessary.

Self-help

Practise the Abdominal and pelvic exercises on page 195 to strengthen the pelvic floor muscles; this will help considerably unless the prolapse is severe. Slant-board exercises are ideal to reverse the effects of gravity. The exercises are done lying on a tilted board, full length, head downwards to reverse the effects of gravity. Exercise regularly but not too vigorously; note that the use of personal bouncers is not recommended.

VAGINAL PROBLEMS

Vaginal discharge

A slight vaginal discharge, or leucorrhoea, is normal, especially before a period. The natural secretions change according to the menstrual cycle and vary from thin and transparent around ovulation to thicker and white before the period: they should not be irritating or smell unpleasant. Learning how to read these signs is the basis of the Billings method of natural contraception. Any changes in colour, smell or quantity signals a problem. The pH (acid/alkaline balance) and ecobalance of the vagina should be in equilibrium, otherwise problems are likely, with poor general health being a trigger. The pH becomes more alkaline at mid-cycle and this is when infection is more likely to occur.

The most common cause of an abnormal vaginal discharge is thrush (see CANDIDIASIS) which causes a thick, white, cottage cheese-like discharge that leads to irritation and soreness, and may smell yeasty though not unpleasant. Other causes of infection are trichomonas, in which case the discharge will be infected, greenish in colour and malodorous. Abdominal pain suggests that the infection has spread and that there is PELVIC INFLAMMATION. Gardnarella, the most common bacterial infection, causes a greyish, thin discharge. Atrophic vaginitis (see page 97) may encourage a discharge. *Note:* Infection is often by a non-specific bacterium and no cause can be found. Diagnosis is by vaginal swab and culture of organisms. Home treatment of infection without a diagnosis is not recommended: follow professional advice.

Any bloodstained discharge should be reported immediately to your doctor, especially post-menopause, as causes include CANCER OF UTERUS and OVARIAN CANCER. It may signal Cervicitis, cervical erosion or cervical cancer (see under CERVICAL PROBLEMS) in younger women. In pregnancy a bloody discharge is an emergency. A watery discharge in late pregnancy may be amniotic fluid leaking from around the baby:

contact the midwife or doctor as soon as possible. (*Note:* A thick white discharge during pregnancy is normal.)

SEXUALLY TRANSMITTED DISEASES such as NSU, gonorrhoea and chlamydia cause discharges, sometimes with pain, and should be treated by a specialist. Tetracycline antibiotics are used, and any damage can be repaired with lactobacilli or probiotics later.

Herbal treatment

Herbs have a lot to offer in treating nonspecific bacterial infections where resistance builds up to orthodox treatment by antibiotics. Some herbal essential oils such as Marjoram, Lemon, Garlic, Thuja, Sage, Clove, Lavender and Eucalpytus are strongly anti-bacterial. *Note:* If these are used, never apply directly to skin and dilute well. They may be added to pessaries or douches (see pages 10 and 12).

Douches: Lady's Mantle, White Deadnettle, Marigold, St John's Wort and Golden Seal tincture in equal parts, dilute one part to fifteen parts water, use daily.

Anti-bacterials: Tincture or tablets of Echinacea, or Usnea (Bear's Lichen), and Garlic, 20 drops tincture three to five times daily. Available individually as proprietary tablets over the counter, 2 tablets two to three times daily.

Cream for irritation: Marigold cream, 50g to which add: tincture of Golden Seal, or Sweet Violet, or Myrrh, or Bayberry and Chamomile, 2ml each and 2 drops of one of above essential oils.

Self-help

Vaginal infections are often spread during sexual intercourse or by wiping yourself from back to front. Sensitivity to deodorant sprays and other vaginal hygiene aids can cause a heavy discharge – the best form of hygiene is daily washing. Avoid perfumed bath products. Avoid using tampons during menstruation as these breed germs; use sanitary towels instead and change frequently. Poor ventiliation contributes to the problem, as organisms thrive where it is damp and warm, so wear only cotton underwear, change it frequently and avoid tight clothing. Use of antibiotics and contraceptive hormones can also cause discharges.

To prevent infections improve general health and hygiene. A good diet plays an important part in building up resistance to infection. Cut out alcohol, sugar and coffee and any unnecessary drugs. Take supplements, particularly Vitamin C for infection (to bowel tolerance levels) and zinc, 25mg, until it clears up. If you take antibiotics or douche, remember to supplement with lactobacilli or probiotics for two to three weeks to restore normal flora. Diluted live yoghurt douches will restore the natural pH of the vagina. Follow suggestions for treatment under specific conditions. If the problem persists consult a medical herbalist.

Trichomonas

This is not a bacteria, rather a single-celled organism or protozoa present normally in the vagina in manageable numbers. When it gets out of control, however, it causes a vaginal discharge like thrush, but which is greenish and thin and smells unpleasant. Orthodox treatment is with the drug metronidaxole (Flagyl). (It can be cleared with herbal douches as well. Both Flagyl and Garlic remove most flora from the vagina. To prevent recurrence take acidophilus preparations to reinoculate the bowel with beneficial bacteria for two weeks and follow common-sense measures for hygiene under VAGINAL DISCHARGE. Avoid intercourse when infected. Be sure to have another test to see that the problem has cleared.

Douches
- Garlic: Make an infusion by adding the contents of 1 capsule of dried garlic powder or 2 chopped cloves of garlic to 1 litre of boiling water and leave to stand covered until cold, strain and use as douche once daily for a week.
- Marigold or Golden Seal: 1 part tincture to 15 parts cooled boiled water.
- Live Yoghurt: 1 tablespoon in 1 litre of cooled boiled water, use as above.

To take
- Echinacea and Usnea (Bear's Lichen) tincture, 20–30 drops of each five times daily. As proprietary tablets available over the counter, 2–3 three times daily, or follow directions.
- or Golden Seal tincture, 3ml three times daily.

Vaginitis

This is an inflammation of the vagina causing soreness and itching of the surrounding area with or without discharge. The normal slightly acid pH of the vagina, created by the doderlein or lactobacillus bacteria, gives some protection against many organisms that flourish in an alkaline environment. Antibiotics destroy the acid mantle of the vagina, as do pregnancy, diabetes, oral contraceptives and frequent douching. During menopause, atrophic vaginitis (see page 97) occurs as the oestrogen-dependent vaginal secretions dry up, the pH changes and the vagina atrophies or shrinks, making infections and inflammation more likely.

Secondary vaginitis occurs after damage or abrasion, as during childbirth or by a retained foreign body such as a tampon. See also SEXUALLY TRANSMITTED DISEASES. Avoid sexual intercourse until it clears up. Avoid sugars and cut down on starches for a while as these create and promote an alkaline environment. Eat acidophilus yoghurt every day and use as a douche alternately with herbs, diluted in boiled water. See other measures under VAGINAL DISCHARGE. Nonspecific vaginitis occurs without any obvious cause.

Herbal treatment

You can use herbal douches or pessaries to treat non-specific vaginitis. Inflammation responds well to herbal douches of Marigold, Lady's Mantle, Comfrey or Chamomile tincture in equal parts, diluted in the proportion 1 part to 15 parts water and used daily until the condition clears. See also VAGINAL DISCHARGE for creams.

Dry vagina

During intercourse dryness and discomfort in younger women are often due to lack of foreplay before penetration, to an unsatisfactory sexual relationship or to anxiety about sex for any reason.

In older women it may be due to menopausal decline of vaginal secretions. Immediate lubrication can be provided by KY jelly, and the general skin condition improved by herbal treatment (see also Vaginal problems in menopause, page 97). The best treatment is a loving sexual partnership.

VARICOSE VEINS

Varicose veins are caused by collapse of the valves in the veins of the legs which prevent backflow. Blood returning to the heart from the legs pools in the veins, stretching the walls, and the pressure causes them to balloon out, becoming tender and sensitive. There is a hereditary connection and other causes include standing all day and having had multiple pregnancies. The first sign is often heavy and aching legs, especially at the end of the day. Later on, characteristic blue knotted veins are seen. Surgical removal of veins is the last resort, but this does not stop other veins becoming varicosed if a preventive approach is not taken.

Self-help

The best medicine is preventive. Take enough rest and avoid standing for long periods if you are susceptible.

Lying with the legs up for short periods during the day, wearing support stockings, and improving circulation by stretching exercises will help. One effective exercise is to lie with legs raised high against a wall and spread, with the back supported on the floor, for ten minutes at a time.

Alternate hot and cold shower treatments directed at the legs – a burst of water as hot as is bearable, followed by a longer burst of cold water – repeated several times will tone up the smooth muscles of the veins as they dilate and contract. Even five minutes twice daily will improve the condition. Exercises that help are brisk walking and swimming, especially using a kicking stroke.

A diet high in lecithin from soya products, and in rutin from buckwheat, strengthens the walls of veins (eat two to three times a week as preventive). Rutin tablets are available over the counter, in which case take 2 three times a day with food. Include foods high in Vitamins A, C, and E and those of the onion family, especially fresh garlic.

Herbal treatment

(Herbs of first choice are underlined.)

- Massage the legs with an ointment containing Horse Chestnut or Witch Hazel (see page 10).
- Comfrey mucilage on a poultice of gauze (see page 9).
- Infusions or tincture of any of the following: Witch Hazel, Horse Chestnut, Marigold, Oak Bark, Comfrey or Mullein, dabbed on several times a day, tincture diluted 1 part to 5 parts.
- Arnica cream to relieve pain and itching.
- *Herbal compress:* Additional benefit can be had from soaking pads of lint or gauze with infusion of above herbs and leaving on the leg for several hours or overnight, covered in plastic to prevent evaporation. Binding with a crêpe

bandage on top of this will help the circulation. Bandage from toe to thigh while lying down. Support stockings or bandaging are best put on in bed before rising in the morning when rest has let the swelling subside.

• Essential oil of Cypress and Lemon added to bath-water, 1–2 drops of each. (Be aware of possible photosensitivity or skin sensitivity to Lemon; agitate water well to disperse oil. Avoid going out in the sun or using a sun-tanning bed afterwards.)

Proprietary herbal creams/ointments for varicose veins are available over the counter: check constituents.

Try taking the following for two to three months to improve circulation and tone veins: Lime Flowers, 2–4ml/g, Prickly Ash Bark, 3–5ml/g, Hawthorn Berries, 1–2ml/g, Yarrow herb, 2–4ml/g, Horse Chestnut, 5ml/g. Total: 100ml/g a week. Dose: tincture three times daily, or infusion/decoction, 1 cup three times daily.

Supplements
Vitamin C with bioflavonoids: 250mg three times daily, when acute. Long-term maximum 250mg daily.
Vitamin E: 400 IUs daily, if acute up to 800 IUs for one to two weeks, or 1 tablespoon wheatgerm daily.

VULVAL PROBLEMS

Vulval warts

Vulval warts or papilloma are caused by a virus, condyloma accuminata. They may be found on the labia, inside the vagina and on the cervix. They are small and irregularly shaped, only 2–3 millimetres across. In men they are found around the head of the penis. They are very contagious and easily transmitted during sexual intercourse. Warts may also spread from the hands to the sexual organs. In their acute stage when they are white they can burn and sting, specially when passing water. Although they appear benign, they can affect the result of a pap smear and are strongly associated statistically with the development of CERVICAL CANCER.

Herbal treatment
Treatment is removal by a caustic wart paint, cauterization or freezing. Unfortunately the warts tend to recur. Although Podophyllum is an effec-tive herbal wart paint and widely used until recently, it is no longer available to the public. Instead you could try tincture of Thuja (Tree of Life), applied neat on a cotton wool bud to the individual warts on the labia twice a day and diluted 1 part to 8 parts water as a douche.

Pruritis vulvae

This is intense itching of the vaginal entrance and labia, which may be due to post-menopausal or other hormone imbalance. A common cause is local irritation by vaginal hygiene sprays, creams, spermicides, etc. Sensitivity to harsh detergent washing powders is not uncommon. Anxiety about sexual intercourse, particularly in younger women, can be a factor. General health may be poor and women with other skin problems are

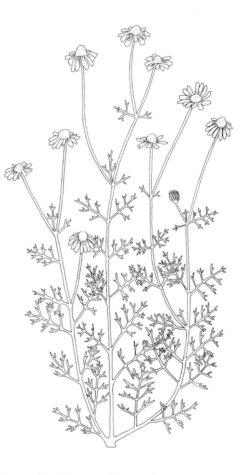

Chamomile (*Chamomilla recutita*)

more prone (see eczema, page 181) and general treatment is often indicated. Have a vaginal swab test to rule out infection.

See also vaginitis (page 189) and CANDIDIASIS.

Self-help
Try not to scratch as this will make it sore. Scrupulous hygiene is important. Do not use wash cloths that can harbour germs or soap, wash gently with clean cotton-wool and warm water with 2ml each of tincture of Marigold and Lady's Mantle added to a small basin of water several times a day. Wear only cotton underwear for ventilation, as this breathes whereas nylon cannot, and do not wear tights. A sedentary life-style contributes to this problem, so take more exercise, and when at work get up from your desk from time to time and walk around.

For menopausal women, see Atrophic vaginitis (page 97) for treatment.

Herbal treatment
• Try creams containing Chickweed (anti-itch) and Comfrey or Marshmallow (soothing). Add 1 drop of essential oil of Peppermint to 50g cream, and apply three times a day or each

time after passing water if very sore. (Do not use ointment as the greasy base can trap heat and irritate.)
• Douche with Lady's Mantle once a day: hold in for ten minutes.
• An old and very effective remedy for itching is a poultice of fresh mucilage of Comfrey on a pad worn next to the skin (see page 9).

Formula for sore, itching skin
Lemon Balm   20g
Chickweed   20g
Marshmallow   10g
Peppermint   10g
Make an infusion with 2 litres of boiling water, cool and strain. Use to bathe affected area morning and night; or use in a sitz bath (see page 12). The infusion can be used two to three times if kept cool.

Vulvitis

Inflammation of vulval area including labia. See vaginitis, vaginal discharge and pruritis vulvae under VAGINAL PROBLEMS for herbal treatment and self-help.

Appendices

Abdominal and Pelvic Exercises

Abdominal exercises
(Leg raises)

Lie on your back on a firm surface with your legs stretched out, arms by your sides with palms of hands on the floor for support.

Breathe in, raising one leg, for a count of four. Breathe out for a count of four while lowering leg. Repeat with the other leg.

Raise each leg six times.

When the abdominal muscles have strengthened, raise both legs together. This is strenuous! Tones the whole pelvic area and flattens the tummy.

Time: five minutes.

Pelvic exercises
(Pubococcygeal (PC) muscle)

A. Lie on your back with knees drawn up, feet flat on the floor. First, imagine you are trying to avoid passing a bowel motion by tensing the muscles of your bottom. (These muscles also surround the vagina and support the uterus.) Next, try tensing the muscles surrounding the vagina. It helps to imagine you are gripping something with the vagina: inserting a finger will help.

Tense hard, breathing in for a count of four, and let go *very* slowly, in stages – imagine a lift stopping on three floors on its way down to the ground floor – then breathe out.

Repeat six times, twice a day.

Time: ten minutes.

Helpful as preparation for childbirth, postnatally, for prolapsed uterus, and stress incontinence.

B. Similar effect is to be had when starting and stopping the flow of urine. Helpful for urinary and stress incontinence. It is easily done each time you visit the bathroom.

Time: two minutes.

C. Using the abdominal muscles, follow stage one of A above. While tensing the pelvic muscles, lift the buttocks a few inches off the floor, supporting your weight on your feet and shoulders.

Repeat six times.

Time: five minutes.

D. *Pelvic rock*. Standing with feet slightly apart, hands on hips, thrust the pelvis forward on the in-breath, and back on the out-breath, achieving a rocking motion back and forth.

Helpful for many gynaecological problems, especially fibroids.

Time: two to three minutes every day.

Breathing exercise

Helpful for increasing blood circulation to all parts of the body, aerating the blood properly; useful method of relaxation if done lying down. Try with the Alexander Technique position ideally after the pelvic exercises. Lie on your back on a firm surface with your knees drawn up, feet flat on the floor, legs slightly apart and head supported on a slim book. Make sure you are comfortable.

Breathe in while counting to ten; try to fill your lungs. Put your hands on your sides to feel your rib-cage expanding; then you will know you are breathing in deeply.

Breathe out while counting to five; force all the air out of your lungs as you do so. Feel the abdominal muscles with your hand on your middle. They should contract strongly to expel all the air.

Repeat five to six times, two to three times daily.

Time: three to five minutes.

Total length of time needed to perform all exercises: thirty minutes daily. Over a few weeks, you should notice the benefit.

Glossary of Medical Terms

Abortus Dead or non-viable foetus.

Alterative Cleanses and purifies the blood; alters existing nutritive and excretory processes, gradually restoring normal body functions.

Allopathy System of therapeutics based on production of a condition antagonistic to the condition being treated.

Amniocentesis Surgical penetration of the pregnant uterus via the abdomen or cervix for aspiration of amniotic fluid around baby.

Analgesic Relieves pain when taken orally.

Antiemetic Lessens nausea and prevents or relieves vomiting.

Anti-inflammatory Counteracting or diminishing inflammation or its effects.

Anti-microbial Destroying or preventing the growth of bacteria.

Anti-mitotic Prevents normal cell division. Anti-mitotic drugs are used in the treatment of cancer.

Anti-oxidant Inhibits oxidation. Vitamins A, C and E are anti-oxidants.

Anti-spasmodic Relieves spasms of voluntary and involuntary muscles.

Anxiolytic An anti-anxiety agent.

Aperient A mild laxative.

Astringent Firms tissues and organs; reduces discharges and secretions.

Atherosclerosis A form of hardening of the arteries in which atheromas or fatty patches are formed within the lining of arteries.

Atopic Clinical hypersensitivity state or allergy with a hereditary predisposition.

Atrophy Wasting away; a shrinking in size of a cell tissue, organ or body part.

Bitter Bitter herbs which in small amounts stimulate digestion.

Carminative Relieves intestinal gas, pain and distension.

Cholagogue Promotes flow and discharge of bile into intestine.

Chromosome A structure in the nucleus of the cell which transmits genetic information. There are forty-six in the human cell plus two sex chromosomes which determine the individual's sex.

Cytokine Small protein produced and released by cells invaded by a virus which forms an anti-viral protein that inhibits viral multiplication (Interferon).

Cytotoxic Having a harmful effect on cells.

Deobstruent Removes body obstructions.

Diastole Period of dilation of the ventricles or chambers of the heart. In the reading of blood pressure diastole is recorded as the lower figure, e.g. $\frac{130}{70}$ mm mercury.

Electromyography The recording of intrinsic electrical properties of skeletal muscle.

Emmenagogue Helps promote and regulate menstruation.

Endocrine Hormonal.

Endometrium Mucous membrane lining the uterus which proliferates during the menstrual cycle and is lost as the monthly bleed or menses.

Epigastric The upper middle region of the abdomen.

Episiotomy Surgical incision into the perineum and vagina during delivery of a baby; obstetrical intervention.

Free radical The process of oxidation gives rise to atoms called free oxidizing radicals which can damage healthy cells. Oxidation of fats, particularly of fried foods, is to blame, as are smoking and pollution.

Galactagogue Promotes secretion of milk.

Glycogen Carbohydrate made and stored in the liver; broken down into glucose as needed.

Gonococcus A bacterium of the species Neissaria gonorrhoeae, causes gonorrhoea.

Hyperfolliculinemia Oversecretion of folliculine, an oestrogen hormone from the ovary; also known as hyperoestrogenemia.

Hyperthyroidism Deficiency of thyroid activity, marked by decreased metabolic rate, tiredness and lethargy.

Hypothalamus Part of the structure of the brain. Among its many functions, it activates, controls and integrates the nervous system and hormonal activities.

Immunoglobulin Human protein with known antibody activity synthesized by lymphocytes and plasma cells and found in blood serum and other body fluids and tissues.

Menarche Beginning of the menstrual function.

Myalgia Muscular pain.

Myxodema Swelling due to fluid retention, associated with hypothyroidism.

Nervine Strengthens functional activity of nervous system; may be stimulants or sedatives.

Neurosis An emotional disorder, manifesting mainly as anxiety, due to unresolved conflicts.

Nutritive Increases weight and density; nourishes the body.

Oxidation To cause to combine with oxygen or to remove hydrogen. The chemical process of oxidation takes place during metabolism of glucose in the body and produces large quantities of energy.

Oestrogenic Oestrogen-producing; having the properties of, or similar to, an oestrogen.

Pap smear Smear taken from cervix to examine cervical cells microscopically.

Perineum Pelvic floor (PC) muscles and associated structures surrounding vagina; region between the thighs bounded by the vulva and anus.

Peritoneum Membrane lining the walls of the abdominal and pelvic cavities and surrounding the organs.

Phytosterol A steroid from plants; plant hormone.

Pituitary Endocrine gland situated in the brain secreting hormones which regulate the thyroid, adrenals and other endocrine organs.

Probiotic Literally, 'pro-life', the opposite of antibiotic; probiotics include lactobacilli such as Lactobacillus acidophilus.

Prostaglandin Naturally occurring group of chemicals that stimulate contraction of the uterus and other smooth muscle; they also affect the action of certain hormones. (The five types are A, B, C, D, E and F with subscripts 1, 2, 3 abbreviated as PGE_1, PGF_2 etc).

Sebaceous gland Secretes sebum, an oil, onto the surface of the skin.

Speculum Instrument used to open the vagina for visual inspection of the cervix.

Steroid Any of a group of chemical compounds containing four carbon rings interlocked to form a cyclopentophenanthine ring system. It includes many hormones, human and plant.

Syntocinon Drug (synthetic oxytocin) used to induce labour or increase uterine contractions during labour.

Syntometrine Drug (synthetic oxytocin) used to contract uterus to deliver the placenta in the third stage of labour.

T-cell 'T' type of lymphocyte or white blood cell, active in the immune system.

Tonic Stimulates nutrition and increases systemal tone.

Urticaria Hives, a vascular reaction of the skin with the appearance of red, slightly raised patches or weals with severe itching.

List of Principal Herbs

COMMON NAME	LATIN NAME
Agrimony	*Agrimonia eupatoria*
Alfalfa	*Medicago sativa*
Aloes, Barbados or Cape	*Aloe vera, A. barbadensis or A. ferox*
Angelica	*Angelica archangelica*
Angelica, Chinese	*Angelica sinensis*
Aniseed	*Pimpinella anisum*
Astralagus or Huang Qi	*Astralagus membranaceus*
Atractylodes or Bai Zhu	*Atractylodes macrocephala*
Bai Shao or White Peony	*Paeonia lactiflora*
Barberry	*Berberis vulgaris*
Bayberry or Wax Myrtle Bark	*Myrica cerifera*
Bearberry Leaf	*Arctostaphylos uva ursi*
Bear's Lichen or Beard Moss	*Usnea barbata*
Betony or Wood Betony	*Stachys betonica, Betonica officinalis*
Birch	*Betula alba*
Birth Root or Beth Root	*Trillium pendulum*
Bistort	*Polygonum bistorta*
Black Cohosh	*Cimicifuga racemosa*
Blackcurrant Leaf	*Ribes nigrum*
Black Horehound	*Ballota nigra*
Black Haw Bark	*Viburnum prunifolium*
Black Root	*Veronicastrum virginicum*
Bladderwrack	*Fucus vesiculosus*
Blessed Thistle	*Carduus benedictus*
Blood Root	*Sanguinaria canadensis*
Blue Cohosh	*Caulophyllum thalictroides*
Blue Flag	*Iris versicolor*
Bogbean	*Menyanthes trifoliata*
Boldo	*Peumus boldo*
Borage or Starflower	*Borago officinalis*
Buchu Leaf	*Barosma betulina*
Buckwheat	*Fagopyrum esculentum*

COMMON NAME	LATIN NAME
Burdock	*Arctium lappa*
Burnet, Greater	*Sanguisorba officinalis*
Calamus or Sweet Flag	*Acorus calamus*
Californian Poppy	*Escholtzia california*
Caraway Seed	*Carum carvi*
Cascara	*Rhamnus purshiana*
Catnip	*Nepeta cataria*
Cayenne or Capsicum	*Capsicum minimum*
Celery Seed	*Apium graveolens*
Centaury	*Erythraea centaurium*
Chamomile, German	*Matricaria recutita*
Chamomile, Roman	*Chamaemelum nobile, Anthemis nobile*
Chaste Berry	*Vitex agnus castus*
Chickweed	*Stellaria media*
Chinese Angelica or Dang Gui	*Angelica sinensis*
Chinese Liquorice or Gan Cao	*Glycyrrhiza uralensis*
Cleavers	*Galium aparine*
Codonopsis or Dang Shen	*Codonopsis pilosula*
Cola	*Cola vera*
Coltsfoot	*Tussilago farfara*
Comfrey	*Symphytum officinale*
Cone Flower or Echinacea	*Echinacea angustifolia/ E. purpurea*
Couchgrass	*Agropyron repens*
Cornsilk	*Zea mays*
Cowslip	*Primula veris*
Cramp Bark	*Viburnum opulus*
Cranesbill, American	*Geranium maculatum*
Damiana	*Turnera diffusa and T. aphrodisiaca*
Dandelion	*Taraxacum officinale*
Dang Gui or Chinese Angelica	*Angelica sinensis*
Devil's Claw	*Harpagophytum procumbens*

COMMON NAME	LATIN NAME	COMMON NAME	LATIN NAME
Echinacea or Cone Flower	Echinacea angustifolia/ E. purpurea	Kelp	Fucus vesiculosus
Elder Flower	Sambucus nigra	Korean Ginseng	Panax ginseng
Eleutherococcus or Siberian Ginseng	Eleutherococcus senticosus	Lady's Mantle	Alchemilla vulgaris
Euphorbia	Euphorbia pilulifera	Lavender	Lavandula officinalis
Eucalyptus	Eucalyptus globulus	Lemon Balm	Melissa officinalis
Evening Primrose	Oenothera biennis	Lemon Verbena	Lippia citriodora
Eyebright	Euphrasia spp.	Lime Flowers	Tilia europea
		Linseed	Linum usitatissimum
False Unicorn Root or Helonias	Chamaelirium luteum	Liquorice	Glycyrrhiza glabra
Fennel	Foeniculum vulgare	Marigold	Calendula officinalis
Fenugreek	Trigonella foenum- graecum	Marshmallow	Althea officinalis
		Meadowsweet	Filipendula ulmaria
Feverfew	Tanacetum parthenium	Milk Thistle	Carduus marianus
Figwort	Scrophularia nodosa	Motherwort	Leonorus cardiaca
Fringe-tree Bark	Chionanthus virginica	Mugwort	Artemisia vulgaris
Fumitory, Common	Fumaria officinalis	Mullein	Verbascum thapsus
		Myrrh	Commiphora molmol
Garlic	Allium sativum	Nettles	Urtica dioica
Gentian	Gentiana lutea		
Ginger	Zingiber officinale	Oats/Oatstraw	Avena sativa
Ginseng, American	Panax quinquefolium	Oak Bark	Quercus robur
Ginseng, Panax	Panax ginseng	Orange Blossom	Citrus aurantium
Ginseng, Siberian	Eleutherococcus senticocus	Oregon Grape Root	Berberis aquifolium
Goat's Rue	Galega officinalis	Panax	Panax ginseng
Golden Seal	Hydrastis canadensis	Parsley Piert	Alchemilla arvensis
Gotu Kola	Hydrocotyle asiatica	Pasque Flower	Anemone vulgaris
Guaiacum or Lignum vitae	Guaiacum officinale	Passion Flower	Passiflora incarnata
		Pau D'Arco	Tabebuia impeteginosa
Greater Burnet	Sanguisorba officinalis	Pellitory-of-the-Wall	Parietaria diffusa
Greater Periwinkle	Vinca major	Penny Royal	Mentha pulegium
		Peony, White or Bai Shao	Paeonia lactiflora
Hawthorn	Crataegus oxyacanthoides		
Heartease Pansy	Viola tricolor	Peppermint	Mentha piperita
Helonias or False Unicorn Root	Chamaelirium luteum	Plantain, Common or Ribbed	Plantago major, P. lanceolata
Herb Bennet or Avens	Geum urbanum	Prickly Ash	Zanthoxylum americanum
He Shou Wu or Fleeceflower Root	Polygonum multiflorum		
Hops	Humulus lupulus	Psyllium Seed	Plantago psyllium
Horsetail	Equisetum arvense	Raspberry Leaf	Rubus idaeus
Hyssop	Hyssopus officinalis	Red Clover	Trifolium pratense
		Rehmannia or Shu Di Huang	Rehmannia glutinosa
Iceland Moss	Cetraria islandica		
Irish Moss	Chondrus crispus	Rhubarb	Rheum spp.
		Rosemary	Rosmarinus officinalis
Jamaican Dogwood	Piscidia erythrina		
Juniper	Juniperus communis	Rose Petals	Rosa spp.

COMMON NAME	LATIN NAME	COMMON NAME	LATIN NAME
Sage	*Salvia officinalis*	Usnea or Bear's Lichen	*Usnea barbata*
Sarsaparilla	*Smilax officinalis and spp.*	Uva-ursi or Bearberry	*Arctostaphylos uva ursi*
Saw Palmetto	*Serenoa serrulata*	Valerian	*Valeriana officinalis*
Schizandra or Wu Wei Zi	*Schizandra chinensis*	Vervain	*Verbena officinalis*
Senna	*Cassia senna*	Wax Myrtle or Bayberry	*Myrica cerifera*
Shepherd's Purse	*Capsella bursa-pastoris*	White Deadnettle	*Lamium album*
Siberian Ginseng	*Eleutherococcus senticosus*	White Horehound	*Marrubium vulgare*
		White Peony	*Paeonia lactiflora*
Skullcap	*Scutellaria laterifolia*	White Poplar	*Populus tremuloides*
Slippery Elm	*Ulmus fulva*	White Willow Bark	*Salix alba*
Southernwood	*Artemisia abrotanum*	Wild Indigo	*Baptisia tinctoria*
Squaw Vine	*Mitchella repens*	Wild Lettuce	*Lactuca virosa*
St John's Wort	*Hypericum perforatum*	Wild Pansy or Heartsease	*Viola tricolor*
Starflower or Borage	*Borago officinalis*	Wild Yam	*Dioscorea villosa*
Stone Root	*Collinsonia canadensis*	Wintergreen	*Gaultheria procumbens*
Sweet Flag or Calamus	*Acorus calamus*	Witch Hazel	*Hamamelis virginiana*
Sweet Sumach	*Rhus aromatica*	Wood Betony	*Stachys betonica*
Sweet Violet	*Viola odorata*	Wormwood	*Artemisia absinthium*
		Wu Wei Zi or Schizandra	*Schizandra chinensis*
Tansy	*Tanacetum vulgare*		
Thyme	*Thymus vulgaris*		
Tree of Life	*Thuja occidentalis*	Yarrow	*Achillea millefolium*
True Unicorn Root	*Aletris farinosa*	Yellow Dock Root	*Rumex crispus*

Useful Addresses

Fertility, pregnancy and childbirth

Association for Improvements in the Maternity
Services (AIMS)
England: Sandar Warshal
40 Kingswood Avenue
London NW6 6LS
Scotland: Nadine Edwards
40 Leamington Terrace
Edinburgh EH10 4JL

Association for Post-natal Illness
15 Jerdan Place
London SW6 1BE
Tel.: 0171 386 0868

Association of Breast Feeding Mothers
26 Holmshaw Close,
London SE26 4TH
Tel.: 0181 778 4769

Association of Radical Midwives
62 Greetby Hill
Ormskirk
Lancashire
L39 2DT
Tel.: 01695 52776 (s.a.e. for list)

British Pregnancy Advisory Service
Austy Manor
Wootten Warren
Solihull
West Midlands B95 6BX
Helpline: 0345 304030

Foresight (The Association for
Preconceptual Care)
28 The Paddock
Godalming
Surrey GU7 1XD
Tel.: 01488 427839

Issue (The National Fertility Association Ltd)
509 Aldridge Road
Great Barr
Birmingham B44 8NA
Tel.: 0121 344 4414

La Leche League of Great Britain (Breast-feeding
advice and information)
BM 3424
London WC1V 6XX
Tel.: 0171 242 1278

Miscarriage Association
Head Office
c/o Clayton Hospital
Northgate
Wakefield
West Yorkshire WF1 3JS
Tel.: 01924 200799

National Childbirth Trust
Alexandra House
Oldham Terrace
London W3 6NH
Tel.: 0181 992 8637

Stillbirth and Neonatal Death Society (SANDS)
28 Portland Place
London W1N 3DE
Tel.: 0171 436 5881

Eating Disorders

Anorexia and Bulimia Care
15 Fernhurst Gate
Aughton
Ormskirk
Lancashire L39 5ED
Tel.: 01695 422479

Childline
Freephone helpline: 0800 1111 (24 hours)
Children and young people up to eighteen years of age

Eating Disorders Association
Sackville Place
44 Magdalen Street
Norwich NR3 1JU
Tel.: 01603 621414

Maisner Centre for Eating Disorders
PO Box 464
Hove
East Sussex BN3 3UG
Tel.: 01273 729818 *(Bulimia only)*

National Association of Young People's
Counselling and Advisory Service
17–23 Albion Street
Leicester LE1 6GD

General

Action for ME
PO Box 1302
Wells BA5 2WE
Tel.: 01749 670 799

Bristol Cancer Help Centre
Grove House
Cornwallis Grove
Clifton
Bristol BS8 4PG
Tel.: 01272 743216

British Association for Counselling
1 Regent Place
Rugby CV21 2PJ
Tel.: 01788 550899
Helpline: 0171 729 2229

Food and Chemical Allergy Associations
27 Ferringham Lane
Ferring-by-Sea
West Sussex BN12 5NB

Institute of Allergy Therapists
Ffynnonwen
Llangwyryton
Aberystwyth
Dyfed SX23 4EY
Tel.: 01974 241376
(Send s.a.e. for list of practitioners)

ME Association
Stanhope House
High Street
Stanford-le-Hope
Essex SS17 0HA
Tel.: 0135 642466

National Endometriosis Society
35 Belgrave Square
London SW1X 8QB
Tel.: 0171 235 4137

National Institute of Medical Herbalists Ltd
56 Longbrook Street
Exeter
Devon EX4 6AH
Tel.: 01392 426022

School of Herbal Medicine (Phytotherapy)
Bucksteep Manor
Bodle Street Green
Near Hailsham
East Sussex BN27 4RJ

Women's Aid Federation England
PO Box 391
Bristol BS99 7WS
Tel.: 01272 633 494
Helpline: 01272 633542

Women's Health Concern
83 Earl's Court Road
London W8 6EF

Women's Health Information Centre
52 Featherstone Street
London EC1Y 8RT
Tel.: 0171 251 6580

Women's Nationwide Cancer Control Campaign
Helpline: 0171 729 2229

Women's Nutritional Advisory Service (PMS)
PO Box 268
Hove
West Sussex BN3 1RW
Tel.: 01273 487366

York Nutritional Laboratory
Tudor House
Lysander Close
Clifton Moor
York YO3 4XB
Tel.: 01904 690640
(Cytotoxic blood tests for allergies)

Suppliers of Herbs

The Dr Edward Bach Centre
Mount Vernon
Bakers Lane
Sotwell
Wallingford
Oxfordshire OX10 0PZ
Tel.: 01491 834678
(Dr Bach's Flower Remedies)

G. Baldwin and Co.
171–173 Walworth Road
London SE17 1RW
Tel.: 0171 703 5550

Gerard House Ltd
475 Capability Green
Luton LU1 3LU
Tel.: 01582 487331
(For stockists)

Herbal Treatment Clinic
6 Beaumont Gate
Glasgow G12 9EE
Tel.: 0141 357 3461
(Herbal formulas used in this book)

Napiers Mail Order
Forest Bank
Barr
Ayrshire KA26 9TN
Tel.: 01465 861 625

Neals Yard Apothecary
15 Neal's Yard
London WC2H 9DP
Tel.: 0171 379 7222
(Chinese herbs)

Optimum Health
Phoenix House
22 Burwood Close
Guildford
Surrey GU1 2SB
Tel/fax.: 01483 301144
(Organic herbs, Chinese herbs, Dr Reckeweg)

Phytoproducts Ltd
3 Kings Mill Way
Hermitage Lane
Mansfield
Notts NG18 5ER
Tel.: 01623 644334
(Fresh plant juices)

Potters Herbal Supplies Ltd.
Leyland Mill Lane
Wigan
Lancashire WN1 2SB
Tel.: 01942 34761

Suppliers of nutritional supplements

Higher Nature Ltd
The Nutrition Centre
Burwash Common
East Sussex TN19 7LX
Tel.: 01435 882 880

Larkhall Natural Health
225 Putney Bridge Road
London SW15 2PY
Tel.: 0181 874 1130
(Cantassium, hair mineral analysis and nutritional analysis)

Bibliography

General medicine

Berkow, R., MD, *The Merck Manual* (16th edition), Merck and Co., Inc., 1992

Davidson's Principles and Practice of Medicine (12th edition), ed. Mcleod, J., Churchill Livingstone, 1977

Dorland's Pocket Medical Dictionary (23rd edition), W. B. Saunders, 1982

Rowley, Dr N. B., *Basic Clinical Science: A Workbook for Complementary Practitioners*, Hodder and Stoughton, 1991

Friedman, E. H. and Moshy, R. E., *Medicine: The Bare Bones*, John Wiley, 1986

Journals
British Medical Journal
Journal of Alternative and Complementary Medicine
Journal of Ethnopharmacology (Switzerland)
Planta Medica (Germany)
The Lancet
What Doctors Don't Tell You
European Journal of Herbal Medicine
The British Journal of Phytotherapy

Herbal medicine

Bensky, D. and Gamble, A., *Chinese Herbal Medicine: Materia Medica*, Eastland Press Inc., 1986

British Herbal Compendium, ed. Peter Bradley, The British Herbal Medicine Association, PO Box 304, Bournemouth, 1992

British Herbal Pharmacopoeia, vol. 1, The British Herbal Medicine Association, PO Box 304, Bournemouth, 1983 and 1990

Christopher, Dr John, *School of Natural Healing*, Biworld Publications, 1976

Grieves, M., *A Modern Herbal*, Penguin, 1977

Hoffman, D., *The New Holistic Herbal*, Element Books, 1990

Nissim, R., *Natural Healing in Gynaecology*, Pandora Press, 1986

Parvati, Jeannine, *Hygeia, A Woman's Herbal* (16th edition), Freestone Collective, 1992

Weiss, R., MD, *Herbal Medicine*, Hippokrates Verlag, Stuttgart 1985

Nutrition

Ballantine, R., *Diet and Nutrition*, Himalayan National Institute, 1978

Cannon, G. and Walker, C., *The Food Scandal*, Century, 1984

Cannon, G. and Einzig, H., *Dieting Makes You Fat: A Guide To Fitness, Energy and Health*, Century, 1983

Chaitow, L. *The Stone Age Diet*, Optima, 1987

Davies, Dr S. and Stewart Dr A., *Nutritional Medicine*, Pan Books, 1987

Gerson, Dr Max, *A Cancer Therapy – Results of Fifty Cases*, Totality Books, 1977

Gibson, R. and S., *The Complete Wheat Free Cookbook*, Thorsons, 1990

Grant, D. and Joice, J., *Food Combining For Health*, Thorsons, 1984

Greer, Rita, *Wheat, Milk and Egg Free Cooking*, Thorsons, 1989

Jensen, B., *Tissue Cleansing Through Bowel Management*, California, 1980

Kenton, L., *The Biogenic Diet*, Century, 1986

Le Tissier, J., *Food Combining for Vegetarians*, Thorsons, 1994

Mackarness, Richard, *Not All in the Mind*, Thorsons, 1994

Marsden, K., *Food Combining in 30 Days*, Thorsons, 1994

Mount, James, *The Food and Health of Western Man*, Precision Press, 1975

Salmon, Jenny, *Dietary Reference Values: A Guide*, Department of Health, 1991

Trowbridge, J. Parks and Walker, Morton, *The Yeast Syndrome*, Bantam, 1989

FURTHER READING

History and philosophy of herbal medicine

Griggs, B., *Green Pharmacy: A History of Herbal Medicine*, Jill Norman & Hobhouse, 1981

Mills, Simon Y., *The Essential Book of Herbal Medicine*, Arkana, 1991

Women's health issues

Achterberg, J., *Woman As Healer*, Shambhala, 1990

Boston Women's Health Collective *Our Bodies, Ourselves* (British edition) Phillips, A. and Rakusen J., Penguin Books, 1978

Breitkopf, Dr L. and Bakoulis, M., *Coping with Endometriosis*, Prentice Hall Press, 1988

Evenett, K., *Coping Successfully with PMS*, Sheldon Press, 1994

Evenett, K., *Everything You Need to Know about Your Cervical Smear*, Sheldon Press, 1995

Grant, Ellen, *Sexual Chemistry: Understanding Your Hormones, the Pill and HRT*, Cedar, 1994

Howard, Judy, *Bach Flower Remedies For Women*, C. W. Daniel Co. Ltd.

Lee, John, R., *Natural progesterone, The Multiple Roles of A Remarkable Hormone*, BLL publishing, 1994

Orbach, Susie, *Fat Is a Feminist Issue*, Arrow, 1989

Orbach, Susie, *Hunger Strike*, Penguin, 1993

Pregnancy and childbirth

Balaskas, Janet, *Active Birth*, Unwin, 1983

Balaskas, Janet, *Natural Pregnancy A Practical Holistic Guide to Wellbeing from Conception to Birth*, Gaia, 1994

Barnes, B. and Bradley, S., *Planning for a Healthy Baby*, Foresight, Vermillion, 1995

Beech, Beverley, *Who's Having Your Baby?*, Bedford Square Press, 1991

Inch, S., *Birthrights – A Parents' Guide to Modern Childbirth* (2nd edition), Green Print Merlin Press, 1989

Kitzinger, S., *Home Birth and Other Alternatives to Hospital*, Dorling Kindersley, 1991

Liedloff, J., *The Continuum Concept*, Arkana, 1986

Noble, Elizabeth, *Essential Exercises for the Childbearing Year: A Guide to Health and Comfort Before and After Your Baby is Born*, John Murray, 1978

Vincent Priya, J., *Birth Traditions and Modern Pregnancy Care*, Element Books, 1992

Menopause

Sheehy, Gail, *The Silent Passage – Menopause*, Harper Collins, 1993

Greer, G., *The Change: Women, Ageing and the Menopause*, Hamish Hamilton, 1991

Hall, Judy, *The Wise Woman: A Natural Approach to Menopause*, Element Books, 1992

Field guides

Phillips, Roger and Foy, Nicky, *Herbs.*, Pan Books, 1990

Phillips, Roger, *Photographic Guide to Identify Herbs and Medical Plants*, Elm Tree, 1987

Schauer, T., *A Field Guide to Wild Flowers of Britain and Europe*, Collins, 1982

Miscellaneous

Bishop, Beata, *A Time to Heal*, Severn House Publishers, 1985

Hay, Louise, *You Can Heal Your Life*, Eden Grove, 1988

Selye, Hans, *The Stress of Life*, McGraw Hill, 1978

Siegal, Bernie S., *Love Medicine and Miracles*, Arrow Books, 1986

Simonton, Carl, *Getting Well Again*, Bantam, 1980

Index

(Page numbers in *italics* refer to illustrations)